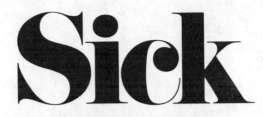

Sick

How people feel
about being sick
and what they think
of those
who care for them

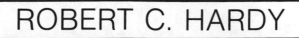

ROBERT C. HARDY

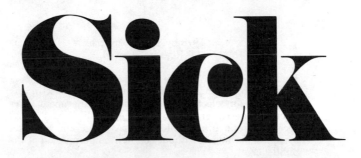

Sick

How people feel
about being sick
and what they think
of those
who care for them

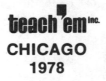

teach'em inc.

CHICAGO

1978

Library of Congress Catalog Card Number:
77-90162

International Standard Book Number:
0-931028-04-3 (Softcover)
0-931028-05-1 (Hardcover)

Designed by Robert Meindl

Printed in the United States of America
by Active Graphics, Chicago, Ill.

teach 'em ᴵᴺᶜ·
625 North Michigan Avenue
Chicago, Illinois 60611

For Chris

Quotations used in this book are from:

Introduction

Medicine is too important to be left to doctors. This kind of statement, which would have been considered meaningless forty years ago and radical twenty years ago, is today widely acceptable. Consumers (sometimes known as patients), fed up with the patronizing attitude of many physicians, are insisting, with considerable success, that they deserve not just a piece of the action, but a piece of the knowledge. The passive role of the patient is passe—and that's what this book is all about.

The sixty cases, divided into nineteen categories, demonstrate that patients have more understanding and more insight into their conditions than generally appreciated by their doctors. They have strong feelings about the care they receive—and the caretakers. They exercise critical judgment, negative and positive, and are willing, indeed eager in many cases, to openly and frankly express their opinions.

This collection of their personal accounts of illness, their encounters with physicians, nurses, hospitals, insurance carriers, lawyers, and the entire medical system, skillfully presented by Robert C. Hardy, makes this book a landmark in the exploding consumer revolt against the secrecy and elitism that has too long characterized the doctor-patient relationship.

Hardy, a hospital and health agency administrator, shows us in this broad-spectrum set of interviews the tremendous range of human behavior when facing doctors, hospitals and illness. Thus, while some choose physicians with care, many others invest more effort in shopping for a new automobile than in selecting a physician. While some are quite satisfied with their hospital care, the accounts of others suggest that a hospital might be regarded as analogous to war; one tries to avoid entering, and once in, the goal is to get out just as soon as possible. Furthermore, in a hospital as in a war, one should never be alone; always have a relative or friend at your bedside for protection against possible damage (usually unintended but nonetheless real) by the "helping professionals" of the hospital staff.

While some patients respond to poor outcomes philosophically, others, in increasing numbers, turn to lawyers. Thus, malpractice and other forms of legal action become valuable methods for changing the behavior not only of specific physicians, but of the medical profession in general. As a matter of fact, one method of insuring special attention on the part of the physician is to drop the word "lawyer" into the conversation.

A remarkable finding of these interviews is the consistently profound base of information patients manifest about their condition. From diseases as common as asthma and cataracts to those as unusual as Bang's disease, the patients are aware of the major aspects as well as the subtleties of causation, diagnosis, treatment alternatives and prediction of outcomes. I am repeatedly reminded of the important rule in medical education: "Allow the patient enough time to talk and he will give you the diagnosis; give him five minutes more and he will provide the treatment." Readers with the conditions covered in this volume will find the subjective accounts of far greater value than the objective medical descriptions in either the scientific or popular publications.

Not only do the patients know their diseases, they also appreciate the victories and failures of their doctors. The scope of reactions to physician error is human, credible and broad-spectrum, ranging from apology to forgiveness to condemnation. The message to physicians is loud and clear—stop talking down to your patients; stop patronizing them as if they were either children or stupid or retarded or all three. These case reports can, indeed should, serve as excellent teaching lessons for medical students and physicians at every stage of training and practice. As a matter of fact, for any health professional who has never been a patient (the best way of learning), this book is next best.

Americans are moving towards two extremes in opting for medical care. On the one hand, they are gravitating in the direction of more technology, more highly specialized institutions and greater passivity as physician dominance grows. On the other hand, an increasing number (still a minority) are moving in the opposite direction—home births, midwifery, breastfeeding, avoidance of drugs, x-rays and surgery; this group is skeptical, sometimes distrustful, of technology and institutions, substituting acceptance of personal responsibility for their own health.

Both groups of patients have at least one common characteristic—an opportunity to greatly benefit from a careful analysis of the patient accounts in *Sick*. This can help them in reaching more intelligent decisions in approaching their own medical care.

Robert S. Mendelsohn, M.D.
November 1977

Dr. Mendelsohn is in the private practice of medicine in Chicago. His column, "The People's Doctor," is nationally syndicated.

Preface

This book is a collection of reactions to the experience of illness — an insight into how some Americans felt about being sick in the 1970's.

There are several reasons why I thought a series of interviews on this subject would be useful. My first objective was to record the experience of a number of patients with common and uncommon conditions so that well people could get a better idea of what it feels like to be sick with a particular disease. I thought this series might be of help to people who are suddenly faced with the problem of adjusting to one of the illnesses discussed.

To be sure, such help may be limited. No one can tell another person precisely how it feels to be sick. There is also the hazard that the reader will assume that what has happened to another person, whether good or bad, will happen to him. It won't. His experience will not be the same.

Still, there are common sensations which can be communicated. There is knowledge which someone who has experienced an illness can impart.

Another reason for this book was to get an idea of how people think about the health care system in America. As the interviews show, people react differently, because their experience is influenced by an infinite number of variables. If the episode of illness is short, relatively painless and brings prompt and positive results at reasonable cost, the patient is likely to feel happy about the people and institutions that took care of him. But if things do not go right, take too long, hurt a lot and the results are worse than expected, the sufferer is likely to have a totally different view of and attitude toward the system.

The process of collecting these interviews took more than two years. I first sought to interview people who had recently been sick and who had been to a doctor or hospital. Thus, the reactions to the health care system which they expressed are totally random. Once people agreed to be interviewed, most wanted to talk at length about their illnesses, though a few needed prompting, as though they had never felt very deeply about any part of their experience.

The names of all people in this book are fictitious. The names of locations and institutions are either deleted or referred to only vaguely. This is to protect the identity of the doctors and other providers of care as well as the patients. Some invented names are used so that the language of the person interviewed will flow in a natural manner. This identity protection was provided so that the patients could feel uninhibited during the interview and comfortable thereafter. Only minimal editing was applied so that each patient's story would come through as he experienced it and described it.

The title of the stories indicates the principal complaint in common language, then the diagnosis, sometimes in common as well as medical language, and finally, the corrective procedure, if any. This use of the complaint instead of a patient's name in the title also causes some necessary depersonalization. However, labeling the patient as a diagnosis or a body part is not an uncommon hospital practice. The patient may be known to the staff on the ward as the gall bladder in 237 or the peptic ulcer in 418. Although everyone decries this practice, it still exists and shows no signs of disappearing.

The viewpoints of the people whose interviews are included in this book are not objective nor are they the result of scientific study of the health care system. These viewpoints cannot be objective because they are personal reactions to the health care received and health care is a subjective, individualized, human service. In addition, each person interviewed based his conclusions on a "series-of-one" encounter with the health care system.

Sick people are submissive people, dependent on their doctor and others to help them. They feel they have to be obedient, subservient and cooperative in order to maintain a good relationship between themselves and the people who take care of them. Patients feel this relationship is essential for their own protection, and they cling to it for this reason.

Sometimes, this reason gets in the way of their better judgment; patients occasionally stick with a physician long after he or she has shown an inability to handle the condition involved. One common theme this book identifies is the tendency of people to select doctors in a haphazard fashion and switch only with great reluctance.

When sick people go to a hospital, they suddenly find themselves in a new, completely foreign environment surrounded by a group of strangers who know each other and know what they are doing but do not always tell the patient what is going on. Patients consequently suffer from a loss of their self-concept, alterations of their body image and a loss of the feeling of confidence which heretofore had enabled them to function effectively in the world of the well. Even their clothes and personal possessions are taken away, leading them to feel exposed and vulnerable. The system has taken over their body. Patients often suffer from acute culture shock as well as a lack of information about what is going to happen next.

Sick people are not in a very good position to question the people who have assumed command of their body, and when they try to find out what is going on, they may be considered presumptive. They can neither evaluate what is being done to them nor tell whether they are treated right or not. While they are sick, they are least able to trust their own judgment or to protest what they might perceive as inadequate care. When the illness is past, few return to their doctor or hospital with constructive criticism. They tend to overlook the apparently unnecessary problems they may have encountered because they must maintain a continuing relationship with their physician and do not wish to be considered ungrateful or disgruntled. Unless they have grounds for a malpractice suit, they just do not bring up the unpleasantries. But they *do* remember them.

The cumulative impression from reading these interviews might be that we are deliberately picking on hospitals or physicians or nurses. This is not the case. It was not my purpose to speak with every disgruntled patient I could find. I selected people with interesting diagnoses; their comments about the health care system are a direct result of their experience. Many of those interviewed for this book did not spend much time talking about what went right during their hospital stay or physician visit. They concentrated on what went wrong. Examples of what went wrong apparently remain uppermost in the minds of most people who seek medical help. The concern, indeed, the fascination with slip-ups seems to be a human inclination, heightened here because, in some cases, errors could have been calamitous or even have resulted in death.

As a former hospital administrator with more than 25 years experience in the health care field, I thought this book might help people who care for the sick understand more about patient attitudes.

Although health professionals are inveterate patient-watchers, they cannot be totally aware of what a patient is experiencing or how he feels about himself and about them. In part, an ill person's feelings and reactions remain unknown to health professionals because they have not experienced the illness personally. In addition, there is often a lack of honest, complete communication. Some patients do not know how to address their doctor-nurse audience. Others do not wish to communicate. And some simply act out the role of patient as they perceive their audience expects them to play it.

These interviews will admit the doctors and nurses and all of the other patient-care providers to some of the numerous informal, clinical pathological conferences (CPC's) which patients conduct in homes, in doctors' waiting rooms, in bars, at cocktail parties, in private corners and all the places former patients gather to talk about being sick. This kind of CPC is usually attended by very few people, often only one, a close friend or relative. The doctor is almost never invited.

Examples of what went wrong or, in some cases, perceptions of what seemed to go wrong, are probably more revealing than success stories. We sincerely hope this book will serve to reduce medical and hospital error by illuminating some of the conditions, circumstances or attitudes that may lead to it.

We also hope health providers and consumers can learn from this collection of patient opinions and that it will provide information essential to the process of improving the health care system in America.

*   *   *

Many accommodating people introduced me to friends who had recently used the health care system. My gratitude goes especially to Ms. Suzan Nesom and Ms. Judy Hisle who provided this link of acquaintanceship.

Particular recognition of the late Ms. Wanda Woodmore's efforts is appropriate because she arranged a number of conferences.

My appreciation goes to Ms. Jeanie Marshall who typed her way through seemingly endless tapes and handwritten transcriptions of tapes.

My special gratitude is expressed for the patience and understanding of Ann, my wife, during the 30 months required to compile this series.

My thanks must also go to the people whose stories this book contains. They were considerate and cooperative, giving their time and commentary willingly. The process of interviewing them was a fascinating experience and considerably enlightening to one who has spent a quarter of a century on the provider side of the health care system.

Finally, a special thanks to Studs Terkel, who through his brilliant series of interview documentaries, *Division Street: America, Hard Times* and *Working* offered me a format and an inspiring level of excellence for this exploration.

Robert C. Hardy

Contents

"Salud, pesetas y amor,
y el tiempo para empujarlas."
—SPANISH PROVERB

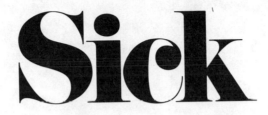

Sick

How people feel
about being sick
and what they think
of those
who care for them

I.
Wild Growth

*When we think of cancer in general terms
we are apt to conjure up a process characterized by a steady, remorseless and inexorable progress in which the disease is all-
conquering, and none of the immunological
and other defensive forces which help us to
survive the onslaught of bacterial and viral
infections can serve to halt the faltering foot-
steps to the grave.*

William Boyd (1885–   )
The Spontaneous Regression of Cancer

1. Lung Cancer

He is 52, slight and totally bald or so it appears because the graying fringe is kept close-cropped. He also seems shorter than average but really isn't. His work environment is the frenetic world of urban promotion, always meeting people, problems and deadlines. He is a dedicated, hard-working proponent of the private enterprise system, carrying out the details of committee plans to attract more industry and build a bigger and better city. He has given up smoking but not the fast-moving lifestyle of the striving, competitive promoter.

- **Sore Throat**
- **Laryngitis**
- **Lung Cancer**

- **Thoracotomy**
- **Radiation Therapy**

My situation began in early May with a case of fairly common laryngitis which kept getting progressively worse. At the time, laryngitis was a common thing around the city, sort of an epidemic, so I didn't give it too much thought until it had gone on two or three weeks, at which time I went to see our family doctor, a general practitioner. I had not seen him before. Members of my family had gone to him, but because of the presence of a doctor in my family who generally looked after my needs and kept me in pretty good straits, I'd never been examined by this doctor. He thought this condition was caused by sinus drainage, prescribed some antibiotics and gave me an injection of penicillin. He instructed me to report back to him in five to seven days if I didn't have some improvement.

In a week I didn't have any improvement so I went back to him, and he gave me another injection and suggested we try two or three more days, which I did. He asked me to call him. I called him when the time was up, and he suggested that I go see an eye, ear, nose and throat specialist. He gave me the names of three or four, all of which I called. It was just before or after the Fourth of July holidays, and I had a difficult time finding them and making an appointment with one of them but I finally did.

I was seen immediately. This specialist examined me, checked my eyes, ears, nose, throat and tested my vocal cords. He found that the left one was paralyzed. He sent me to have an x-ray, told me to wait for it and bring it back. He checked the x-ray and without being too specific, indicated that I had a rather serious problem and that he would like for me to see another doctor right away. He didn't tell me what the problem was. That alarmed me because

I had no idea what he was talking about whatsoever. But apparently, it was something more than just a routine case of laryngitis.

To back up — he said he wanted to talk with my family physician by noon the next day. I tried to reach him without success. The EENT man called me about one-thirty or two o'clock the next afternoon and said that *he* had not been able to reach my family physician, either, and that my condition was such that I should immediately see this surgeon he would like to refer me to. He made the appointment.

This surgeon came to his office between operations to examine me. It was a day he normally didn't see office patients. He examined me and told me there was a tumor present in my left lung.

He said I should go into the hospital of my choice and that he would proceed to study the case from that point. He was very open and very frank. He tried to remain neutral and without giving any particular indication of fear or anything else, he said, "You have a serious condition. We don't know too much about these things but I feel that we can do good. I want to do everything I can. We need to run some tests, evaluate them and then see what our program should be from that point on."

That was on Thursday and he suggested that I report to the hospital the following Monday. His reasoning was that they would not accomplish much the remainder of the week. The waiting didn't help my weekend much.

The first day in the hospital, they gave me some routine tests, drew blood, urinalysis. Then the next day, they began a lengthy series of tests, the names of which I can't describe — pulmonary function tests, blood tests, several varieties of x-rays, scannings. Number one was a liver scan and the second series was a number of scans, particularly the bones and skeletal portions of the body.

The tests were concluded on Thursday afternoon, and I saw my surgeon that evening. He indicated that the tests were generally in my favor, that there had been no spread or additional tumors. The exact nature of the tumor was not known to him at that time. He wished permission to do a thoracotomy to get a biopsy of the tumor and determine its exact nature and to dictate what kind of treatment should be indicated from that point on.

The operation was done at ten o'clock on Saturday morning and it took an hour and 45 minutes. First, they made an incision at the upper part of my chest — I don't know what this region is — just under my collarbone to obtain a lymph node to see if there was any infection there. He found none and then proceeded with the thoracotomy, came up and got a biopsy of the tumor. He made an incision in my side, came into my chest cavity and got access to my lung and the tumor that way. They just skin up there and get a biopsy of the upper lobe. He had already done an optic fiberscope examination of that part of my lung. This instrument provides light and vision into the lung. The doctor looks through an eyepiece and can introduce the instrument into the various passages of the lung.

He inserted it down my throat. This optical procedure was done under a light, local anesthetic, just to keep it from irritating my throat. He just jammed it down my neck but there was no pain, no unpleasantness. In fact, it was surprising how pleasant and interesting it was to watch him.

The most interesting thing was my introduction into the surgery itself in preparation for the thoracotomy. They gave me a hypo or some sort of sedative about eight o'clock in the morning. And this is still a mystery to me, believe it or not. I got to surgery about 9:30 or 9:45 and was left in a holding area. The anesthetist came by and introduced himself, asked if I was comfortable, which I was. He was a very kind gentleman; pulled the blanket up over me a bit more. He came back by a couple of more times. Pretty soon, he brought one of his nurses by and asked her to take me to outside the door of operating room 17, which she did. I lay there a few minutes, and in the meantime, personnel came by to determine if I was comfortable. Then they took me into the operating room, asked me if I could get over on the surgical table myself and I said I could. They guarded me, of course.

The anesthetist came by and said, "Well, if we just had a surgeon, we could get started." And I thought to myself, "Oh, my God, the old Army game, hurry up and wait." (*Laughs.*) I kinda crossed my arms against my chest and lay my head back. Pretty soon, I heard my surgeon's voice. I was anticipating that he was going to tell me we were ready to begin when, in fact, we were in the recovery room, and he was telling me that it was all over and in a few minutes I would be taken to intensive care. I have no idea how the anesthetist did that because I don't remember a thing after he said if we had a surgeon we could go ahead. Maybe my memory was just that hazy, maybe the sedative they shot into me had done more than I thought, but it's still a mystery to me. I look back and laugh.

I was taken to intensive care, saw my family on the way and felt reasonably good. I had no pain, no nausea, nothing from the anesthesia.

Intensive care was a little more baffling. You go in and here is a bunch of compartments, a pleasant-looking atmosphere but obviously a very busy, businesslike place. They hooked me up to a monitor, the contacts of which were put on me before I even came up to intensive care. (*Coughs vigorously to clear throat. Voice is raspy and not too clear.*)

They came around frequently, looked after my comfort, took my blood pressure. I couldn't have any liquids so they gave me crushed ice. They were very good. I had an I.V. running.

I had no pain from the surgery but I did have a pain in my back. The first two shifts in intensive care were fine, I had no problems. There was one nurse I didn't get along with well. I asked for assistance trying to relieve my back pain and I got some rather rough and uncooperative treatment. I kept asking for a pillow to put under my back. They said I could have a painkiller, but all I really wanted was a pillow under my back. But this particular nurse wasn't too cooperative at all. She shoved the pillow under me, pulled on one of the drains, a sizeable drain I had in my left ribs, and was just generally rough.

I put up with that for a little while and when I tried to call her again, I couldn't find the call button. Finally, I flagged somebody down and they came and got her again. We had another round. Pretty soon my wife came, it was one of the visiting periods, and I complained to her about it. She got the nurse again, and that irritated her even more. My wife, after she left, called the doctor immediately who apparently called the hospital and raised a little thunder. Without any choice, I was given a shot for the pain, which did help. If I knew then what I know now, I would have asked for a shot to start out with.

The attitude of that particular shift was quite appalling. After that shift went off, we went back to the finest service I've ever seen.

I was there in intensive care until Monday, slightly after noon. Then they put me in a semiprivate room. I accepted a double room on the premise that I'd be given a private room. My roommate was a little bit radical. He was the assistant pastor of a local church and was very outspoken on certain religious matters, not unpleasant, just talkative. You'd like to have a few moments rest without somebody beatin' your ear and he just kept on going. He was fussin' and complaining to everybody, too. I don't know what his problem was. Primarily a heart condition, I think. He was undergoing tests. I had to live with him half a day, which wasn't too bad, but it was long enough under the circumstances. I had to prevail on some influence in the hospital to get a private room readied for me later on that evening. Otherwise, I don't think they would have gotten me a room to myself. I know the administrator and he rustled me up a room. Perhaps I should not have imposed on him. I think they had a room all along but they may have been too busy to ready it.

I left the hospital three days later having been there 11 or 12 days. While I was taking the tests, I ate the food like the world was coming to an end. I couldn't get enough to eat and I enjoyed it all. After the surgery, what I got was not what I would have chosen if I'd had free choice. The soft diet was not too appealing and it was an effort to get it down. They were urging me to eat, and maybe it was the anesthetic or the surgery, but it just didn't have any taste to me. I think it was primarily due to my condition.

"Did you ever smoke?"

Yes. I smoked until about four years ago and I had been smoking since I was 18. I'm 52 now so I smoked for 30 years. Incidentally, that was the first question the surgeon asked me. I used to smoke cigarettes, about one-and-a-half packs a day, sometimes more. Later, I smoked these miniature cigars. I inhaled the cigarettes but not the cigars.

"Why didn't they take the lung tumor out?"

They considered it risky because of its proximity to the aorta and a certain nerve. They indicated to me that their choice of treatment for this particular tumor would be irradiation by linear accelerator. No chemotherapy. The radiologist wanted to start the day I left the hospital but my surgeon said no, he preferred that I start on Monday, so there was only about a three-day lapse there.

I reported back to the hospital on an outpatient basis and had a conference with the radiologist, in the presence of my wife. He told me what they were going to do, what the effects would be, if any, what would be involved. He said although I would not have severe side effects, I would experience some unpleasantness which probably wouldn't be too bad. After that, they fluoroscoped me and marked out an area on my chest to receive the radiation. It was an area about five inches long and four inches wide, irregular in shape, on the upper left part of my chest. A secondary area spanned around the side of my neck here, missing my Adam's apple. They blocked that out in the machine. On one day, they'd give me radiation in the main chest area, and on alternate days, they would give me that plus the neck area. This was five-days-a-week, Monday-through-Friday, for 31 treatments, about six weeks. I got exposed from the front and also the back side.

For the first three weeks, I had no side effects whatsoever except the inconvenience of not bathing that area for fear of washing off the field marks. I could bathe, but I had to avoid getting that area wet. About the fourth or fifth week I noticed the onset of listlessness and weakness which they kept telling me I would have. It was not anything serious but I just didn't feel like getting out and threatening a bunch of wildcats. I had a light skin irritation and a little thickening of the throat which made it a bit difficult to eat and to swallow certain kinds of food, particularly if they were dry. My skin reddened but it didn't itch much. The treatments themselves were like x-rays, no feeling at all.

I finished these treatments three weeks ago yesterday and I'm feeling better every day. The full effects of the radiation won't be observed until 12 weeks after the termination of treatment. Then they'll x-ray me and they're hoping they'll find that the tumor has shrunk. They feel at this point that the tumor has been deactivated.

When the doctor told me I had this tumor, frankly, it alarmed me, but he did it in such a way that left me with a feeling of confidence. He was outright and open about it, told me I had a serious condition but they felt they could do something for me, at least give me comfort, and they were going to try everything they knew how. Now, I feel it has been a very interesting and enlightening experience. I don't feel like the end of the world has come. It hasn't been at all unpleasant. Of course, I am concerned, both for myself and my family, about what the future may be. I've talked to other people who have had similar experiences and I get encouragement from them, so I don't feel too badly about it. The doctors seem to be more concerned about my general level of health than they are about the tumor. I have a weight problem; they tell me to eat anything and everything I can get my hands on. The radiologist gave me some medication to decrease the irritation on my lung, but he also said, as a side effect, it would probably increase my appetite, which I think it has done.

"Many people are shocked when they are told they have cancer. How did you feel?"

I think, in this instance, the doctors avoided using the word "cancer" itself. All except one and he was just in on a substitute basis. That may have had some psychological effect. They refer to it as "a tumor" or "your condition." I've wondered about this. The substitute radiologist kept using the word cancer and that sort of gave me an abrupt reaction which I'd just as soon not have had. Otherwise, I really don't think of myself as having cancer. Maybe I should.

I had a very pleasant surprise when I came out of surgery. I figured they'd have some gloomy kind of news for me. They didn't say I was going to be well in 30 days but they did say, "Well, we are ready to proceed and put you on the next phase of the program." I felt like they were going to make progress from that point on. Somehow, they just inspired confidence and I appreciate that.

I think if there is any inequity in insurance coverage, it's in the schedule of allowances for physicians' services. It doesn't seem to be quite adequate. Of course, with major medical as well as basic insurance, I'll recover more.

My biggest question about the health care system is the referrals between doctors. Not the basic referral from my family physician to the EENT man to the surgeon. That was all in good order. But, for example, perhaps a petty example, the EENT sent me to get an x-ray and bring it back. He looked at it, apparently saw what he needed to see and referred me to the surgeon. The surgeon saw the same x-ray, read it, showed me what was there and what it indicated to him. This seemed to satisfy the need. But, not only did I get charged for the x-ray, which I expected, but I also got charged for an interpretation by a radiologist, which probably wasn't necessary. The radiologist's interpretation cost me $25.20 over the cost of taking the x-ray, which was $25. My physicians had already made their interpretation so I can't see why I had to pay the radiologist, too.

I think overall, I can complain very little, but I think the cost of medical care is extremely high now. I'm thankful I had major medical insurance. Without it, I'd have been completely lost. And people in a lower economic stratum could not have come through it at all.

"Are you advocating national health insurance?"

Not necessarily. But I think if we do not find some way of moderating medical expenses there's going to be a problem with the public in general, at least among the lower half of our income families. They won't be able to afford adequate care.

I think I got a reasonable charge from my doctors. The EENT man only charged me $12.50. The surgeon's charge was $900. The radiologist will probably charge $250 or $300, but that's not for the treatments. They were $790 and that was completely covered by my insurance.

I'm concerned about my future, but I don't feel like I'm destined for doom right away. I keep thinking that it is not near as bad as it might have been. I understand my case parallels Arthur Godfrey's almost identically. Of course, he smoked for a long time, too. I'm very definitely opposed to cigarettes, any kind of tobacco. I can't help believe that the cigarettes were a major factor in my getting this tumor.

"What made you quit smoking?"

I had a chest pain, actually a little bit lower down. About that same time, several prominent citizens in town had discovered that they had lung cancer, so the combination of those factors scared the hell out of me. I gave up those miniature cigars immediately. I went to a physician and had a general examination, including my chest, but he pretty well gave me a clean bill of health. So why I came up with this tumor four years later, I don't know, but I believe that smoking for 30 years had something to do with it.

> *Tobacco surely was designed*
> *To poison, and destroy mankind.*
>
> Philip Freneau (1752–1832)
> *Poems*, "Tobacco"

2. Cystic Fibrosis

While not all lumps that grow in the breast are cancerous, the medical profession must assume they are malignant until proven benign. This dark-haired lady is married for the second time. She is not yet 40, but she has had so many health problems—a hysterectomy and loss of hearing, as well as what she refers to as "cystic fibrosis"—that she feels she is "falling apart." Her greatest difficulty, though, is living with the knowledge that the next lump she finds in her breast may turn out to be cancer. The actual medical term for her condition is most likely fibrocystic disease of the breast.

- **Lumps in the Breast**
- **Needle Biopsy**
- **Cystic Fibrosis**

I asked my doctor, "What keeps causing these lumps in my breasts? Why do they come back? Am I doing something or is there something I'm *not* doing? Is it because I've had the hysterectomy? Maybe I'm on the wrong kind of hormone or the wrong kind of thyroid or something."

He said that I have what is called cystic fibrosis disease, and chances are, I'll continue to develop these cystic-type growths in my breasts until one, I have a double mastectomy, or two, I have cancer which necessitates a double mastectomy.

He suggests that I have a double mastectomy after I'm 40. I'm 38 now. But I say, "No, no way!" Again, that's vanity, I guess.

The doctor calls these hard growths which appear . . . he calls these lumps "benign nodules." All of them were benign except this last one. He said it was definitely a tumor, and he'd done the needle biopsy and all. I had even signed the consent papers to do the mastectomy and if you don't think that doesn't put you through it mentally. But I went through it and it came out all right.

He did the needle biopsy in three or four places and couldn't get any fluid out of it. Yet it was different than the others, larger, and it wasn't the kind which would move away when you touched it. It wasn't a "floating cyst"; it was attached. The first time he measured it, it was one size and when I went back two weeks later, it had grown. These things, along with my past medical history, made the doctor think it was a tumor.

"Did they do a frozen section while you were on the operating table?"

Evidently they did and evidently they found it wasn't a tumor. I've had three of these in the left breast and two in the right breast.

I've had these nodules on the inside edges of my legs and on the underarm, on the back shoulder part. I don't know what you call it. Back in here. *(Places arm over left shoulder and points to shoulder blade.)*

The doctor said these could have been connected all of the way back to the time I had all my trouble previously, the hysterectomy, the bowel resection and the thyroidectomy. Those cysts may have started out as something as insignificant as a cystic-type growth and gone undetected. They could have started 15 years ago when I was having so much medical trouble.

I asked him, "Do you mean I have to look forward to going through this every two or three years? Every time I take a shower and find a lump, am I going to have to go into the hospital and go through this?" It is not a time-consuming thing because you just go in one night, have it removed and go home the next day. But it's the constant fear of wondering if it's going to turn into breast cancer, if there's one in there so deep that I don't know it's there until it turns into a malignancy. I worry about breast cancer constantly.

The doctor said, "There is no way to tell. You may go for the next six or seven years without having any trouble, or you may be back in here next year and have to have it done again. In six months, you may be back."

"Are you taking any medication for cystic fibrosis?"

No. In fact, he took me off all my hormones and my thyroid pills. I was taking Premarin, 2.5 milligrams a day. I'd been on that ever since my hysterectomy. So I've been off all medication for the past six months, since last March.

I don't know just what that's done for me. I do know that I am more nervous now, but whether that's due to being off the hormone pills or the fact that I've been through so many medical problems recently, I just don't know. I've noticed an increase and fluctuation of my weight, which may be due to not taking thyroid any more. I don't know a whole lot about medical, but I think that has something to do with it because ordinarily, I don't have a weight problem. Now, I'll put on 15 pounds, take off seven or eight of it, and the next thing I know, it's right back on again. Today, sitting right here, I'm probably 12 pounds heavier than I was six months ago when I had that breast surgery and he took me off the medication. And I haven't changed my eating habits so there's nothing else I can attribute it to, unless it's just the "middle-age spread" getting me.

"Now that you have this diagnosis, do you ever think about getting a consultation from another physician?"

Well, I haven't done anything. He's the same doctor who did my thyroid; he's the same one who did the bowel resection; he's the same one who did the other breast operation. He's a very competent surgeon, in my opinion, and if he says that's what I've got and I can't take pills for it or can't take shots for it, I go along with that.

Medical people are like policemen, you take them for granted. If you don't need them, they are out of sight, out of mind. But, boy, when you need 'em, they are the most beautiful people in the world.

> *What I call a good patient is one who, having found a good physician, sticks to him till he dies.*
>
> Oliver Wendall Holmes (1809-1894)
> *Medical Essays,* "The Young Practitioner"

3. Cancer of the Colon

He is obviously ill and having great difficulty coping with his problems. He is a tall, thin, pallid-complexioned man, probably in his middle 40's, who works as an inspector for a neighborhood renewal project. He relates his experiences quietly but seems to be reaching out for help. He is bewildered by his many problems, unsure of the steps he should take to regain his health and to reestablish his relationship with his estranged wife.

- **Weakness**
- **Cancer of the Colon**

- **Surgery**
- **Peritonitis**

Everything began with my first visit to my family doctor in January of this year. I went because of a slipped disk in my neck which was causing a lot of pain in my left arm. Through the treatment, we worked that out, but he did notice my blood count was a little bit low. He prescribed some iron pills for me to build my blood back up and told me to come back and see him later.

I went back to see him but I wasn't doing any good. My blood count wasn't coming back up. Along about February, I began feeling weak, couldn't walk up steps without being pretty well winded. I continued my visits with my doctor until finally, the latter part of February, he sent me to one of the local clinics there to have x-rays made of the abdomen area and the chest to see if there was anything wrong. They took these x-rays and found nothing.

"Did they do a lower G.I. series?"

No, no. Where they introduce fluids into your ass? No, they did not. All I did was drink a fluid and then they took the x-rays. Nothing through the rectum.

The report came back everything was fine, but I continued going down and down and got so weak that finally he decided to send me to a specialist here in town, where they gave me everything. That was about the first of March, five days before they put me in the hospital, because when they found what was wrong . . . . The specialist did two days of testing and readily found the tumor. And it was quite some size. Located on the right side of the colon. He said chances are, of course, that it would be malignant and suggested that I go back to my family doctor and have him suggest a surgeon. The doctor who did the testing specializes mainly in the cancers. In fact, my wife's daughter, who died of leukemia when she was eight years old, went to the same doctor.

Anyhow, he said I should go into the hospital immediately, so I went back to my G.P. who suggested a surgeon and told me to go over to his office and talk with him right then.

The surgeon said I was to go into the hospital immediately. At that point, I didn't take the thing very seriously. After my talk with the surgeon that first day, my wife and I returned home and I called my parents and told them I was going to have to have an operation. It didn't seem to upset me at all. It did my wife; she cried on the telephone. But for some reason or other, while I took it seriously, it didn't seem to upset me. The surgeon said I had a 75 percent chance of 100 percent recovery.

When I was admitted to the hospital on Saturday, they began blood transfusions because they had to build me up before they could operate. I believe I had a total of seven quarts of blood. I'm sorry, pints.

The operation was performed on Monday. But when the doctor opened me up, he found there was a great deal more than he realized. This tumor, he said, it was about the size of his fist, had eaten through the wall of the colon and gotten into one of the loops of the small intestine, adjacent to the colon. I don't know how much; I think a third of the colon was removed and one loop of the small intestine was taken out.

"You said the first symptom you had was weakness, but one of the seven danger signals of cancer is a change in bowel habits. Did you have any such change?"

Absolutely not. No indication. No loss of appetite. No loss of weight. Nothing except the weakness. However, this weakness I didn't notice too much until I suppose two or three weeks prior to my testing when they found out what was wrong with me. But no, I still ate quite heavily. I always did eat quite a large amount of food. At the time I went into the hospital, I weighed 198, and when I left the hospital 12 days later, I weighed 167. Now, because of a second trip back to the hospital, I weigh 147.

The first time, I was out of the hospital for a little over a month and this temperature stayed with me, approximately two degrees, sometimes less than that. Otherwise, I felt fairly good. I stayed at home, didn't do anything. I felt strong enough to do for myself, but the temperature seemed to be bothering me, emotionally, I suppose, a little. With impatience with my wife.

My biggest problem was the soreness. I didn't actually have any pain in the abdomen area and I didn't feel hot.

The reason I had to go back to the hospital a second time was because one Friday night I woke up with an enormous pain, approximately below the stomach, I believe. The pain was so severe that all I could do was sit. I didn't say anything but I was sweating profusely, all over. After about two or three hours, it let up, and I went back to bed.

The next day, the same thing occurred and I detected a dark-reddish color in my urine. I immediately went to the hospital again, thinking perhaps the urine had blood in it. They tested it, and it did not. I don't know what it was that colored the urine, but it wasn't blood.

But I was terribly sick. I vomited at the hospital. They put me in a room and they put in the stomach pump and the I.V. and I was quite ill, looked pretty bad, really. Wife said my color was fairly yellow.

After I'd been in the hospital about a week, the doctor, after checking me through the rectum . . . . But let me back up a bit. Before I got sick, the doctor said that I had an infection, could feel the cysts, one or two of them in there, pretty good sized. He gave me antibiotics, hoping that perhaps my system would absorb them, but he didn't have much success. He said there was a possibility that he would have to lance them, open them up. Before he had a chance to do this, I got terribly sick and back into the hospital where I stayed a week before he performed the operation. He went through the rectum and lanced a couple of cysts, each a bit smaller than an egg, he described to me. He withdrew the fluid and cleaned everything out. He gave me a saddle block and I talked to him through the whole operation; didn't seem to be nervous, I didn't fear it because I'd already been through the worst part. I asked him what he was doing from time to time. Can't say that I enjoyed it. I was awfully uncomfortable.

The operation was apparently successful because I felt pretty good when I returned to my room that night. During the next few weeks in the hospital my fever went down and my appetite picked up. After 22 days of my second round in the hospital, I was dismissed.

Since then, I've felt fine. My appetite was fairly wild; I had an enormous appetite. I wanted to eat okra and melon. I didn't ordinarily have a craving for okra but I just went wild over it after I got out of the hospital for some reason or other. Boiled okra! My tongue was somewhat parched, a little tender, and there were some things I didn't like, but now, a couple of months later, I'm completely back to normal as far as my original tastes are concerned.

My second trip cost me another approximately 25 pounds. I went down to a bottom weight of 138 when I left the hospital the second time. I've gained back about eight pounds.

The doctor said I had peritonitis when I got sick and went back in the second time. He explained that there was more wrong with me than he had expected at the original operation and that's the reason that this infection had occurred. This was where the cancer had gotten into the small intestine. They cut out a piece of my small intestine and sewed it back together again.

When I got out of the hospital the second time, I felt pretty good, emotionally and mentally. I felt that this was it, temperature was down, everything was fine, big appetite. Awfully weak and sore, but everything was doing just fine until about 10 days after I got out of the hospital. Something happened which has deteriorated me, I believe. My wife left me. She walked out and took everything I had.

My parents were with me. They stayed with me about a month to get me on my feet, set me up in my apartment. I'm not divorced yet, but I believe the mental part of it has broken me down quite a bit. I know that if my wife had stayed with me, I would have recuperated better. Mentally, it has hurt me. Right now, as I talk to you, I'm probably the weakest I have been since I got out of the hospital the last time. *(Unable to go on, he stops to rest for several minutes.)*

I've always slept good at nights, without pain. After lying in bed for several minutes, the soreness seems to go away. But now, recently, I wake up. Last night I woke up about three o'clock with a great deal of pain. But I would say that all in all, the operation was completely successful.

I go back to my general practitioner every three weeks now for a checkup.

"Were you given any follow-up radiation therapy or chemotherapy?"

No. No therapy at all. The doctor didn't mention anything about it. The best he could tell, everything was pretty clean. It wasn't necessary to have follow-up therapy. The operation was pretty successful with the exception of the infection which set in later on. But I might add one thing. I've been concerned about this because so many people have talked to me and wondered what kind of follow-up therapy I'm having. Most of them are friends or family who have had follow-up therapy with their cancer. I'm going to ask the doctor tomorrow. I don't know if it is ever too late to have follow-up therapy. Yes, I am going to ask him.

"How long were you off work?"

Well over a month, and after that, it was only an occasional visit to the work area. My sick leave finally ran out at the end of July. Fortunately, I had quite a bit of annual leave built up, which I'm using now. Then if that runs out, I've got disability insurance.

These days I'm working half days. I go home about noon and get flat on my back. The doctor said it would take a long time for me to regain my strength and my weight. This has been my main gripe, the soreness and not gaining weight, but the doctor says this will come, to be patient. It may be six months or more before I can do most anything I want to do. I get rather impatient because I'm limited in what I can do, especially now, being separated from my wife and living in an apartment by myself. I can drive, which I have to do in my job, but there's no physical labor involved. Before all of this I was pretty active. Everything was normal, and I noticed no change in myself until less than a month before I went into the hospital.

I'd like to have all of my weight back. Even though I weighed 50 pounds more than I do now, I was considered slender for my height, maybe a little bit of tummy on me but not much. I'd be tickled to death if I could put on 10 pounds in the next couple of weeks because there doesn't seem to be much progress in my weight gaining. I check every morning on my scales and there's been no change. I'm not on a special diet; he told me I could eat anything I like and as much as I want. The doctor also said he didn't think there was anyway I could hurt myself by overdoing. He said when I got tired to sit down or lie down and rest for a while, so apparently there are no restrictions on what I eat or what I do.

"What is your attitude toward your physicians?"

Well, *(chuckles)* as long as I get well, absolutely excellent. I think they did a wonderful job. They knew what they were doing. After all, we've come a long way in this type operation over a few years ago. Perhaps there should have been a bit more investigation as to exactly what was wrong with me. In other words, the fact that the cancer had gotten into the small intestine. Whether this is detectable or not I don't know, but it seems to me it could have been found out, possibly. Not being a doctor, of course, I wouldn't know. I think the first doctor they sent me to didn't look far enough. There was nearly two months between the first visit to the clinic for x-rays and the one where the specialist found the cancer. And that is quite a long period for cancer to grow. This upset me a little.

Last summer I had a physical here at the Medical Center but it must have not been a thorough physical. They detected nothing at all.

"Did you have any complaints at that time?"

No, just a checkup. They gave me the EKG and blood test and the doctor went over me, but if it were thorough enough I suppose they would have detected the cancer then, almost a year prior to my operation.

There must be different types of physical examinations, light, medium and heavy, and if I had asked for the works, perhaps they would have found something then. But then I had no reason to suspect that I needed the works.

Now, in the future, perhaps three, four or five years from now, I'll go through the same examination I did when they found out my problem originally. I'm returning to the doctor every three weeks now, but he told me when I'm feeling okay, he wants me to come back in six months, then a year and then three years. He said, "Long after you've forgotten me, I still want you to come back and see me."

In general, I would say that anyone who goes through this type of operation should have a good wife who is going to stay there with him and take care of him, see him all the way through. It means a lot.

> *In the hour of sorrow or sickness,*
> *a wife is a man's greatest blessing.*
>
> Euripides (484-406 B.C.)
> *Antigone,* Fragment 164

4. Cancer of the Thyroid

Men seem to have health problems in their 40's or 50's. Maybe it is the male climacteric, an often unrecognized phenomenon, bringing on times of crisis. This 50-year-old appears totally secure, financially, socially and educationally. Yet he underwent the torture of extensive teeth problems and, shortly thereafter, was hit with cancer of the thyroid, for no apparent reason. But then, cancer doesn't need a reason.

• Neck Cancer
• Carcinoma of the Thyroid
• Surgery

When I first felt a lump in my neck, around my thyroid, I was concerned enough to call my family doctor the same day I made the discovery. He also was concerned and he had me get an appointment at a tumor institute for iodine uptake tests.

I had to wait a few days for that appointment and I remember being very apprehensive during that interval and commenting to my wife that if there was something else major wrong with me that I didn't think I was going to be able to stand it.

In due course, the report from the tumor institute went back to my doctor and he appeared to be concerned; suggested that I see a surgeon whom I had known for a number of years and had great confidence in. Incidentally, I was very well treated at the tumor institute. They seemed to understand that people who came in there were inclined to be apprehensive and they went out of their way to show kindness.

After being examined by the surgeon, it was recommended that I have an operation. I wanted to wait until our daughter had graduated from high school, which was to be in a matter of weeks so there was a period between the time I knew I had to have an operation and when it was actually performed that we had a good deal of apprehension. Mine was related to the fact that I'd lost quite a bit of weight over the previous year so I had a foreboding that the difficulty which had been discovered was very likely malignant.

The time of the surgery arrived and the operation went well. Malignancy was discovered in two areas of my neck but the surgeon assured me in the next day or so that he thought he had removed all of the malignant tissue and my chances of full recovery were extremely good.

After I had been out of the hospital a couple of weeks and hadn't had a great amount of pain, apparently the nerves were regenerated and the pain began. It was intense for a period of some days. I remember going several nights without sleep, even under medication.

But, in general, the recovery went well and after about a month's time, I was back at work. I did, however, lose the mobility of my right arm and had to have several weeks of physical therapy to regain the use of it. I think this might have been avoided if I'd been cautioned that too much inactivity might bring about that condition and if somebody had suggested along the way that I give my right arm some exercise.

My medical insurance eventually paid for most of my bills, which were sizeable. But I had considerable difficulty with the hospital in their billing procedure. I think there ought to be some way to simplify this three-cornered transaction between the patient, the hospital and the insurance company.

There doesn't seem to be any standard way to go about it and I got all loused up with the hospital.

The care they extended to me for the few days I was in there was excellent. I had no reason to feel they were not a first-class institution.

After I had been back at work for about three months, I discovered another lump in my neck, in the same general area where the surgery had been performed. This time I was not just apprehensive, I was really scared.

I made an appointment with the surgeon immediately and he recommended fast action. Within a couple of days I was back in the hospital, had a biopsy, and fortunately the result was negative, to my great relief.

I've not had any problems since and I look back on my entire experience with a very favorable impression of all of the doctors, nurses and institutions I came in contact with. I think we are particularly fortunate in a large metropolitan area to have the kinds of facilities that are represented at the tumor institute and the hospital which is associated with it.

The surgeon is a man I've known for 25 years and had great confidence in to begin with, so I found his presence in my case to be one of great reassurance.

> *Some patients, though conscious that their condition is perilous, recover their health simply through their contentment with the goodness of the physician.*
>
> Hippocrates (460?-377? B.C.)
> *Precepts,* IV (translated by W.H.S. Jones)

5. Skin Cancer—Lymphoma

A hospital administrator in his middle 50's, he has spent some three decades as a health care provider. We talked about the impact of this sudden reversal of roles, the advantages and disadvantages of inside knowledge of the workings of the system and the shock of learning one has cancer. He said he appreciates the value of being able to pay for his medical care but also recognizes the futility of long years dedicated to advancing his career and becoming financially secure only to face the specter of an untimely death.

- **Skin Cancer**
- **Basal Cell Carcinoma**
- **X-Ray Therapy**
- **Lymph Gland Cancer**
- **Lymphoma**
- **Reticulum Cell Sarcoma**
- **Surgery·**
- **Cobalt Therapy**

I've had cancer twice. When I stop and think about that, which I don't very often, it occurs to me that most people never get cancer. They just worry about it. Maybe I got it because I was born under the sign of Cancer, birthday July 3. A crab. I remember when I was taking my cobalt treatments, we were talking about it, and I mentioned to a friend the fact that I am a Cancer, that is my zodiac sign is Cancer. I remember my buddy saying, "Look, that's a sick joke." Of course, cancer is nothing to joke about, and the internist who got a hold of me when I got the lymphoma made that pretty clear. On the other hand, everybody who gets cancer isn't about to toddle off this mortal world, either, which is the kind of thing you have to remind yourself of if you think about it at all.

I don't think about it much. It's been three years since I was operated on for lymphoma in my right axilla — the polite word for armpit you know — and it's been even longer than that since I had skin cancer, I guess two years or longer. I can't remember precisely. So for five years I have lived with the knowledge that I can get cancer. And that's not just useless worry; that's a fact, substantiated twice. But I almost never think about it. I read an article, oh, several years ago now, about some research which indicated that people who had cancer aren't anymore liable to get it again, statistically speaking, than people who haven't. This was very comforting, but I think it's bogus because speaking with a radiophysicist the other evening at the Faculty Club, he said that people who have had cancer are much more likely to have it again. Maybe the fact that I've had it twice already would support what he's saying. Of course, they say that skin cancer is just different from other kinds of cancer and that it is really not the same sort of thing as cancer of the colon or the liver or something like that. In any event, I don't plan to waste much time worrying about it. Frankly, I think about it only at the three-month checkups I have at the internist's office.

The word cancer will strike panic in your heart. When the doctor tells you you've got it and even if it's only skin cancer and even though you know, *you know* it's controllable. The first time this happened, I wasn't even in a doctor's office. The announcement came about very casually, and I'm sure the doctor meant it to be that way, but it had the same effect: panic! There were four of us sitting at lunch in a twentieth floor restaurant that revolves and you can see the whole city. It was very pleasant because this doctor, whom I had known years before in another city when he was an intern and I was the hospital administrator, became the medical consultant to a development company building nursing homes around the country. They were interested in building a rehabilitation facility, an experimental kind of thing, related not only to their nursing home business but to the health center in which I was interested. So everything was very positive and pleasant and life was beautiful until right at the end of the lunch, when the doctor said, "That's a cancer you've got on your cheek there. Why don't you come on over to the office and we'll take it off." He was so casual about it all.

Well, I'd had this bump on my right cheek which didn't heal, didn't seem to want to go away, but having had acne in my youth and subsequent problems ever since, I didn't pay any attention to it. I'd occasionally get infections and they'd ordinarily go away, but this one didn't. At the time, I didn't have a regular dermatologist and only went to see my internist once a year, probably less than that, so I figured that it wasn't anything and that it would go away sooner or later.

Needless to say, I was more than a little shocked by what the doctor said at lunch and made my way directly to the clinic where my internist had his office. I knew they had a dermatologist there so I just went in and asked for him. He saw me that afternoon. As I recall, I didn't even wait very long, maybe an hour.

"There are two things we can do," he told me, "We can scrape it off or we can burn it off. I prefer excising the lesion (I think these were his words) because it doesn't leave as much of a scar." So he stuck it a few times with a local anesthetic and carved away. It didn't hurt and didn't bleed much. As I recall, he cauterized the area, stuck a small bandage on it, and I figured that's all there was to that. My panic of the preceding lunch hour subsided rapidly after the dermatologist assured me that it was no big deal and that the small procedure he had just performed would probably handle everything.

Well, it didn't. What seems now like a year later, maybe it was six months, maybe it was 18 months, I don't remember, there it was again. In the meantime, the dermatologist had taken off to Atlanta, moved completely, so I couldn't go back and confront him with his poor choice of procedures. It was necessary to find another dermatologist and resort to Plan B, radiation therapy. Well, finding a dermatologist wasn't any trouble because the clinic which was fresh out of dermatologists was referring all their patients to another man in town who was in solo practice of skin cancer and dermatology. That's what the sign on his doors says. He, indeed, resorted to Plan B and burned off the lesion in a series of x-ray treatments. He would adjust a lead shield so that it had an appropriate size hole in the center and direct the x-rays onto the lesion which was exposed in the hole when this lead doughnut was laid over my cheek.

The procedure didn't hurt. I just had to go back for half a dozen treatments and wear a bandage over the place on my cheek which got bloody and ugly but after a while it healed up. Now I have a scar on my right cheek the size and shape of the ball of my thumb.

"What happens if this radiation doesn't work?" I asked the dermatologist. He said, "Well, it will probably work. It usually does. In some cases it doesn't and then we have to do skin grafts and other things." He didn't elucidate and I didn't worry. He did give me some stuff called PreSun to apply on my face every day between April and October. "Your skin is sun-damaged," he said, "and there is no point in getting it more sun-damaged. Put this on every morning in the spring, summer and early fall and, hopefully, that will keep you from having any more of these." So I use the PreSun religiously. Oh, I forget once in a while, but most of the time I protect my skin with it, wear sun glasses, wear a hat, all those good things. I don't go swimming.

Well, most of the time for most of the people skin cancer is no big deal. It's out there where you can see it and when you go to the dermatologist, he can do something about it. Of course, you have to be able to recognize that you've got it, which I couldn't, and then you have to get to someone who can do something about it. Of course, everybody can't do that. Either they don't know enough or they don't have the money or something. I'm sure there are some skin cancers which are tough to heal. But if you have to have cancer, skin cancer is the very best kind to have.

Other kinds of cancers are bad news. Lung cancer, cancer of the rectum, things like that. Again, I was lucky. I had a kind of cancer I could identify, at least I knew it was there, and it was one which the doctors could do something about. This one showed up as a lump in my right armpit. But at first I didn't even know that it was there.

You know what saved my life? A pair of grass shears, for goodness sakes! I have an electric-powered edger which I ordinarily use to edge the grass around the sidewalks and the driveway and so forth, but three summers ago, it was on the fritz. It had a short or something in it and just wouldn't work. We were expecting out-of-town guests and I wanted to spruce up the place and make it look nice, so I decided I would do the edging with the hand shears. Well, it's not ordinarily all that much work, but it was this time. At first, I thought I was just out of practice or out of condition because the squeezing motion necessary to operate the shears caused my hand to get stiff and numb and painful.

This pain continued up my arm and persisted for a few days after I had done the edging with the hand shears. I was naturally curious about this unexpected side effect of using the shears and began to feel around my hand and arm and it was then that I discovered the lump in my armpit. I could see it and feel it when I raised my arm. It didn't quite look or feel like the other armpit and although I had never noticed it there before, it didn't seem to be all that important. You know, you always hear about the seven danger signals of cancer and strange lumps is one of those. But when you raise your arm, there's a sort of lump instead of a hollow there anyhow. And even though I compared one side to the other side, I wasn't ready yet to admit that I was anything more than a little lopsided.

As I recall, the discomfort in my hand diminished although it didn't go away all together. The lump bothered me. Not physically, understand, as it didn't interfere with anything I was doing, but I was conscious of it. It just sat up there, silent and painless, except for occasional funny feelings down my arm and in my hand.

All that happened in late August, and early the next month I drove my daughter to college in Colorado and took a side trip to the Santa Fe fiesta. I was by myself. My wife couldn't go on that trip. I enjoyed myself at the fiesta, wandering around the Santa Fe square during the day, but restless and alone and wide awake in a strange hotel room, I spent much of two nights worrying about the lump under my right arm.

When I got back home, I looked up my internist only to learn when I called the clinic that he was off on a trip to England. Fortunately, this particular group practice has a way of accommodating anybody who just calls up and wants to see a doctor. They can handle anyone the same day. At first I thought, well, I'll wait 'til my doctor comes back, but when I learned that he'd be gone another couple of weeks, I decided to go on in. It was ten o'clock in the morning when I called, and at 1:15 I was being seen by an internist. Before three-quarters of another hour had elapsed, I had been seen by a surgeon. The internist had looked at the lump, took a brief history and said, "Well, I don't know what that is but it will have to come out." Bingo, just like that. I think doctors are very intolerant of strange lumps. Anyhow, he sent me down the corridor to see the surgeon. The surgeon didn't know what it was either, but he came to the same conclusion. "We'll have to just snake that right on out of there, whatever it is." I think he knew all the time what it was, but, of course, just looking on the outside, he couldn't tell for sure what was on the inside. He scheduled me for admission to the hospital and surgery in about a week.

Admission to the hospital was no problem. Because the hospital administrator was an old buddy of mine, I got the only room with a private bath and shower in the whole hospital and he visited me a couple of times during my two day stay.

The surgery itself was nothing. They gave me a sedative to dope me up, and I was carted merrily on to the operating room. I joked with the nurses and conversed with the nurse anesthetist until she put me under. That was nine o'clock or so in the morning and by supper time I was gradually coming back into the world of the conscious, no pain, no strain.

Of course, at that time I didn't know what the lump was and neither did the surgeon. But he zipped it on over to the pathologist so he could slice it up and look at it under his microscope. I was in the hospital in mid-week. The surgeon called me at home on Saturday about noon to tell me that the lump was malignant. The lump, I learned later, was reticulum lymphoma, grade III, and I'm not sure to this day just what that means.

The panic was there again. The doctor had reassured me that he had removed all of the ping-pong ball size lump in my axilla and said that they would probably give me a course of cobalt radiation for "the mantle," which I learned is the upper torso. He said, "I'm going to turn you over to an internist, a hematologist, who is experienced with these things and let him give you a thorough examination and then decide what to do." My own internist was still out of town, still in England, so the surgeon turned me over to a man who used to be with the clinic but now is in his own private practice.

The appointment with the internist wasn't until the next week, Tuesday or Wednesday, I think, so I had the entire weekend to think about all the other lymph nodes in which cancer might be growing. The surgeon didn't say a whole lot. He implied that the radiation would take care of anything that the surgery didn't. If there had been metastasis hither, there or yon, radiation would handle it. But the panic was there. Half of my mind was struggling to believe it was no big deal, that the surgery and the radiation would handle it but the other half of my mind couldn't stay away from the idea of imminent death. How much cancer have I really got? Where is it? What will it do to me? How sensitive is it to radiation therapy?

The panic didn't last long. Before I was ready for my appointment with the internist, the positive half of my mind had taken charge and I was resolved not to worry about it. The internist, though, was a very serious-minded person, a great personality, a doctor's doctor. He was a person in whom I had great confidence and whom I had known in the medical field for a number of years in connection with the development of a new building for the hospital in which I had been the previous week. He gave me to understand immediately that I had a serious disease, that I should not wait to take the next step, which was a complete diagnostic work-up for cancer in lymph glands elsewhere throughout my body. He said, "Now we're going to do it all, and we're going to do it now." I heartily agreed with his approach. Strangely, though, despite his discourse on the seriousness of my disease, I had the feeling that everything was going to be okay.

The doctor said, "Now, we can do this work-up on an outpatient basis or we can put you in the hospital. It's easier to do in the hospital but we don't have to. It will take about a week." "Fine," I said. "Let's do it in the hospital." It was not hard to decide. This way I would get a week off, a rest cure in the hospital, you know, and besides that, I had two insurance policies, Blue Cross-Blue Shield and major medical, both of which would pay if I were in the hospital and wouldn't if I were treated on the outside. So there wasn't much question about how we were going to handle this little ol' diagnostic work-up.

By Thursday I was in the hospital again, scheduled for blood tests, x-rays, G.I. series, upper and lower, and lymphangiography. Now that's a fascinating procedure. Apparently, lymph nodes in the upper part of the body are either easily felt or seen on x-ray but the lymph nodes in the abdomen and those parts have to be outlined by a dye and then viewed by x-ray in a process they call lymphangiography. The radiologist introduces this dye into the lymph system by cutting a hole on top of each foot, probing around for a tiny lymph vessel with an even tiner needle and then allowing the dye to drop slowly into the lymphatic system by gravity. This is not a painful procedure because they use novacaine or some other pain killer to deaden the pain when they do the cut-down.

Threading a very fine needle into one of the lymph vessels is a delicate procedure because the lymph vessel is even smaller than a blood vessel and very hard to find. As a matter of fact, on one foot (it has to go into both feet) it was so difficult to find a lymph vessel that the radiologist had to make two or three cuts. These cuts are made on the top of the foot immediately behind the toes. Apparently, the lymph vessels surface there, and if they can be found at all, that's where they're easiest to find. It is a tedious procedure and you have to lie very still. As I said, the dye goes in by gravity, and it takes half or three-quarters of an hour for the dye, once it starts, to ascend the legs through the lymph system and thus outline the glands in the area of the groin. I spent much of the afternoon getting that procedure done on me. There was a radiologist and I think a radiology resident and a technician or two running around. I was lying on a very hard x-ray table during the procedure and it was difficult to lie perfectly still.

When the dye had gone to all the places it was supposed to go and they did a series of x-rays, they found some nodes in the groin area were "suspicious." Lymph node analysis by x-ray is a rather inexact science but there was enough of a suspicion of possible involvement that the radiologists decided to give me a total course of cobalt therapy, not only for the mantle but also for the groin.

That's what this week in the hospital was for, to check all of the areas of my body by numerous methods to see if they could find cancer anyplace else. They checked the lungs, stomach and the lower G.I. tract. The upper and lower G.I. series is always a bunch of fun, where you swallow the barium for the first procedure and you get a barium enema for the second procedure. They're not done on the same day, fortunately. For the upper G.I., they just take a bunch of rapid x-ray pictures, but for the lower G.I. series, after you've had a regular enema, got cleaned out and have been given a barium enema to outline the gut, the lead-aproned radiologist takes over. He looks into his fluoroscope and moves you around the table, punching your full abdomen, shoving you this way and that, always looking into his magic-mirror fluoroscope. He takes pictures along, also, so he has a record of all these maneuvers.

I was in the hospital seven days for this complete work-up. I really had to be there about a day and a half. If the health care system had been organized, geared up for outpatient care, I could have gotten most of the stuff done outside the hospital. As it was, it was very convenient for the internist. He made rounds every day, he knew where I was, and he could schedule the work according to his requirements and those of the hospital. I got a rest cure and I got the whole bill paid. These are all strong motivators for him and for me but this is also one of the reasons medical costs are so high. I even got a couple of passes to leave the hospital to go home Saturday night for supper and to church on Sunday morning. It was like I was in the Army again. I could get a short-time pass as long as I reported back for duty.

My internist was a very practical kind of a guy. The first time he visited me in the hospital, he said, "Have you got any whiskey?" I said, "No." He said, "That's the thing to do, you know, to make your hospital stay rather pleasant. You just order up some ice about 4:30 (they serve dinner early, about five). Then you reach inside your bedside cabinet, pull out a fifth of Jack Daniel's or whatever you happen to like and have yourself a toddy." As a hospital administrator, I could see how this procedure might be frowned on. As a current and very obedient patient, I followed my physician's advice to the letter. My wife went to the liquor store, got a fifth, and it was indeed an enjoyable stay in the hospital. The one exception happened one evening when a snoopy night nurse supervisor came around about six or seven o'clock, opened the drawer to my bedside cabinet where all my personal stuff was, including my fifth of Jack Daniel's. She held up the bottle, looked at me and said, "We try to keep this out of the hospital." I looked at her and said, "Yes ma'am." But believe me, I kept it there for the duration.

As I said, I had a rather pleasant stay during that week because I was spending more time resting than testing. Oh, there were little irritants, like the fact that I was sharing a bathroom with the patient next door and the traffic wasn't bad but quite often the joker in the next room would lock the door on my side and forget to unlock it. Then when I needed to use the facilities, I couldn't get in and had to call the nurse. But this was just minor. I had no real criticism about the hospital or the people or even the food, and as a hospital administrator, you can be sure I looked around and I was prepared to be critical.

At the end of the hospital stay, the cobalt therapy began. With the test reports in, and the suspicious nodes down in the groin showing up as a result of the lymphangiography, I was turned over to the radiotherapist for a round of cobalt that last 106 days. This was the elapsed time between the first treatment and the last one. I'd get a shot of radiation two or three times a week.

Cobalt therapy is really a painless process. You feel nothing when you're irradiated. The cobalt source is in a great massive ball suspended above the treatment table. A door in this lead ball lets the radiation out when the machine is adjusted at the appropriate place above the area to be irradiated. No wires, no noises. The radioactive cobalt is just sitting in that big ball doin' its thing and when the doors open, the radiation comes out and hits you wherever the radiologist says it's supposed to go. Well, there is a noise, too. It's a sort of hum when the timer comes on and then at the end of the two-minute exposure period, the characteristic clunk of the door as it swings shut in the lead ball stopping further exposure to the radiation.

It's interesting how they direct the radiation to the right spot. First, they mark the skin where they want the radiation to go so that in successive exposures they can put it back in the same spot. They do this with indelible ink so that you have permanent tattoo marks, little dots where the radiation boundaries are placed. Then they focus the machine by turning on an electric light which simulates the radiation and then they can adjust the ball up and down over your body until the light covers the area which they want to irradiate. Whatever the light covers, the cobalt radiation will also cover.

During the period of the first few treatments, you feel nothing and you think, "This is a breeze." About that time you begin getting a white blood count prior to every treatment. The radiation knocks your white blood count down from around 7500 to a third of that or lower. In fact, that's the way they tell whether you're getting the radiation too fast. When your blood count gets around 2100, you get a holiday. They will postpone a treatment or so until your count comes back up to around 2500. The longer the treatments go on, the lower your blood count goes, and the worse you feel. You feel dragged out, totally enervated, on the edge of nausea; your energy is gone.

I felt like hell, but I continued to work every day because you might as well feel bad at work as at home. Some people can't do that. But I never lost my appetite or lost my dinner. But I never got conditioned to the odor of the x-ray department. I couldn't define the odor or describe it to anybody but it's a characteristic smell. The minute I would hit the door of the department, I'd become nauseated. Maybe this was psychosomatic but that's the way it worked.

During all this time, I lost pubic hair and hair under my arms. I don't grow hair very well anyhow and the radiation therapy essentially did in all the hair follicles in those regions. The skin on my back got rough and red as though it had been sunburned. It itched and for a while I had to apply a lanolin-based cream several times a day. Finally, in late January, it was over. Front, back, groin, armpits, neck, the works. My daughter, still in school in Colorado, sent me a "Happy Last Cobalt Treatment Day" card as a celebration of that joyous day. The radiologist said it would take about six weeks to recover, to feel myself again and he was pretty accurate in his estimate. It was two months before I could start to exercise regularly again and six months before I got back to the mile and three quarters jogging distance which was part of my exercise routine several times a week.

All and all, I'm lucky. I have passed 60 percent of a five-year cure. You know, that's the way they figure cancer survival. If you survive for five years, they figure you've got a pretty good chance to keep going. I didn't suffer all that much in the process and my insurance paid all the costs. As a matter of fact, the major medical permitted me to make a small profit on the follow-up visits. Major medical benefits have now expired after two years and my Blue Cross-Blue Shield which covers seven dread diseases including cancer in a special deal called "extended benefits" is also about wiped out. The only thing left now to pay for follow-up visits is the hospital care which will accommodate the cost of my x-rays every three months. For me, the system works just fine, but having been in the health care field for 25 years, I can appreciate the fact that I'm in a lot better position than most to make it work.

As I said when I started out, I hardly ever think about cancer any more. The assurances which I've had about my disease have come from people who ought to know what they're talking about. One is a doctor who had leg cancer some years ago and got over it, hasn't had a recurrence and is probably the best tennis player in the whole medical center. He was very kind and his reassurances at the appropriate moment while I was going through the cancer treatments were welcome and very much appreciated. All of the medical faculty was good to me. One doctor indicated that having lymphoma at my age, then 52, meant that the odds were pretty good against a recurrence. Evidently, had I been a bit older I might have had more problems. These are the things which you appreciate particularly from people who have experience and who know, people whose judgment you trust.

Cobalt radiation is cumulative so once you've had a round, you can't have another round because it builds on itself and there's a limit to how much radiation therapy one can tolerate. Fortunately, standing in the wings, is cancer chemotherapy. So if I have to go over this route again, the medical profession won't be completely out of therapeutic resources.

As one of my physician friends likes to say, living itself is a terminal disease. Personally, I'd rather be alive than dead and that's why I like to lengthen the odds wherever possible. That's the reason I don't smoke, I exercise, I watch my weight, do all those good things the doctors tell you to do but don't always do themselves. With cancer, though, you are just a sitting duck. The opportunities to prevent cancer aren't really very good. You can stay out of the sun. You can give up smoking and you can watch for mysterious lumps but that's about all. So after you've done that, there's no point in worrying or even thinking about it. So I don't.

> *While there are several chronic diseases*
> *more destructive to life than cancer,*
> *none is more feared.*
>
> Charles H. Mayo (1865-1939)
> *Annals of Surgery* 83:357, 1926

II.
Bumps, Bulges
and Droops

Dermatology is the best specialty.
The patient never dies — and never gets well.

Anonymous

Is not . . . plastic surgery an art and the plastic surgeon an artist? The plastic surgeon works with living flesh as his clay, and his work of art is the attempted achievement of normalcy in appearance and function.

Jerome Pierce Webster (1888-   )
Forward to Sir Harold Gillies and Dr. Ralph Millard, Jr.'s *The Principles and Art of Plastic Surgery*

6. Plantar Wart

We sat in the director's conference room; he was out of town. It was just after lunch. This vivacious, raven-haired Cuban girl in her early 20's is an appointment secretary for a specialized health facility in south Florida. Bilingual, she can shift instantly from English to Spanish and back again as she speaks with patients calling in to make arrangements to see one of the doctors in the clinic. In fact, she relates so well with Spanish-speaking clients that they ask for her personally, address her as "Doctor Marquita." She is friendly, attractive, outgoing, strongminded.

- **Wart on the Foot**
- **Plantar Wart**

Actually, the doctor didn't tell me it was a plantar wart. I asked him did he think this was a plantar wart and he said, "Well, I think so."

I've had this wart two years. It's on the inside of my heel on the right foot. It is not where I step on it but it rubs a lot, like where I put shoes on.

The first time I had it treated was about a year and a half ago and it was by a doctor at the beach. I was working in a hospital at the time and they told me to go to this dermatologist.

He took me in the office and gave me a shot, which numbed my foot, and with a razor blade, he cut it off. Yes, a razor blade. Not a scalpel.

He didn't look too professional, you know. He looked kind of grubby. The only thing that looked half professional was his coat, a white lab coat. Other than that . . . . And he was supposed to be a very good dermatologist in private practice on the beach. He was in private practice but he's not practicing any more.

Yeah, he chopped it off with a razor blade and the thing started bleeding like crazy and he put a patch on it. He said to come back in six weeks. But it kept hurting, you know, so I went back the next day and I said, "Look, this thing is bleeding. What should I do for it?" It wasn't bleeding that much but it was bleeding pretty much and he said, "No, it'll stop. Just come back and see me in six weeks."

It stopped bleeding. Four weeks went by and I called him from work and told him it still hurt, what should I do? He didn't say anything about taking a shower or not getting it wet. So I asked him, can I go swimming, because it was in the summertime and he said, "Just don't get it wet because I'm doing a study on it!"

That was a year and a half ago and about six months after he cut it off, it started growing back again. He didn't cut it off, he just cut the surface off. He didn't dig or anything. Like if I take a razor blade and just cut — like when you shave, you just cut the surface hair. That's all he did. And it started growing back again. He sent me a bill for $60.

First, he didn't tell me what it was and he didn't ask me if he could go ahead and treat it. He just took me in the office, looked at it, gave me a shot, cut it off and made an appointment for six weeks. That's all! That's all he did.

I haven't paid him yet and I'm not going to. I could have done that at home. He didn't give me any information. You know, he didn't say, well, this is what I want to do, is it okay? I thought at least he'd have to have consent.

Maybe a week ago, it split. It was pretty big by this time and maybe the dry weather and the salt water caused it to split. I'd been going swimming a lot.

Then it began to hurt. Monday morning it hurt a little bit and I didn't think about doing anything about it. Tuesday morning I asked a couple of the girls here in the institute what to do. You're supposed to have access to any medical services at the county hospital. Whenever their employees or their doctors need the services here, they come and there is no charge to them. And we get courtesy treatment at the county hospital.

So I called their dermatology department and they asked me if I had a clinic card for the county hospital. I said no and they said I had to have one. So I called "credits and classifications" and they said it would cost me $18 for a clinic card and then the examination is free. I said, "I don't understand why if *your* people get seen here for free, we don't have the same privilege. It's not the matter of paying the $18, it's the principle. We don't charge your employees for coming here." And she said, "Well, I'm sorry, but that's the way it is."

So I got a clinic card and then I had to call the chief of dermatology for an appointment.

"You start at the top and work down, don't you?"

Oh, I always go to the top. When I have a problem here, I always go to the director. I've been working here, it's going to be a year in June.

So I called the dermatology chief's office and found that he was out of town for a month, so I asked who was taking his place. It was the assistant chief or another doctor in the department, so I called the assistant chief's office. I couldn't get an appointment with him for two weeks. So I said, "Well, this thing hurts. I would never have called unless it hurt. I don't want him to do anything. I just want him to look at it and then tell me what I can do. He's not going to have to put me in the hospital, or even take 45 minutes. I just want him to look at it."

"Oh, we can't do that," she told me, "He can't see you for two weeks." When I told her I'd have to go see somebody else, she said to call the other dermatologist. So I called his office and told the secretary my problem and she said, "Oh no, the first appointment we have open is in a week and a half."

When I said I didn't want to wait that long, she said I could come to the clinic that afternoon or get an appointment to be seen by a resident at 7:20 that evening. I asked her how long I'd be there because I was working and wanted to arrange to be seen during my lunch hour. "Oh, no, you'll be here most of the afternoon."

I told her I couldn't come and stay all afternoon and by 7:20 my foot would fall off. She started laughing and I laughed but I told her I'd have to get it taken care of somewhere else.

By then, I almost started crying because it really started hurting. So I went to one of the doctors here at the institute to see if he could use his influence to get me in to see one of the county hospital dermatologists sooner. A couple of the institute doctors looked at it, thought it looked like a plantar wart and said the assistant chief of dermatology ought to look at it. When I told them what a time I'd been having getting an appointment, one of them said, "Aw, that's stupid. We'll call his office. If the county hospital employees can get seen right away here at the institute, you should get seen right away over there." He had a secretary call the dermatologist's office. He talked to the dermatologist, explained the circumstances and the dermatologist said, "Well, gee, send her right on over."

I was there about an hour and a half. I went straight to his office, didn't have to go through the clinic, get a card or anything. When I got there, they said, "We've been expecting you."

It's the same thing that happens here. If a doctor calls and talks to a doctor, the patient has a 99 percent chance of coming in and being seen the same day.

So the doctor looked at my foot and he said, "Aha! How long have you had it?" And I said I'd had it treated about a year and a half ago. "Who treated it?" And I told him and he said, "Ha ha! Oh yes, I know him well. He's out of practice now."

I said, "Oh really? Why? What did he happen to do? Did he just retire?" He was real young, about 45, so I knew he didn't retire. "No, no," the doctor said, "He just all of a sudden dropped out of practice." And I said, "That's interesting. I'm glad my foot's still there."

The doctor said, "What you have here is the sort of wart we treat by freezing it. It takes more than one treatment. You'll have to come back several times." When I asked him if it would hurt, he said it would and I said, "Will you give me something for the hurt?" And he said it doesn't hurt bad enough for anesthesia and yet it hurts enough. I didn't understand that because if it hurts at all they ought to give you something for it.

It killed me! He did it there in his office and I was there about 45 minutes. I don't know what he used. It's a liquid and then vapors. It hurts like heavens. It hurt a lot. That whole night my foot kept throbbing and I couldn't get to sleep. I can't believe it. I went on Tuesday and here it's Friday and it still hurts. I can't walk on my heel. I have to go back in three weeks. The treatment is supposed to eventually kill it. He says it's a virus and I said, "What do you get it from?" And he said, "We don't know." I said, "Well, how do you avoid it?" And he said, "We don't know." "Is it contagious?" "We don't know." "Can you spread it by contact. That is, if I touch it and then touch my leg higher up, will I get another one?" "We don't know." "Well sir, are you sure that it's a plantar wart?" "We think so." Real positive reinforcement there. But he seemed to know what he was doing. I guess.

The doctor said it would take about three freezing treatments to shrink it. It looks big now and it hurts big. I doubt if it's as big as it hurts. (Laughs.) Then they can take it out and I asked him if it had roots and he said no, it didn't have roots. So I asked him, "Then what are you going to take out?" My impression is that you have to dig it out if there is something deeper in there and he said, "Well, no, we're just going to take out what's surrounding it so it won't spread." So I said, "Okay" because by that time I was in too much pain to keep asking him about it and let it go. I'll probably go back but every time I think about how much it hurts, I say I'm not going back. I told him if you're going to treat it with a razor blade, you're wasting your time.

The first time, when the first doctor worked on it, he put this like sulphur on it and the whole back of my foot turned black. When he put it on my skin, it smoked. This is just part of burning it, he explained and I said, "Oh, God, this could go through to the bone. I'd like to be able to walk." But at least it didn't hurt. He gave me a shot that numbed it.

But this freezing treatment, whooo!

I don't know whether I'll get courtesy treatment because I was so nervous, I didn't think of asking. I don't know if it'll be free because the doctor here called the dermatologist or because we're entitled to it as employees of the institute. He didn't mention it and I didn't ask because I was too shook up.

We have hospitalization insurance here at the institute but I didn't take it because I'm covered by my father's insurance and my mother's too, so I don't worry about these visits costing me, but it's just a lot of hassle trying to arrange for them yourself.

"It's better if you know somebody?"

Yeah. And that's so! 'Cause you have the same problem, no matter who you know. If I know President Ford, and I say, "Look Jerry, I have this problem with my foot. Who can you call for me to get me in right away?" It's the same problem whether I call Jerry Ford or my mom. If my mom calls and the doctor doesn't have anything open, they won't see me today, but if Jerry Ford calls, boy, you bet I'd be in there within 10 minutes and probably be served coffee while I'm there.

> *The custom of giving patients appointments weeks in advance, during which their illness may become seriously aggravated, seems to me to fall short of the ideal doctor-patient relationship.*
>
> James Howard Means (1885-1967)
> *Daedalus* 92:701, 1963

7. Fat Abdomen

Her black hair is piled high on her head, forming a frame for the fair, very white skin of her face. She is 40 and rather plump. Her husband is a retired military officer, and she works in a downtown city government office. They have a teenage daughter.

- **Fat Abdomen**
- **Tummy Tuck**
- **Panniculectomy**

I have had a history of being heavy and, of course, gaining weight and then losing it causes loose skin. I had very often thought, "Wouldn't it be nice to take a knife and cut off the fat, you know, and get rid of it." Through the years they finally have improved upon this method of removing fat from your stomach.

I had gone with a girlfriend to see a plastic surgeon and I asked him about it: were they doing this kind of surgery, was it perfected and would a person find it advantageous to have it done? He said that in the last seven years they felt they had improved on this method and it would be to my advantage to have it done if it was that important to me to remove what I felt was a disfigurement. It's called an apron.

"What does he call this surgical procedure?"

Panniculectomy. What they do is cut through the . . . sometimes they do a "W" cut and pull from all four directions and take the loose skin off and it makes you have a tight abdomen again. Some women do it to get rid of old scars from other surgery and some women do it to get rid of stretch marks from having babies or gaining weight. Myself, I did it to get rid of loose skin where I had carried weight and then lost it. The doctor said he would recommend it to me, that he thought I would feel better by it.

So I went back to see him later and he explained exactly what he was going to do. I have always wanted it so it was right quick-like. Within two weeks I had made up my mind and was scheduled for surgery.

I went into the hospital one morning at nine o'clock and was operated on at eleven. At the same time, I also had breast implants. In another operation,

I'd had my breasts removed and asked this doctor if he could do both operations at the same time, the panniculectomy and the breast implants. He said yes.

"Silicone?"

No, it's much improved over silicone. It is something of a lubricant-type material which was manufactured to begin with to lubricate real large drilling tools and things like that. It's clear. And it's in a clear bag, but it's all made out of this . . . it's some kind of a rubber product but it's not silicone and it's not plastic. In that other operation, they tried putting inserts in and they were silicone and they get hard. Of course, my body rejected them. The doctor said that these would not get hard and agreed to do the breast implants at the same time. I'm very satisfied with the breast implants.

Well, I'm really satisfied with what he did on my stomach except the mistake that was made here *(points to left side)*, and I can't say it was his fault any more than mine. Mostly, it was lack of knowledge of what was expected of me and I suppose I expected more of him, at least to tell me and I think doctors neglect this.

I was in surgery for I think it was three-and-a-half hours, and I came out of it real well. I didn't have any problems in or out of surgery. I think my family said I was in recovery for about an hour but I don't remember. It must have been pretty late when I woke up. I came on and off, you know. I remember waking up and seeing someone with me there or someone saying something to me. All I remember, it hurt like the dickens *(laughs)*, and I really hadn't planned on hurting that bad. Of course, I was so sick when I had my breasts removed and in such pain, I was tolerable of pain. But this time, it really hurt. It was a real burning pain. I couldn't move because I was cut from about two inches behind where my arms hang down clear around to the same place on the other side. You're not going to roll over, and you can't move in any way and I wasn't supposed to use my arms on account of my breasts, you know. So it was pretty painful. They tell you to cough and, of course, anything you do centralizes in your stomach. I didn't know that everything you do actually affects your stomach muscles and when that happens, it pulls on them and, gosh, that was painful!

They kept me pretty well out on pain pills or shots, maybe for a day and a half. I was in the hospital a week and during that time I had problems with lack of oxygen. I couldn't breathe. I actually hyperventilated and they thought something had gone wrong with my heart. They called in this special doctor and ran some tests and he said I didn't have enough oxygen in my blood. I was using the oxygen up. The strain of the operation on my heart was causing it to use the oxygen up faster. So they gave me oxygen. They brought some kind of machine in and used it two or three times.

The pain kept up for about four days. I remember on the fourth day the doctor came in and asked me how were my breasts, and I said to him, "Who has breasts?" They should have been painful but I hurt so bad below, you know, I didn't even think about what was happening up top. After my stomach quit hurting, I could tell that my breasts were also painful but that pain was insignificant compared with my stomach.

I was awfully weak. Of course, I'd never had major surgery before. I didn't think I'd be that weak. I thought that within a week, I'd feel good. Maybe, I expected too much, but I was so weak, so weak. I couldn't get up at all. Just coming up out of the bed took everything out of me. They didn't tell me to get up and walk while I was in the hospital. I did because I'd heard of gas pains with hysterectomies and that sort of thing but you also have them with this. And I didn't know that. I thought that if they didn't go into the intestinal wall, you would not have gas, but you do. That was quite painful and I sat up a couple of nights because I thought it would be more comfortable to sit up but it really wasn't. After I was up, though, it took a lot for me to get back into bed so I stayed in this chair they had there rather than try to make the effort to get back in bed.

When I came out of surgery, I asked the doctor how many stitches I had. There were 284. Because I also have fat deposits here on the high hip, right below the waistline, he wanted to go back here (points to the hip toward her back) to remove some of that, and so to cover the whole circumference of my abdomen and the incision in the back took 284 stitches.

They had it covered up with thick gauze pads and then ace bandages wrapped around there real secure. The doctor has an assistant who comes in every day, and when they were putting on the dressing every morning, he'd say it looks fine and he'd rewrap it. Of course, they kept my breasts wrapped at the same time and the third day they let me put a bra on.

But he never did tell me what the ace bandages were for and, not knowing, I thought it was to keep the drain tubes in place — they were in there for three days — and to keep the incision covered. When they released me, of course, I came home.

Well, I don't know if you've ever tried to put ace bandages on. It's kind of a big roll, and it's rather difficult to get them tight and try to hold big pads on at the same time. My daughter stayed with me and helped me with the bandages after I was discharged on Friday.

Tuesday, I was supposed to go back to the doctor's office and Monday I was home by myself. I got along pretty well but the thing about the ace bandages; it was so difficult to get them on and off and I still thought it was just to cover my incision, and because I have pretty rounded hips, everytime I would move in bed or even just laying there, they'd slide up. They are elastic-type bandages, you know. They'd end up practically around my waist or very deep and tight around the lower section, you know. It kinda aggravated one side of the incision and I thought, well, if it is just to cover the incision and I am on clean linen, it wouldn't hurt just to leave them off. So I took 'em off and left them that way one whole day.

When I went in to see the doctor the next day, I was wearing the ace bandages because I had to keep my outer clothing from touching the incision. It was more comfortable, actually, with the pads on there because I still felt insecure, like my stomach was going to fall or something. (Laughs.)

The doctor had me come in the back door (laughs), and I had a feeling that he didn't want anybody to see me. I thought, "My God! Do I look that bad?" My family was really worried about me, said I looked terrible. In fact, they thought I was going to die. They were scared to death.

This girlfriend who went with me to the doctor that day had really encouraged me to have the operation, and my daughter said she just stood there and bawled, said she wished she hadn't talked me into it. So I really must have looked bad. Of course, I'm 40 years old and I guess a person who is not 40 wouldn't need it. It took me 40 years to get in that bad o' shape, I suppose.

I really felt bad that I was going in the back door. He told me how to use the back elevator. Of course, it might have been for my comfort, but you feel sorry for yourself after an operation, anyway.

"Did he ever tell you why he had you come in the back way?"

No, *(much laughter)*, no, no. Well, I teased him about it. I said, "I know why you didn't want me to come in the front. You didn't want anybody to see me." Of course, he is the nicest thing. He treats you like you are in his home. He acts like you are the only patient he has.

When I went in that day he said, "You are not keeping those ace bandages on correctly." And I said, "Are you trying to tell me something?" And he said, "Yes, you are not keeping those ace bandages on correctly."

"What's 'correctly?' " I asked him. And he said, "Young lady, don't you know what these are for?" I said, "Really, no!" And he said, "Well, what do you think they're for?" I said, "Well, I thought they were to keep the dressing on the incision." He said, "Not at all! There is not a place on your stomach I have not cut. I lifted your top skin up and I cut fat from all over your stomach. There's not a place from your waist to your pubic line that I haven't cut on. It's all like raw meat, underneath and the top skin. If they are not pushed back together, like gluing furniture back together, and held there, your body will put off a fluid which is a protective type thing and it won't heal."

The protective fluid collects and, of course, it has to have someplace to go to. So it settles and forms a pocket and the doctor takes a syringe-type needle — looks like something they'd use on a horse because it is about eight inches long and as big around as a quarter and has a needle about three or four inches long — and uses that to draw off the fluid. He'd take two or three of those tubes of fluid out at a time. He said if I'd start using the ace bandages right it would heal and stop throwing off that fluid.

So he wrapped it up real well but I was aggravated about it because I had planned to be back on the job within two weeks. I told the doctor, "You have made me lose one week of healing by not telling me this. You're the doctor. I'm the patient and I don't know what it takes to get me well. You have that knowledge and you should have told me that."

For a month I had to go back and have fluid drawn off. He said that if there's any in there at all, fluid draws fluid, and it will just keep on collecting. That's why he's going to operate again. The way he explained it to me was that the tissue healed down hard and formed a pocket because it wasn't pressed down evenly by the ace bandage. Now, my right side is perfect. The fluid went to my left side. Whether it went there because it had to go somewhere, I don't know, or whether it was because I didn't have it wrapped as well on the left side as I did on the right side, but the two weeks following my first visit to the doctor after surgery, I wore that ace bandage day and night. It was just like being in a cast, you know. It itches and it stings and you have different sensations from it. But in my mind I was healing so it really wasn't that bad. Finally, I was doing what was right and I knew I was going to get well. I kept looking forward to getting my strength back, which took me almost a month. I felt that if I could get my strength back, this other wouldn't be so hard. I would get so disgusted because I couldn't get up and stay up. I couldn't cook dinner without feeling like I had everything taken out of me. I enjoy being well and it was a month before I could be productive again, so I felt like I could do something.

The doctor said he feels like he didn't take out enough on the left side, so what he'll have to do is go from the middle of my abdomen back out to the left and correct the pocket formed by the fluid as well as take out more fat.

I'm almost sure, although I can't swear to it because I don't have any proof, that the assistant who is studying under the doctor did my left side. I'm sure he is a very fine breast surgeon because I know two girls who had breasts done by him but I think this stomach deal is something real new. They don't do it as often and the boy who is studying under my doctor maybe wasn't as experienced at this operation. But it was funny because my right-side incision was real rough and it stuck out, looked like it was puckered, and my left side was just laid down so smooth and had real fine stitching. One day I was teasing this younger doctor when he was tapping me, drawing off the fluid. I had to go in everyday except on Sundays for a month. At first you think it won't be long but towards the end you get sort of paranoid. I held the tray for him at times, but at the end I hated it so bad. It just really got on my nerves.

But I asked him one day, "Who sewed up this right side?" And he said, "Dr. John did." And then I said, "Well, who sewed up this side? The same person didn't sew up both sides." He said, "I did this side." I said, "Boy, this right side really looks a mess. It really looks ugly." And the assistant said, "Well, he takes a rougher stitch than me." The left side looked good but, of course, that's the side that turned out bad. But the young doctor was trying harder and probably took more time.

When this assistant first saw it — Dr. John had gone on vacation for a month — he was real upset and said, "That looks horrible. What happened?" And I said, "You tell me." I also told him, "Dr. John is not happy at all. In fact, he wants to redo it."

I told the young doctor that my left side looked like the "before" and the right side like the "after." The left side has a pocket. You can see it. It's a bulge. He said it's hard to tell when you're lying down how much to take out and he turned, kinda like he was sick over the whole thing, so I felt like maybe he actually did it, although I never did come right out and say so.

Then when I went back last week and Dr. John said he was going to redo it, his assistant was in there, and he said, "If you could lie down all of the time, you'd look perfect." And I said, "Well, I'm not that lucky." But you know, after they put you out, you have to trust these people, the physicians, like you do God. You're all in their hands, and if they don't take care of you, who's going to? It's God and them. It is really a responsibility and I think a doctor should have a little more dedication to the patient. I took him at his word because I know his reputation, being a very fine surgeon. I trusted him not to let an inexperienced person mess up my life. I have lost one month at work. I liked to have lost my job because of the time I was off and now I am going to have to go back into the hospital.

He says that this time will not be as bad. I keep going, "Oh, please, don't let it be," and I hope it won't. But I am going to have to take off again and this time without pay because I used up all of my sick leave and my annual leave. And my job is in jeopardy, I feel. I had to talk with the director of the company I work for, and he promised me I would not lose my job, but they called me before I went back last time and told me I didn't have a job. Although I trust the director, there aren't really any guarantees. He really doesn't have that much say if it came right down to the nitty-gritty. If somebody said, "Get rid of her," she'd go, you know?

I mentioned before that in the hospital they thought I had something go wrong with my heart. I thought I did, too. I thought I was going down for the count. This was the fourth day after surgery and my doctor was getting ready to release me. I passed out. I hyperventilated is what happened and, of course, tried harder to breathe and hyperventilated.

About six years before, I had gone to a reducing doctor and he took my blood pressure and he said, "Don't you feel awfully tired?" And I said, "I haven't even been to work yet. What do you mean, am I tired?" He said, "We can't find that you have any blood pressure." And I said, "So? I'm doing great." But they couldn't find much of a pulse, either.

I don't know how he tested me to find out, but he said that I had a leakage, that my bad blood was leaking into my good blood and it was using up my oxygen. So I asked him how I would be able to tell when it became dangerous and he said I would turn blue. So I said I'd always carry a mirror around with me. (Laughs.)

A doctor once told me that if I learned to breathe properly, that I would not hyperventilate. He said if you take real deep breaths and you are not exhaling, you take in too much oxygen and that causes you to pass out. You'll notice this starting to come on when you start sighing a lot. Well, I don't do that anymore. I practice not doing it. So this hyperventilating hadn't happened to me for probably five years, and when I did it in the hospital, it scared everybody and they called the doctor right away. I couldn't even talk, I was so short of breath. Just a few words would exhaust me and then I'd get scared and start trying to get my breath and that's when I'd run into trouble hyperventilating.

Anyway, my doctor said he was going to send another doctor to see me and he did. This doctor comes in and orders a test; I didn't know you had two channels of blood, venous and vascular.

This little girl who come in to take my blood was shaking. She said, "I've got to take a vascular blood test and I've never done it before and I don't know whether I can or not." She was stretching my arm out and I said, "You mean you don't know what you're doing? What's the difference?" And she said, "Well, you have venous and you have vascular veins. The one we get your pulse from is the one I've got to hit, and don't know whether I can or not but I'm going to give it a try." Well, she poked me once and she didn't make it and then she did it again. Then, I told her, "I'm going to tell you, honey, that really hurts, and if you don't make it this time, you're not going to get another chance. They think I had a heart attack, and if you think I'm going to sit here with you punching me and not knowing what you're doing, you're wrong."

There was a guy standing behind her, a young man. Of course, by then, I was quite touchy. And I asked, "Well, who is he?" And they said, "He's applying for a job." And I said, "The hell he is! This man doesn't even know me and he's standing in my room. Get him out of here." You expect the nurses in a hospital to see you nude, but this man walked off the street to apply for a job. I sure didn't care for him experimenting with me if he didn't have any experience. He left, but I thought I had my right of privacy in that room, you know.

I must have passed out again because the next thing I knew another young man was sitting beside my bed. He said, "Ma'am, I've had three years experience taking blood tests." And I said, "Oh, you mean what that girl did wasn't good?" And he said, "No, ma'am." Then I said to him, "I'm going to tell you something. I'm just going to give you one chance." He went ahead and stuck me and evidently he did it right.

But I called my husband practically in hysterics and said for him to come get me because I'd had a bad experience before in another hospital and I wasn't going through that experiment stuff again. I told my husband I thought they were trying to kill me. They were trying to find out why I was having a heart attack and I thought they were going to give me one in the process.

In a little bit, this specialist doctor came in and stood at the foot of my bed and told me who he was. He said, "You don't have enough oxygen in your blood." And I said, "I don't?" And he said, "No." Then he pulls out his card and he said, "If you ever need a doctor, call me." And he turned around and walked out.

Later, my doctor called me and I told him what the specialist had said. This was really a big strain on me because I couldn't talk very well and I felt really helpless. And my doctor said, "The hell you don't! Didn't he tell you why you don't have enough oxygen in your blood or how you're going to get some?" I don't imagine my doctor will ever call that man in to consult again.

That's really why I fear this operation. It's not so much what he's going to do. I just don't know what the danger is. All I know is that the doctor a long time ago told me I'd turn blue.

My husband was real upset. He and my family don't want to lose me. I've been a mother for a whole long time. He told me I couldn't go through this operation again; he just wasn't going to put up with it. He's afraid that I won't come out of it. I said, "Well, there's one thing about it. I'll never know it. That's the kind thing about being put to sleep. You don't know it." But, of course, your family does and I guess I should have been more considerate before I had the first operation and the chances I was taking. But I really didn't think it could affect you that serious, that those kind of complications could come up.

"How do you feel now?"

Physically, I feel great. I've got all my git up and go back. But as far as the incision and things, it's still very tender. And the side where the pocket is, by the evening it is very sensitive. And it fills up, kinda like a balloon. I don't know what happens to the fluid, now that he quit draining it. It's probably just absorbed because I'll notice after a couple of days, it's not swollen, and then in a couple of more days, it will fill back up again.

The people who knew me and knew I was going to have this operation expected me to go down like in sizes. Well, this is not true. I had fallen fat up in here *(points to her abdomen)*, but here I had a roll of skin, like a lap, that sat down on the top of my legs. Well, I've never seen the top of my legs. When I bent over to tie my shoe or put on a shoe, I had to bend over this roll of skin and it was miserable. Actually, it wasn't for you to see the results of the operation and say, "My goodness, she has a nice looking stomach" because you would never know and even the people I work with and my family wouldn't necessarily know. Of course, my family tells me I look better but I think that is just to make me feel better. But they can't appreciate the change like I do because I know it's not there anymore. I don't have that uncomfortable feeling when I'm sitting down. Before if I didn't have on something tight, it wasn't held up, you know? To me it is a personal satisfaction. It's not for anybody else's benefit, it's just mine.

"Since you had all of these problems and if you had known what you now know, would you have made that same decision?"

No, I don't think so. Of course, I have this other operation staring me in the face. Now, you ask me that a month from now, if this left side looks as good as the right, I'll say, "Yeah." If I held something so that I can't see my left side, I think I really look a lot better. Of course, I didn't have any scars on my stomach before and now I have scars to live with. But nobody gets to see the scars but me and they could see that roll, but I don't say that this operation is the answer to a fat stomach. You have to get rid of it the other way. My stomach isn't that much smaller although he took four and a half pounds of fat out of there, which should have made a whole lot of difference. Of course, this one side is swelled, but I can't tell any difference in my clothes. I can just tell I'm flat here *(points to lower abdomen)*, and I don't have to bend over anymore because I don't have this bulge down here. Unless you've had one, I don't think you can appreciate what I'm talking about.

I know several women who want to have it done. In fact, my boss's wife is going to have it done. She called me several times when I was home and I really did feel rotten. I thought I was never going to get my strength back. Of course, if you have had surgery before, you know what it takes out of you, but I hadn't. And she told me, "You are absolutely scarin' the hell outa me, but I'm still going to have it done." And she is.

Once when I was in the doctor's waiting room after the surgery, a lady got up and offered me a seat on one of the soft, low divans, but I refused it. I said, "I really do appreciate it, but I don't think I could get back up." Finally a hard chair which had arms I could use to raise myself back up became vacant and I sat down. This lady leaned over and whispered to me, "What did you have done?" because everybody in there don't want the others to know what they are there to have done, a face lift or a breast job or what. After I told her, she said she was having the same thing tomorrow. When I asked her if she really knew what she was doing, she said, "Yes, I want it real bad." I couldn't tell that she was needing it as bad as she was wanting it, so I said, "There's more to it than meets the eye. Unless you can talk to someone who's had it done." "Well, I don't know anybody," she said. I said to her, "Let me tell you one thing. Be ready to give up one month of your life and have people wait on you. And keep those ace bandages very tight. From the moment they put them on you, do not ever take them off for at least three weeks." I explained to her why.

A week or so later, I seen her in there again and she was sittin' there just so perky and I said, "How are you doing?" She said, "Fine. I'm going back to work next week." And I thought, "Oh, God!" Because I'm still going in and being pumped every day and still had the darned ace bandages on 'cause he had to put a tube in to help drain it. I was getting pretty aggravated with it all. She said, "I really appreciate you telling me about those ace bandages. You know, they didn't tell me a darn thing."

I felt sure they wouldn't. I don't think they do it on purpose. I just think they take their job so for granted that they do a good job but they fail to inform a person. They don't realize we are so ignorant as to what we are paying for.

The other day the doctor said to me, "Really, you don't look that bad." And I said to him, "If I wore a girdle, I didn't look that bad before I come to you, and for $2,000, you're supposed to make me look better."

The next operation is on him.

Anybody who is anybody seems to be getting a lift — by plastic surgery — these days. It's the new world wide craze that combines the satisfactions of psychoanalysis, massage and a trip to the beauty salon.

Eugenia Sheppard
New York Herald-Tribune,
February 24, 1958

8. Drooping Eyelid

She and her husband live in a surburban apartment complex in a Southern city. They are retired but comfortably well-fixed and enjoy traveling and social activities. She is small, has white hair, smokes rather heavily. Though the results of her surgery were not what she expected, it did not affect her sense of humor.

- **Drooping Eyelid**
- **Plastic Surgery**

I made an appointment with the doctor about a week before Thanksgiving. Jim had wanted me to go to Acapulco and I didn't want to go. So I told him to go to Acapulco and I'd go get my eye fixed.

I was already blind in my right eye. My left eye had a water sack down below and a thick upper lid, so I went to have that taken care of. I went to Dr. Grady because he'd been recommended to me by a friend. He made arrangements to operate on me the day after Thanksgiving. He was going to repair the upper lid and the lower lid, I suppose, to release that water. He didn't tell me why the water had accumulated. It just happens. He said it happens often.

Two days before Thanksgiving he called me and said he wouldn't be able to take care of me but this other doctor would. He said this man was a very good plastic surgeon, so he took me up and introduced me to him. They both told me there was nothing to it; it was done through a local and it would just take a short time.

I went in the day before Thanksgiving. I was supposed to have a local but I didn't get anything to eat that night at all. The next morning they came in and wrapped my head and took me down. I waited a little while and finally the doctor came and we went into the operating room. He introduced me to another doctor whom I didn't know. I said, "Let's get going. I'm tired of waiting."

The first thing I knew, I was dead to the world. They gave me some kind of a shot that knocked me out completely. I hadn't anticipated that. I expected hypodermics around my eye, which I'd had before.

When I woke up, I was in my room. I asked what time it was. They had taken my watch off me. It was two hours later and I asked how come it took so long and they said they'd kept me in intensive care for an hour. "Intensive care? For what?" I asked.

Oh, before that, he came in and begged me, pleaded with me to let him operate on the eye I was blind in because the upper lid was drooped. He said I would get that water sack in the lower part of my blind eye because after the operation on my left eye, the water would transfer over to the other one. Well, I didn't know whether it would or it wouldn't. He sat there for an hour and pleaded with me to pay him another $300 and have both eyes done. So finally I said, "Okay."

When I woke up in my bed there was a nurse there, standing beside me. Both eyes were bandaged. I didn't think both eyes should be bandaged because the eye itself hadn't been operated on and I had to see. Twelve years ago when I had my cataract removed, my eyes were never bandaged. I just had aluminum shields on them.

The nurse said I had to lay very quiet and told me someone would be in to feed me. She showed me where to press the button if I needed anything and said I couldn't go to the bathroom by myself. They didn't want me to rip a stitch or anything.

The other doctor in the operating room was an anesthetist. His bill was $96 over the $600 for the surgery and the charge for the room and everything.

The doctor came in the next morning, took off the bandages, signed me out and I went home.

A week later, I went back to the doctor to get the stitches taken out. I looked fine. Both eyes were up and fine, but when he went to take out the last stitch from my right eyelid, the one next to my nose, he couldn't get it out. He said to me, "I'm so nervous I don't know what I'm doing and you're nervous, too, so lay down!" The nurse made me lay on the table; I was sitting on the edge of it. That stitch must have been caught in the bone because when he pulled it, it bled and it hurt like the dickens. But it hadn't hurt the other eye. I asked him about the stitch and he said, "Oh, that'll be fine."

Well, it wasn't. It left the upper eyelid up there so that, as you can see, I've got an open space there. A week later, my husband took me back to the doctor's office and we showed it to him. He said he couldn't see anything wrong with it; it looked fine to him. He said both of my eyes have that opening on them. I said, "My left eye doesn't have it." That's all he said. He didn't do anything about it. He bid us good-bye and we had to leave.

From then on, I went around looking like a maniac. I called Dr. Grady and at first he wouldn't see me. Then the second time, he told me not to come into his sitting room but to come direct to his office. I went in and sat there 35 or 40 minutes and he came in and said, "I think it looks fine," after looking at my eye. But it didn't match my left eye.

I was going to sue him. We went to an attorney who told us to go to some other doctors. We went to three others doctors and none of them would do anything about it. My eye didn't look good but they didn't want to get into any malpractice suit.

The first doctor sent me to the second one who said he'd operate on my eyelid. He said he'd repair it for $400 but he wouldn't appear in any suit. And he wouldn't show us the letter the first doctor sent him when he referred me. He told us that the operation I had was a long operation and the doctor who did it might have gotten tired and this could have caused the effect I have.

Then I went to a third doctor, and he wouldn't commit himself one way or another. I didn't go back to the attorney because he said he couldn't do anything unless we had some other surgeon who would corroborate that it was a bad deal. I was fed up.

I had beautiful blue eyes and my artificial eye looked just like my other eye, until this operation. Now, the lower lid is low and bent in and the eye lashes on it grow in instead of out. And do you know what the doctor said? "It's a false eye. It won't hurt anything."

Husband: When we saw that the first doctor sent us to a silly son-of-a-bitch like that, there was no use talking about it. What we're talking about is, what does a guy do for $600? He knew he had a false eye there and he could screw it up and nothing would hurt. And he could get another $300. My wife doesn't want to sue anyone. All she wanted to do was get enough money so she could have that eyelid lifted so she wouldn't look like she was goofy.

The ophthalmologist we saw first after all this happened was very emphatic about the silliness of going to a plastic surgeon for an eye job. He described the doctor he referred us to as a this, that and the other in medical terms. He said he knows all about eyes and all about plastic surgery and *he's* the kind of man it takes to do an eye job.

"How did you learn about the plastic surgeon in the first place?"

Patient: The daughter of a friend of mine had her stomach made smaller by this plastic surgeon. The doctor who did operate on me is a burn specialist. A plastic surgeon for burns. But he thought he could make $600 on my eyes.

When I was in the hospital, it was Thanksgiving day. Everybody was talking about the Thanksgiving dinner we were going to have, but I don't know what I had. My eyes were bandaged and I couldn't see. The nurse told me I could eat it with my fingers, they weren't going to feed me. I fiddled around with the plate. It was stone cold, as if it had just come out of a freezer. I didn't know what it was, so I pushed the tray right off the table onto the floor. I was disgusted.

I had an intravenous, I don't know why. There was a needle in my left arm but there was nothing to hold it down, to keep the needle from coming out. When I reached for the phone once, and dropped it, I bent my arm. When I did that, I broke the intravenous needle off in my arm. I heard the needle crack. I grabbed ahold of it and held my arm up. The nurse and the doctor came in and put tapes around my arm, above and below, real tight. I didn't want that needle going up or down in my vein because that could have killed me. When I removed my hand, where I was holding my arm, the doctor said, "Well, I'll be damned. That needle *is* broken. I didn't believe it."

Oh, I've had some weird experiences in hospitals. When I had my second cataract operation, years before, they tied my head up in a sheet, just like the first time, and poured distilled water over my eye before they began the surgery. And I just couldn't resist saying to the doctor, "Well, here I am in the 'sheet house' again." *(Laughs uproariously.)*

It is no part of a physician's . . . business to use either persuasion or compulsion upon the patients.

Aristotle (384–322 B.C.)
Politics, VII, ii (Tr. by H. Rackham)

III.
Breath of Life

*Some folks seem glad even to draw
their breath.*

William Morris (1834–1896)
The Earthly Paradise, "Bellerphon at Argos"

9. Emphysema

The dining room of the suburban house had been converted to a bedroom because the patient could not make it up the stairs. I sat in a chair at his bedside and he sat, fully clothed, on the side of the bed. On a table within reach was a mist-making machine to which was attached a long tube. On the end of the tube was a mask. As we talked, he would stop occasionally to breathe for several minutes through the mask, inhaling medicated mist so that his breath would come easier and he could continue.

He is a retired newspaper man in his early 60's, blonde and very thin. He speaks with the ease of a person who has spent a lifetime putting words together. He is ambivalent about his doctor, trustful and at the same time suspicious.

- **Difficult Breathing**
- **Pneumonia**

- **Tracheotomy**
- **Emphysema**

About a year ago in September, I thought I had a bad cold or something and stayed home for two weeks. About the fifteenth of September, when I planned to go back to work, I woke up one morning and just couldn't breathe.

So I called my doctor and he told me to meet him at the hospital. It was a Monday morning, and when I got out there, he didn't think I had pneumonia, but anyway, that's what it turned into. Sometime during that first week in the hospital, I lapsed into unconsciousness and the next thing I knew, I was in intensive care.

"How long were you unconscious?"

Maybe a couple of days. I woke up in intensive care and this was on a Sunday. I don't guess the doctors knew I could hear them, but I heard them talking and they were going to do a tracheotomy. I remember that. I was in there three weeks and, oh, it was just like being in a cell. There was only one window and they had the bed arranged so that the head of the bed was on the window wall and I couldn't tell whether it was day or night. There was a clock but I couldn't tell if it was seven o'clock in the morning or seven o'clock at night. So I asked them what I had to do to get out.

Well, they had me rigged up to some kind of a machine to breathe; I don't know enough about it, but it was an accordion-type thing that went up and down. They said if I could stay off that for 24 hours, I could go into a private room. So I told them, "For God's sake, let's get that thing started!" So they took me off and a day later I made it back to a private room. But I couldn't walk.

To cut a long story short, I was in the hospital two months and I came home the day after my birthday, which was the 16th of November. I was 59, that was last year.

My doctor told me when I came home that I had almost died. My doctor didn't tell me much but he did tell my wife I had emphysema. Of course, I had known that for some time. Ten years ago, I had bought a piano, a baby grand piano, from my next door neighbor and I refinished the case. A friend of mine who tunes pianos and works on them came over and picked up the big part that has the harp in it, and he was going to clean that up and restring it and so forth. I went over to his shop one Saturday to see how he was doing and he was spraying that harp with lacquer. It was in his garage, but it was really more like a house; it was all closed up. When I woke up the next morning, I couldn't breathe so I went to the doctor — I had a different doctor then — and he told me I had a chemical-induced emphysema which I had got from that spray. He told me he had had patients who had died from inhaling those fumes off of those sprays. I don't understand it because the fellow who was spraying the harp didn't have a mask on.

But anyway, that's how it started. And, of course, my smoking didn't help it any. I smoked all my life, up until a year ago, up to three packs a day. But it wasn't the cigarettes that started it, so my doctor said. Course, that didn't help any.

When I was in the hospital for two months with oxygen, I couldn't have smoked even if I wanted to. So when I came home, I had two months under my belt. Well, after you've gone through what I went through, you don't go back to smoking. Have you ever had a tracheotomy and had to be . . . what do they call that when they dip out the phlegm that you can't cough up?

"Suctioned out."

It's pretty painful. After a few such sessions, a cigarette isn't worth it. Oh, there are still times I want one, don't misunderstand. But it has made a difference. I don't drink coffee any more because I guess coffee is too clearly associated with cigarettes. The coffee just doesn't taste like it used to. I think it is all associated in my mind with a cigarette. It's the same way with a drink of booze. I just don't have any desire for a drink because that, too, is associated with cigarettes.

I'm retired now. I had to. I'm not able to work now. It was my doctor who suggested that I file for disability under Social Security. He told me that I could have qualified three years ago, but he didn't say anything to me about it then. I was working, I didn't know any better and, of course, it wasn't near as bad then.

I've been back to the hospital five or six times since I got out last November. Just for three or four days. At first, I went back because I just couldn't breathe at all, with the oxygen and medication, I still couldn't breathe. But now, I think I've learned to control that. I don't know, I haven't read that much about it, but I think emphysema must have some psychological aspects that I wasn't aware of. I know now that if I lie here and try hard enough and concentrate on it that I can regulate my breathing. When I wake up and can't breathe, I don't get upset about it. I don't panic because I know that if I lie there and breathe through my mouth for a while, pretty soon I'll get the rhythm back and I'll be all right. The more you panic, the less you can breathe. Which stands to reason.

The last time I went back, I had pains in my chest and my stomach and my wife thought I had bronchitis and I guess my doctor thought so, too. But after he got me out to the hospital, he found out that I had been breathing through my stomach more and that I had sore muscles.

But I don't know why I've gone back so many times. There are some things the doctor has done which I don't understand and I don't mean to find fault, but he's never told me.

I don't much believe in taking a whole bunch of medicine. One day I was so spaced out, I felt like I was on dope so I went to the doctor for a checkup and I told him I thought I was over-medicated. I dropped some of it. I knew that the tranquilizers didn't do anything particular so I quit taking them. And I knew that the sleeping tablets didn't help so I quit them. And I wondered if there wasn't some of the other medication I could eliminate and he said yes. This was a different doctor. My doctor was on vacation and this one was substituting for him. You see, I'm on Bronchosol and he said to cut that back about a third. So I cut it back a third and I felt fine. Then I cut it back to half and it worked fine, so I cut it back some more. The doctor told me I cut it back so far that my breathing got out of kilter again.

Course, I know that the weather has got an awful lot to do with the way I feel. When I first came home from the hospital last November, I got up and went Christmas shopping and went back to work for two or three weeks. But I think I could do that because the weather was cool and the humidity was low and there wasn't any pollen or dust in the air. It's in the spring, during the rainy season, that I have difficulty. Right now, for the past few weeks, I have been feeling pretty good. We've just recently had our house fixed, siding put on and the windows caulked and it's airtight, so that may be another reason that I haven't had too much trouble lately. Oh, I've been out. I was out and worked in the yard an hour this morning. It is in the evening that I seem to clog up.

Every time I went back to the hospital, I had to go in an ambulance because I had to have the oxygen except the last time when I had chest pains. That didn't have anything to do with my breathing. My wife took me out there then. Once I had to go back during an electrical storm. You know, a front was passing over and it was so close that I couldn't breathe.

In time, I learned that if I don't panic and I lie there and breathe through my stomach and my mouth, why, I'll get my breathing back. Because when I went to the hospital and they took me out of the ambulance and took me into the emergency room, they just laid me on that table and I had to lie there and wait for an hour. So I decided, "Shoot, if I'm going to do that out at the hospital, I can do it here at home."

Back in September, when I first went in the hospital, I was having a chill, so I asked the nurse for a blanket. She told me I wasn't having a chill but my teeth were chattering. She never did bring me a blanket and wouldn't pay me any attention at all. The doctor came and read the nurse the riot act. I remember the doctor telling me that this is one hospital where the nurses never listen to the doctors. He said there was nothing he could really do because there is a shortage of nurses and the hospital won't fire them.

I had difficulty with their accounting department, too. Because we have two policies, I just signed my insurance over to the hospital, like I always do, and they wound up owing me $480 or $500. This went on for six months or so. Fortunately, I didn't need the money, but finally I began getting these nasty letters. I owed them $50 for an emergency room visit and they were going to charge one-and-a-half percent interest a month. And the reason I owed the $50 emergency room charge was because they had applied a payment to the wrong bill. My insurance companies had already paid and when the hospital sent them a bill, they wouldn't pay it a second time.

Finally, what really blew my stack was that when my daughter came to get me, they weren't going to let her take me home until she'd paid that $50. My daughter said that our policy pays all. "All you have to do is look on the ledger sheet," she told them. And he said, "There's no need for me to look on the ledger sheet. I know what it pays. I've read the policy." Then my daughter said, "Well, why don't you just deduct that $50 from what you owe him?" With that, it shocked him so much that he did look on the ledger sheet and he let me come home.

Oh, that made me furious. I called the hospital and asked one of the secretaries, "If you have a board of directors, I want to know who the chairman is." I've been in public relations long enough to know there's no need to mess with the peons. So I called the chairman, and the very next day the accounting department called me. He apologized and was very nice. He cancelled the emergency room charge and sent me my check. He also explained to me what had happened.

That's all my complaints. They've been very nice to me and I've had excellent service out there.

It was very depressing there in intensive care. One night, I called the nurse because I wanted her to suction me. I got this little black nurse's aide so I asked her if she would suction me and she said, "Yes, if you show me how, I sho' will." I just can't imagine having . . . I wasn't in that position, but supposing my life depended on that girl's knowledge. Where would I have been?

And there was one nurse there, oh, she was mean. The pain she put me through when she suctioned me. I didn't know until I got upstairs in a private room and still had to be suctioned that the nurses could do it where there was no discomfort at all. But every time that nurse in intensive care did it, boy, it was awful. And I didn't know any better. It wasn't unbearable but I waited until I couldn't stand it any more before I'd call anybody to suction me, it was that uncomfortable. But upstairs, there were times when I thought the nurse hadn't even started and she was already through.

One day something happened in intensive care that I needed a nurse and it was just about time for them to change shifts. I rang the bell and turned on the light and nobody came. I could see that nurse out there standing, and she'd wave back to me but she never did come in. It wasn't very important because I lived through it but, you know, when you're down and you're sick and you get panic-stricken, it's a pretty hellish experience.

When I got in a private room, the care was much better. They were more considerate, I'll put it that way. But while we're on the subject, let me tell you something. There was a water fountain in my room that wouldn't work and one day when I was having so much trouble breathing, they came in there, brought this jack hammer and every thing else and worked on that damn water fountain. It about drove me out of my gourd, the dust flying, the racket.

Once when I was in intensive care, they had a patient who died. Man! That liked to scared me to death. All of the whistles went off and everybody went running. That's kind of a shock, too, to have somebody working on you and all of a sudden they drop everything and run off and you hear all of this stuff going off. That's depressing because I knew somebody died. I was at the end of the hall and I could see clear down there.

Overall, the service was very good and I have nothing really to complain about.

"What did the doctor tell you about your problem?"

He really has told me very little. I don't know what he told my wife but when I came home from the hospital in November, I thought I'd be just like I was before. I made arrangements to go back to work the first of January, the way the doctor said I could and I was upset because I could only work two hours a day. I just didn't have the strength. I'd get tired and my mind would get tired and I just couldn't think. And I couldn't walk the different places I had to go. I had a very bad spring and that's when I went back to the hospital about every month.

Now that the weather is cool and the humidity is low, I am feeling pretty good. Somedays I go shopping or to the bank, or go get a haircut and these are things I couldn't have begun to do in the spring. Some days last spring, I couldn't even walk into the kitchen to eat. I was breathing on this thing *(bronchial mist machine)* and was on oxygen all day long.

The doctor doesn't say much except that I'm never going to get any better. The day I came home from the hospital this last time, I got provoked with my doctor. He was talking with a resident physician who makes rounds with him, a young doctor, and I heard him tell that doctor I've only got 16 percent and he didn't see how I could do as well as I did. Fact of the matter is, he said he didn't see how I felt like getting out of bed. Well, it made me mad and I was very depressed. The more I thought about it, the madder I got and I thought, "Well, hell, if he doesn't know any more than that about it, how does he know whether I'm going to get well." So I was determined I was going to show him.

I don't mean to find fault with him. God, he's been wonderful to me. I'd never go to another doctor because, in the first place, he's done things for me no other doctor would do. If I need anything, he'll come. That's the reason I quit going to the other doctor I had. He didn't have the time to see me. Of course, that doctor didn't tell me, but his nurse said to me that I'd have to make an appointment to be sick, six weeks ahead. If I can't see him, it doesn't do me any good to have him, so I just never went back.

I have an awful lot of time to read and I was reading in *Reader's Digest* about a survey of emphysema patients. They had done some autopsies and found that people who had quit smoking for two years, their lungs had begun to restore themselves. And I asked my doctor if he'd read it and he said no, he hadn't read it but he didn't believe it. He said there are some parts of your body which will renew themselves but the lungs aren't one of them. I thought that was a strange thing to say. When you are grasping for hope and you read a scientific paper . . . how can you say whether . . . . At least, I think it bears looking into.

"I guess you have smoked for your entire lifetime."

I started when I was a freshman in college, when I was 16, so it was 40 years.

"Do you think the public understands the role of cigarettes in emphysema?"

I don't think I understand it. Of all of the people I know who have smoked, I only know three or four who have suffered any ill effects, so I don't know whether it's that or heredity. I think alcoholism must be inherited. A drink or two doesn't bother a lot of people but it can kill somebody else. I think it must be that same way with cigarettes and I just happened to be one who couldn't take it. It may be that if this chemical-induced emphysema hadn't come along, maybe I wouldn't have it now. I don't know. Cigarettes don't do you any good but a man I know is in his 70's and he smokes more than I used to. And my uncle smokes cigars and I understand now they're as harmful as cigarettes. No, for everyone you can name who's got emphysema or suffers, I could name you a dozen smokers who don't. I don't know.

"How would you advise people?"

Well, if you don't smoke, for heaven's sake, there's no point in starting. And if you can quit, I would quit. I tried and I quit for as long as two months. A lot of people I know who have quit say they didn't enjoy it to begin with. But I did enjoy it. I would still enjoy it. There are days that I don't even think about it and then, for no reason at all, I think, "God, it would be great to have a cigarette."

I have a friend who quit and she said to me, "Well, you know, it just dawned on me one day that I went to bed at ten o'clock and did without a cigarette until I woke up in the morning." I didn't do that. I'd wake up in the middle of the night and smoke a cigarette. I think it's a psychological thing. I think some people need 'em and some don't. If you don't start, you're better off.

And it is offensive, I've learned that. I've been places recently where people smoke and I have had to get up and leave. And if we have friends over to play cards and they smoke, I either have to ask them to quit smoking, which I don't like to do, or I just come in here and breathe on my machine until I can face them again.

I certainly wouldn't advise anyone to learn to smoke.

The patient's family will never forgive a guarantee of care that failed and the patient will not let the physician forget a pronouncement of incurability if he is so fortunate as to survive.

George T. Pack (1898–)
Annals of Surgery 127:1105, 1948

10. Asthma

The curly-haired redhead moved quickly into the room, was detained by his mother just long enough to be embarrassed by being introduced, and dashed out again. He is a handsome youngster, about eight years old. His mother, also a redhead, is on the high side of the childbearing age and obviously worships this beautiful child of her later years. The boy's father is the manager of the local branch of a New York-based firm of maintenance contractors. The mother insists that her son adhere carefully to the rules of living which will prevent asthmatic episodes. The boy plays football and does everything else his medical problem will permit, which delights his father.

- **Rattled Breathing**
- **Bronchial Pneumonia**
- **Asthma**
- **Tonsillectomy**
- **Adenoidectomy**

We're talking about our son, Jim. He's our fourth child.

I commented to the people in the hospital that he was rattling, that is, when he breathed he rattled, there in the hospital, just after he was born. Of course, I may have been a little bit more particular because he came to us late in life, because our other children are quite a bit older.

I commented about his rattling to the pediatrician, who said to me, "Now you are a mature mother and you know that babies sometimes have mucus in their bronchial tubes and that will clear up."

Jim was allergic to all kinds of milk. When we brought him home from the hospital we went from one kind of food to another and finally came up with soy beans. That was the only thing he wasn't allergic to, didn't throw up and which didn't cause a skin rash. I kept taking him to the pediatrician until I finally decided that I was old enough and smart enough to know that there was something terribly wrong with this child. So I started taking him to an internist, a general M.D., a family doctor. I said, "This child is sick. He's a year and a half old and there's something wrong with him." And the doctor said, "Yes, there's something wrong with him. He's got bronchial pneumonia." That was just the beginning of a long period of visits to doctors.

When Jim was two years old, I said to the doctor, "Don't you think this child has asthma?" And he said, "Yes, I do, and I suggest you take him to the allergy clinic, the asthma clinic."

"Then you made the diagnosis?"

Yes, I did make the diagnosis, because I asked. I could hear him wheezing and was more conscious of it because my brother has two daughters who have it so I had been exposed very lightly to someone who has asthma. My brother doesn't live here in town. The doctor did not volunteer it; I was the one who asked about whether Jim could have asthma, so you could say I put my finger on what was wrong.

I took my baby to the allergy clinic for the tests and it was pathetic. A two year old doesn't understand all of the things that happen to him, all of those needles under the skin and everything. When it was all over with, they gave me a nice, big report on him, how asthmatic he was, how it was unusual to find a child that young that had as many allergies as he had. They listed them out and they said this child needs to come in twice a week for desensitization shots.

But the catch to it was, if your child is taking desensitization shots and by the time you get home, he has an asthma attack, you don't take him back to the allergy clinic for the treatment of the asthma attack. You have to have your own doctor do that.

I took this little booger down there and, two shots, one in each arm. Twice a week. The first time I took him, by the time I got him home, he was vomiting, he was so sick. This was in the afternoon and I had to take him to the regular doctor who said he must have had some reaction to whatever they gave him.

So then, we went again and I told them about the reaction Jim had and they said not to worry about that because that wasn't the first time that had happened. So they gave him two more shots and by the time I got Jim home, he was sick, real sick and then he went into an asthma attack and I had to rush him to the doctor again. Oh, yes, he vomited. This attack was a severe one and didn't go away the way it should have gone away, and the next thing I knew, he had bronchial pneumonia.

I called the doctor and he said Jim didn't have to be in the hospital, that I could do as much for him at home. He said Jim didn't need to be under oxygen, just a vaporizer.

I called the allergy clinic back and I said my son will not be down because he is sick, he has pneumonia. They told me that when he got over it to bring him back down. And I, like a ninny, took him back down there when he got over it. He had been sick for two weeks.

I went back there because I thought it was the thing I was supposed to do. He got a shot and before I got him home, he had vomited all over my car. I had stopped at a service station to get some water to bathe his face and he threw up there, in the driveway. And of course, he was so small.

I called my regular doctor and said, "Jim's sick again." And the next day, when I took the child to see him, Jim was still vomiting. That's when I decided I was doing this child an injustice by taking him to the allergy clinic. I called the doctor at the allergy clinic and said, "Look, you should change the shots. You've got 'em too strong. My child is sick again." But he said, "No, it takes time for them to build up this immunity."

Being as old as I was, I decided this was for the birds, this was all wrong, that I was hurting my child. It took about three months for all of this to transpire and besides the shots, they'd given him other kinds of medicines, antihistamines, for him to take, and between that and the shots, he was just sick. So I quit taking him to the allergy clinic. I said there must be a better way.

Jim has had pneumonia three times in his eight years. By going to the clinic and having all of these tests made, I did find out what he is allergic to, which I didn't know before. We tore out our heating and air conditioning and had a new one put in and had a Honeywell electronic pollenator put in. It burns up all of the pollen in the air. This helped him because he is very allergic to Bermuda grass and, although we live in the city, I can't pave the entire city.

I went to my internist then and told him that they're killing Jim at the allergy clinic and I can't take that any more. He said, "I don't blame you. Now, it's just going to be trial and error until we find out what helps him and what doesn't help him."

The wind and dust and the grass and the pollen have been real rough for him. I've tried to keep him in a controlled atmosphere as much as I can, but he's an active child and that's hard to do.

I carry a prescription for the amount of ACTH and adrenalin which Jim needs when he has an attack. Sometimes we have to take him to a hospital emergency room for a shot and I have these amounts written down on a paper I carry with me. It's not a hard decision to know when to take him in for a shot. When your child goes, "Haaaa," (*demonstrates by noisily sucking in her breath*), you can see his chest contracting, his lungs aren't getting enough oxygen. You know when your child is bothered by a little bit of asthma, you can hear his wheezing or whistling up a storm in his lungs.

You don't want to rush them in to the doctor or the emergency room unnecessarily, I know that. The adrenalin is hard on their heart. It has the tendency to enlarge their heart. The doctor told me that but he didn't tell me anything I didn't know because one of my nieces has an enlarged heart from taking so many adrenalin shots. Then our internist had a heart attack and was trying, as graciously as he could, to cut down on his practice. Also, his office was almost downtown and sometimes it was pretty hair-raising to get Jim down there when he was having an asthma attack, so he could have his adrenalin, ACTH, etc. So I went shopping for another doctor.

I asked the internist's nurse what to do once when Jim had an attack and she asked if there was a clinic up beside us somewhere. When I told her there was, she said she would call them. The doctor I took him to at this new clinic wasn't going to give him any shots until he had found out about Jim's trouble. He was very gentle, and acted like he had treated an asthmatic person before.

When our internist did get out of the hospital after his heart attack, he told me, "I just can't keep it up." He meant his heavy practice. So I decided right then and there that Jim had too many years to live, that I had to find someone to take care of him.

I went back to the other doctor at the nearby clinic and said, "Here I am. I won't call you unless I need you. I never call for a cut or a fall, but when I do call, I need you." He said, "I can understand that."

This doctor is a general practitioner, not a pediatrician. I left the pediatrician when I tried to tell him Jim was asthmatic and he wouldn't listen to me. He's been treating Jim now for a little over two years. That's right, it has been that long. He has been just great with him, just great, and Jim has improved.

Jim had bad tonsils and before when he had tonsillitis, he'd always go into an asthma attack. Of course, they said there is not any doctor in town who'd touch him, taking them out. The doctor he has now kept saying, "They've got to come out, they've got to come out. But I don't think it's just the right time."

Well, Jim kept having problems and in January of this year, he started having kidney infections and was just going down hill and the doctor said, "Now's the time. Somebody's got to take this kid's tonsils out."

So I said to him, "Who do you recommend? I don't want anybody that doesn't know what they're doing because this is an asthmatic child."

I took Jim to the surgeon my doctor recommended and told him Jim was asthmatic and gave him the list of things he is allergic to. But, as far as medication goes, they do not test children in allergy clinic as to what medication they are allergic to. The skin tests are not for medicine. They are for all of the things you live with. So to find out what kind of medicine an asthmatic child is allergic to, it's trial and error. And it can be rough. And when you encounter a medicine they're allergic to, boy, you stamp it on your mind, right then and there.

We discussed the medication I knew Jim was allergic to and I told the doctor, "He has never been put to sleep." I told the doctor to be sure the anesthetist he uses knows that this is an asthmatic child. He said yes, he would.

Well, whatever anesthetic they used, Jim was allergic to it. He had several seizures in the hospital.

"Wasn't there any way you could test for that?"

This was what I wondered about. But how do you tell your doctor, "Look, I want you to do some tests to see what kind of anesthetic he's allergic to." The guy would just look at you and say, "You idiot! I'm the guy who's spent 10 years studying. You don't know anything about it." How do you tell him?

Anyway, it was a very hair-raising experience in the hospital. The surgeon later told me the name of the anesthetic Jim was allergic to. But Jim was so violently allergic to it that he vomited and vomited and had diarrhea and became dehydrated. He had three seizures that first day after he had his tonsils and adenoids out because the vomiting and all brings on the asthmatic attack. He was also allergic to the Demerol they gave him, I found that out.

I called the nurse, told her he was vomiting and that I needed some help. She came into the room, and his Daddy was there and Jim went into his seizure and it's a very traumatic thing to go through. Here's this child who has just had his throat cut open and his nose cut open, and blood running out of this nose. They don't want him vomiting. They don't want him "Haaaaa," gasping for breath through his mouth.

Really and truly, this nurse acted as though she didn't know what was going on. I said, "He's having a seizure. We need some help." The child was flat. An asthmatic child cannot breathe when they're flat on their back. The first thing you do is get him up, not all the way up, but you have to prop him up so he can breathe. She says, "Oh, no, he has to be flat. He's just had this operation." But I told her, "You go get some more help."

Jim was laboring awfully hard to breathe and I told the nurse to get the doctor because we've got to give Jim something to relax him and calm him down. Previously, when I told the doctor that my son was asthmatic, I don't think it impressed him but when he came in, he was shocked, let's put it that way, and he was almost apologetic. This kind of got me thinking, "Well, you know, you didn't listen to me. I wasn't saying this to get sympathy for him. When I said he's asthmatic, I mean he's asthmatic."

After they gave him a shot and he got sicker and sicker, and the nurse came in to give him another one, I made her stop.

When the doctor came in the next morning, he had a very pathetic look on his face again and agreed when I said Jim had been very sick. The doctor said, "I'm going to give him one more day on glucose. He's dehydrating." Jim's veins are hard to get a needle into, they roll or move around.

I said, "Jim's going to tough it out. If you give him more Demerol, it'll kill him. He's a fighter and you're just not going to give him another thing. We'll get all of this out of his system and he'll just have to tough out the pain from his throat and his nose." And the doctor agreed with me.

It took Jim two weeks to get over this operation. I knew it wasn't going to be easy. Doctors are very reluctant to put an asthmatic person to sleep. They breathe through their mouth and trying to breathe through a sore throat from a tonsillectomy and having your adenoids out and when your nose is swollen, it's twice as hard. And then if they have an attack with the throat swollen, that's why they labor so hard.

He was operated on on Monday and on Thursday he was still throwing up and having diarrhea. Well, that must have been the last in his system because he started recovering, he got his appetite back, and since then he has been doing great.

His regular doctor was right. His tonsils were rotten from the inside out. The surgeon who took them out cut them up to see and said they were rotten on the inside and this was what was causing the pus on the kidneys and the poisoning. He has not had an asthma attack since then.

Doctors do not tell you all of the things to look for. It could be that they don't have time but then there's something terribly wrong with our society. They should have time to tell the characteristics that go along with an asthmatic person.

To begin with, Jim was born with a "cross bite" instead of an "over bite." A lot of people call it "bulldog mouth." He drooled all of the time, never had his mouth closed. He was breathing through his mouth and it was a continuous slobber, all the time. I was taking our oldest child to the orthodontist and had Jim up there one day. He looked at Jim, who by then was about two, and said he had a cross bite. He said, "I'd like to make a retainer to pull his chin back in. He really needs to have it done." I said all right. The orthodontist said this bulldog chin is pretty characteristic of asthmatic children. So we had this brace made. The dentist said if you can just get him to suck, give him a bottle, anything. But Jim never really liked the bottle. Now that I think about it, he didn't want to do the sucking because it interfered with his breathing. He was trying to breathe through his mouth and suck a bottle at the same time and that's hard to do. Well, if I'd been told that, I think I'd have been able to cope with it a little better.

Jim is very active, very strong-willed. For a while, I thought he was hyperactive and then I thought no, it's just me. I found out that asthmatic children's metabolism is higher than ordinary because they're taking two or three breaths for every one breath that a normal child takes. Jim's adrenalin is pumping faster and he is more active. If I had known that or I had been told that at the asthmatic clinic, you know, I could have coped with it more mentally, instead of worrying about whether there was something wrong with my child because he was busy, busy, busy all the time. Jim doesn't walk, he runs. He's been running through this house ever since he started walking. He never did walk, he ran.

If this had been told to me, I would have expected it. My pediatrician told me that, out of a hundred children, there might be one bigger than he was for his age. He was just a big, active boy with asthma.

"Some asthmatic children tend to outgrow their asthma. Is Jim one of these?"

Well, now, they say that if children are going to outgrow it, they outgrow it by the time they are 12 years old. Jim has not outgrown his. He's better, but he hasn't been over his tonsillectomy long enough to really know how much he'll improve.

Springtime, with all of the pollen around, the Bermuda grass and the leaf mold, is hard on Jim but the fact that he's doing so much better this spring thrills me to death. You know, an asthmatic person is very subject to upper respiratory ailments, sore throats, colds, bronchitis, you know, viruses. You get that, and then it goes into asthma.

And something else. After the surgery on his tonsils and adenoids, the doctor said to me, "Now, this child is going to have to learn to breathe again, through his nose. His adenoids are bigger than his tonsils, if you can believe that, but now he can breathe through his nose." It's awkward for him to breathe that way, but he's working on it. When I see him with his mouth open, I pat him on the chin and say, "Close it. You've got two big holes up there to breathe through now."

I also found out that it's pretty common for asthmatics to be fair-skinned, blondes or redheads. Jim's a redhead.

A medical chest specialist is long-winded about the short-winded.

Kenneth T. Bird (1917–)

11. Hyaline Membrane Disease

She is a petite, brown-haired woman in her early 20's, reserved but friendly. Married, she works as a secretary to help support their one surviving child who is cared for in day school.

It is only after talking with her and understanding the trauma she endured in the death of her twin babies, that her quiet strength becomes apparent. This experience has changed her attitude toward childbearing and has made her quite bitter about the deficiencies of one institution in the health care system.

- ● **Difficult Breathing**
- ● **Lung Disease**
- ● **Hyaline Membrane Disease**

"You mean you didn't know you were going to have twins until two days before you delivered?"

I suspected but the doctor didn't. I'm small-framed and two months after I got pregnant I was in maternity clothes. I was already uncomfortable in regular clothes. By the time I was five months pregnant, I was ready to pop.

There is a history of twins, even triplets, in my family. None in my immediate family, but there were a couple of sets of twins in my grandfather's family and my grandmother had one set of twins in her family and in the next generation back there was two sets of triplets. So I wasn't really surprised.

I kept asking the doctor because I was gaining an enormous amount of weight, seven pounds two months in a row. And I was eating meats, vegetables and fruits and that was it. He said, "No, you're eating potatoes, something you're not supposed to."

By the time I was four or five months pregnant I had gained 20 pounds.

In the meantime, we moved and I was closer to the small town where my family used to live and to the doctor who delivered my entire family so I changed doctors. He asked me how far along I was and measured me. I thought I was five months along but he said I measured seven and a half. He set the date a month ahead, said I'd deliver about August tenth, instead of September tenth. I thought, "Fantastic! I'll get this over a month before I thought I would."

Two weeks later, he checked me, pressed on my sides and all and then decided he ought to x-ray. "It's not because I hear two heart beats," he told me.

They laid me on my stomach on the x-ray table, which I thought was ridiculous, and took a picture. The doctor looked at the x-rays and announced that I was having twins.

This was on July eighth. He told me to go home, go to bed and rest; thought I'd go another 10 days to two weeks. He said the babies looked pretty small.

Instead of going home and going to bed, my mom and my sister took me to Sears to shop for twin baby clothes. That took two or three hours and I got pretty tired.

I had in my mind that my husband would be mad at me because I was having twins and that made me upset. We wanted two children, a boy and a girl, and we had our boy. And we didn't have the financial capability to add on two more children. My husband was out of town but he called that night and I told him we were having twins. Ecstatically, he came through the phone at me, "Fantastic! I love it!" So I relaxed.

Two days later, when I awoke, it was raining and I didn't feel very well and that's the day I went into labor. It was Thursday. The babies were born about six weeks premature.

Their lungs were not completely formed. I was told that there is a coating on the lungs which keeps them from collapsing every time you exhale. The twins' lungs did not have this coating so every time they exhaled, their lungs would collapse and they would have to struggle to inflate them again. This put a strain on their entire system. They call this hyaline membrane disease.

The first one was born at 8:40 in the evening, a normal birth. They got him into an incubator and hand-pumped him when he needed it but he breathed by himself — he could draw a breath. It was a struggle but they kept a close watch on him.

"What do you mean 'hand-pumped'?"

They had a tube down his throat and a doctor there hand-pumped oxygen into his lungs.

Then I had two more severe contractions and stopped labor. At 9:25, I finally had the other baby; he was a breech, he came down the birth canal and was hung; his arms were up instead of down at his sides. His navel cord dropped out completely and the doctor held it up to keep him from losing oxygen to his brain. I finally had another severe contraction and the doctor grabbed hold of his legs and started pulling. Ten minutes later I finally had him.

He never did really breathe by himself. He was either hand-pumped or on a machine from the time he was born. They told me when they left to take the babies to the university children's hospital in the city, early the next morning, "We don't hold hopes for 'Baby B' because he can't breathe by himself, but 'Baby A' is able to hold his own and has an 80 percent chance, or better, of living." They said 'Baby B' had only a 40 percent chance.

They left about 2:30 in the morning. Children's hospital has their own special ambulance staff and they came down and picked them up. They have an attendant, they have a nurse and a driver. The attendant is a physician's assistant, something like that. The ambulance is supposed to be equipped just as a nursery would be.

Earlier, I saw the children in the nursery. They put me on a guerney and let me look at them through the nursery window. That was about one or 1:30 in the morning. I stayed for about five minutes. Michael, Baby A, had no problems and he was in an incubator by himself. But Daniel, Baby B, was having trouble and there were two doctors and a nurse standing over the incubator. They stepped aside so I could see him.

The nurse's aide who was with me had been on duty for about 12 hours. She was holding my I.V. bottle. I felt sorry for her and after five minutes I suggested that she roll me back to my room. Of course, I thought I'd get to see my babies again.

The ambulance took off to the city without further delay because Baby B was too critical. About three a.m. my folks took off to go home and as they drove up the highway they saw that the ambulance was pulled off at the side of the road. They stopped and were told that the ambulance had busted a fan belt and the motor had heated up. They had to wait for a fan belt to be brought out.

In the meantime, they had called another ambulance, a commercial one, in the city and one from Johnsonville, a small town nearby. The Johnsonville ambulance got there first but the attendant decided they shouldn't go in that one because it wasn't as well equipped as the one from the city would be.

An hour later, the children's hospital ambulance got a radio call that the city ambulance had broken down on the way and wouldn't be able to make it.

They got the children's hospital ambulance fixed and went another 20 or 30 miles toward the city when the ambulance broke down again, the same problem. My folks had followed them and the Johnsonville ambulance did too.

The nurse insisted that the babies shouldn't be transferred to the Johnsonville ambulance because it didn't have a "mixer box" on board. I don't know what a mixer box is.

They called the city ambulance company and they decided they'd send another one of their ambulances, a regular one.

When the city ambulance got there, they found out that its siren wasn't working so they spent another hour changing the children's hospital ambulance siren to the city ambulance! My dad had tools in the back of his car so he helped them change it.

You mean they had to have a siren at six or seven o'clock in the morning?"

I don't know. Instead of transferring the children to the Johnsonville ambulance, which was still sitting there, they changed the siren and put the babies in the city ambulance. My mom and dad said they didn't understand it because the city ambulance was the same kind which Johnsonville had sitting there all that time.

Finally, they arrived at children's hospital at five minutes 'til eight. What should have taken an hour and a half took over five hours.

The ambulance attendants didn't have the right size tubing to go down the children's throats so they could use the positive-pressure breathing machinery so they had to use oxygen and hand-pump them. They said that the strain of hand-pumping and the wrong size tubing had cut down their chances of survival.

"How long did the children live then?"

Daniel, Baby B, died at quarter 'til twelve Friday morning. Michael lived until five or six o'clock Saturday morning. They told me that the first three days is the critical period. Some of the doctors at children's hospital said that sitting on the side of the road cut Michael's chances down from 80 percent to 30 percent. The transportation itself weighed against them but sitting on the side of the road cut their chances down severely. By the time Daniel got to the city he had only a 10 percent chance of living.

When I called the children's hospital Friday evening about Michael, they told me he was progressing twice as fast as they had expected but they were going to keep him in to see that he got along all right, to be sure.

That night the nurses gave me a muscle relaxer so I could sleep. The next morning, I woke up about 7:30 feeling really good because I had slept well. My husband was sitting by the bed. I sat up and began rattling off all of the things the doctor had told me about Michael the night before, how much he had breathed by himself, how they had decreased the pressure, how they had compensated for his white blood count which was up, how everything was going along just fine. Suddenly, it hit me the way my husband was just sitting there. He said, "He died about six o'clock this morning." I couldn't believe it, so he called the hospital and they told me over the phone that Michael was dead.

They wanted to do an autopsy on them but I said no. I said, "They had problems being born, they had problems living and I'm not going to have people cutting on them now that they are dead."

The funeral was set for Monday. Sunday I made arrangements with the funeral home, called quite a few people, got ahold of the people I wanted to come to the funeral, took my nerve pill, went to bed and cried for the rest of the night.

The next day was a blur. I had family pressures from both sides — to please each one. I was caught in the middle and it just didn't work. And the funeral was another big hassle. We were told that we could not bury the babies in the same grave, that we would have to buy two separate plots, buy two different caskets and have two different ceremonies, everything. I told them, "No, they came into the world together and they'll leave together. They'll be in the same casket, in the same plot. If we can't get it here, we'll go some place else."

"And did you prevail?"

Oh, yes, I did. That was something I stood firm on. They were born together, they left together.

"When did you decide that you would seek the advice of an attorney?"

In September. We made a trip to New Mexico in August and I had a lot of time to think. I knew that the ambulance had not been inspected for the year. The inspection sticker called for reinspection in June and here it was July eleventh when it broke down, so it had been out of inspection for more than a month. I know that things break down but this was just pure negligence on the part of the hospital. I didn't know whether they had even looked at the motor during the previous six or seven months. I felt like it should have been checked over.

I gave the lawyer all of the facts I could, doctors' names, witnesses, etc. I didn't hear anything for eight months and finally got in touch with my lawyer and asked him what he had found out about the case. He said, "Well, Kathy, we're not handling that any more," and told me they didn't have the time or the ability to take care of a case like that. He had turned the case over to another law firm without even notifying me, which came as quite a surprise.

I called the new law firm and gave more information to the lady lawyer who was now handling the case. I called her about every two weeks to ask her about it and finally she said it didn't look too good. First, she said, "Children's hospital calls me about once a day. They have decided that if you are going to sue the hospital, they want payment in full or they're going to turn it over to a collection agency." We had been told not to pay anything on it. She said they were doing it as a threat to her.

Finally, she told me, "Children's hospital doesn't have liability insurance; therefore, we're suing thin air. There's nothing there to sue. It is a state-supported institution. There is nothing we can do."

So I took her word for it and told her to drop it. I still don't understand why I did that. The lawyer said that they requested the state's permission to sue, but I saw nothing in writing, no copies of letters or anything. We really don't know if they did or not. We took their word for it.

There is a two-year statute of limitations which runs out in about three more months.

"What are you going to do?"

I'm not sure. I am thinking seriously of consulting another law firm, one that handles these kinds of things specifically. It sounds like I'm money-hungry but really, I'm not. I just want satisfaction to know they're not going to do it again. You've got to admit there can be mechanical failure, but they don't have to be so lax. They've got to take care of their ambulances. I just want to make sure they are going to do that. I just don't want someone else to go through the same thing we did.

"You said the lawyer originally proposed to sue for $225,000. How did you feel about that?"

(Sigh.) I felt like, "Fine, if he wants to, great. If he can get it, fantastic. I can get out of debt, pay my hospital bills. But all I really want is for them to take care of the bills which I felt like they were responsible for, the hospital bills, the ambulance bills and the funeral costs.

It's beginning to be a personal vendetta now. I don't want this to happen to someone else. For a long time, I kept a mental record of the deaths at children's hospital. They do have a high ratio of deaths there. I know that they have a lot of sick children there and a lot of those deaths can't be prevented, but I feel that one of my twins could have lived. I had no hope for the second baby but I still think the first one would be alive today if their equipment had not been defective.

I want the personal satisfaction of knowing that they are not going to put anyone else through the mental anguish I had.

I will not have a baby again. I have been turned completely against it. If I could find one, I'd take it. I'd gladly have a dozen and a half running around me but I'm not going to have any more.

"Did you decide to be sterilized?"

I haven't yet. *(Laughs.)* This is in my mind. But I'm taking severe preventive steps and I have this nagging urge to have a ligation. I build up a dependency on a child while I am carrying it. I was dependent upon those babies. I was dependent on my first one. I need them terribly. I need to hold them. I need to feed them. I need to know that I am needed for them. I need to know that they need me.

I nursed my first one because I was then the only one who could feed him. He had to have me. I had already decided I was going to breast-feed the twins.

I cannot build up this emotional dependency on a child again and then just have it ripped away and forget about it. I just don't want to get pregnant again.

No woman can call herself free who does not own and control her body. No woman can call herself free until she can choose consciously whether she will or will not be a mother.

Margaret Sanger
Parade, December 1, 1963

IV.
Listening

Within a bony labyrinthean cave,
Reached by the pulse of the aerial wave,
This sybil, sweet, and mystic Sense is found—
Muse, that presides o'er all the Powers
of Sound.

Abraham Coles (1813–1891)
The Microcosm, "Hearing-Powers of Sound,
   Music of Nature"

12. Stapedectomy

She is 38. She married young and has one daughter who is also married and another who is in high school. Because she was divorced while her daughters were still very young, she has had long experience as a working mother. She currently works in a city government office. Recently remarried, she and her husband live in a subdivision on the outskirts of the city, where cars clog neighborhood driveways and streets almost like jackstraws. She is friendly, cooperative, verbose.

- **Loss of Hearing**
- **Stapedectomy**
- **Inner Ear Transplant**

My hearing loss was not caused by an accident of any sort as far as I know. I just noticed a loss in the ability to hear well. It was quite some time ago. I worked as a police dispatcher and had a headset on my good ear, my left one when I was on duty. I couldn't hear people with my right ear so I learned to read lips.

This problem got progressively worse. When I first started noticing I couldn't hear very well, it wasn't bad and I assumed, like so many people did, that I had a slight cold that had settled in my ear or a slight ear infection or something. I was single at the time and didn't think I could afford to have anything done about it. I was vain enough, being a woman, that if I thought something couldn't be done, I didn't want to resort to a hearing aid, so I just overlooked it. I compensated for it by reading lips and making sure I was in a position to read people's lips or be close enough to hear and making sure that my good ear was available for that purpose.

"Did your friends notice?"

No one knew it. When I had the first operation last November, I called my father and my mother to tell them that I was going to go into the hospital. My mother said, "I didn't know you were hard of hearing."

My stepmother had this same operation back when I was a teenager living at home and I remember how hard of hearing she was and how the operation helped her. But I also remember how expensive it was, so I waited a number of years before I did anything about it.

I went to the same doctor who operated on my stepmother, knowing that he was very good, and also, he operated on my ex-husband for ear problems.

"What do you understand a stapedectomy to be?"

The way I understood it, he removed the defective stapes bone and replaced it with a kind of metal or wire antenna. He said it would react somewhat like a TV antenna does — receive the sound waves and transmit them through where I could hear them, cause vibration of the hammer or something of that sort. I don't know the exact details.

I was in the hospital one day. I went in on Wednesday evening, had surgery on Thanksgiving day and went home that day. I was awake for the entire operation. They give you shots right in your ear, much like a dentist does in your gums. The shots hurt but the surgery didn't hurt at all. It was frightening, basically because I was awake. They had my head draped, so I couldn't see anything but a nurse holding my head and taking my pulse reading. You hear all of the talking between the doctor and the nurses. You hear the instruments he's using, the drills and the little saws. You notice the extreme increase in the volume of hearing when he removes the defective bone. Then he did something to my eardrum and even the little clicking of his fingernails sounded like a bomb going off.

I was really surprised. If I hadn't been awake, I'd have thought they had just rolled me down to surgery, left me there an hour or two and just brought me back. I had no pain; I had no nausea; I had no dizziness. Evidently, they gave me something to make me sleep after the surgery and it was several hours later when I woke up. I was just starving to death. All I wanted was some food.

I ate a real good meal, I rested well and I waited. They keep you propped up for the first four or five hours after surgery and you are no supposed to lay on the operated ear. As soon as that was over, I lay down, slept all night, got dressed and was ready to go when somebody came to get me the next morning. I had no pain at all.

I had instant improvement in my hearing. Even with all of the packing and everything he had in my ear — they use a little remote-control TV camera or some sort of an instrument that's kinda like an x-ray machine and he operates by osmosis — well, they had this covered up with a big plastic bag. One of the technicians took the cover off of this thing and I nearly cleared that table. The sound scared me to death. And the wheels on the stretcher clicking. There were so many things I could hear after the operation that it made me very nervous until I got adjusted to it. And I was extremely sensitive to sounds. What woke me up in the hospital the next morning was that a maid had started a vacuum cleaner and was running it two or three doors down the hall. That noise woke me up and I had to go ask her to turn it off. Of course, now, as soon as the swelling started, the sound subsided somewhat.

I have just had this ear redone. It was three weeks yesterday. I don't feel, at this point, that I am hearing near as well as I did the first time. The first time it was just super. That was ten months ago and along about a month and a half ago, the last of July, I began noticing that if there was any other kind of noise at all in the room and someone was talking to me, I'd have to say, "Wait a minute, wait a minute." Even if there was water running in the kitchen and my daughter would say something to me, I'd have to turn it off to hear what she was saying. It bothered me but I thought maybe I was just readjusting my hearing levels and so forth so I didn't get too concerned until my husband noticed a significant difference. I was laying in bed, on my good ear, and he said something to me and I didn't respond. He knew I wasn't asleep so he tapped me on the shoulder and I raised up and said, "Do you want me?" And he said, "Didn't you hear what I said?" So then I realized how bad it was getting again.

I told my husband, "Well, let's wait and see if it's a piece of scab breaking loose or whatever." I knew I hadn't done anything to damage it. We scuba dive but I hadn't been all summer. I had not been in a plane or done anything the doctor told me not to do. So I couldn't see any reason for it to deteriorate that rapidly.

We waited a week or so. We have our own business and do things on the weekend which make it important for me to hear. I noticed that my hearing was worse than it was before the surgery. My husband said, "I don't care what you do but you call the doctor Monday and go back in," which I did.

He gave me a hearing test and it showed a negative reaction. In fact, it was worse than the one he gave me prior to the first operation. He said there wasn't any way he could tell what the problem was, what had caused my hearing to deteriorate, without going in again. So we made the arrangements to do that.

This time, he said he did a complete inner ear transplant. I went back for my checkup a week after surgery and they removed the packing and the stitches. It was late in the evening when he saw me, after five o'clock when I got off work, and I didn't take time to talk with him so I really don't know what he did this time. The main thing I do remember him saying during the surgery, "Gosh, look at that massive bone growth. How could it have grown that quick." So I know I had some kind of bone growth over the hearing canal. He had to chip and grind that away. I could hear him chipping and grinding.

He said he couldn't give me any guarantee that it wouldn't happen again. Once you have a problem like this, and I don't know whether it was the bone actually growing or it was calcium deposits, it could happen again. If I'm lucky, my hearing will stay at a relatively level tone.

"Have you detected any change in your hearing since the operation?"

I can tell that it is some better but it is considerably worse than it was after the first operation. I'm not up to standard by any means yet. Of course, it's only been three weeks.

With this second operation, I had pain, loss of equilibrium, dizziness, nausea, upchucking, severe ear pains, headaches, sore jaw, swelling. This time, I had the whole thing. So maybe I'm expecting a little too much, too quick. I'm hoping that my hearing level now has something to do with the swelling. I am still getting scabby deposits out of my ear. But it isn't painful anymore. Once in a while I'll have a sharp pain, like maybe if you stuck a toothpick in your gum, but it is instantaneously there and gone. It doesn't linger at all.

"How long were you in the hospital this second time?"

Ordinarily you go home the next morning but he kept me two days. I had surgery at one o'clock in the afternoon and I was there all of the next day and went home about noon on the following day. At that, he didn't want me to go home then. I was still having nausea and dizziness but I was ready to go home.

They were very good to me in the hospital, though. While I know they can't foresee these kinds of problems, I was in one of their new modern wings which has a console which you pull out of the bedside table that has your phone and your nurse call button and all of this. Unfortunately, this console was on my right side and I wasn't allowed to lay on that side. So I had to lay on my left side and I couldn't reach the phone or any of those buttons. I was extremely nauseated and very ill all night long. The other lady in the room had to call the nurse for me because I couldn't reach the button. When I got sick, I couldn't find the call button and when I lifted my head up, I'd get sicker. It looked like they might have taken that into consideration and put me on a bed where I would have been facing the console, but I'm sure they have other things to think about. They were very good to me. I probably wasn't the best patient in the world.

The cost of all this was approximately a thousand dollars the first time. The doctor's bill was $650 the first time and of course you have no anesthetic bill because he administers his own, which consists of five shots directly in the ear. The hospital bill was about $324.

Now the second time around, the doctor did something I thought was very admirable, something I certainly didn't expect. When I went to him the second time he said, "Well, there's no reason for this to have happened and I feel that it's probably my fault." So he redid it, without any charge to me whatsoever. Except the hospital bill, of course. I thought that was extremely unusual. He's the only doctor I know who gives guarantees with his work.

This is much better than a hearing aid, much better for my vanity. Particularly if it works. As you are aware, some kinds of hearing aids can't help; some kinds of surgery can't help. My particular hearing problem probably would not be helped by a hearing aid, anyway, so my doctor is hoping for good results from this operation.

I still have hopes. I think it probably will improve later, but right now, I am extremely apprehensive because of the difference between the first one and the second. And I'm apprehensive that the improvement may last four months and then my hearing might go out on me, again. Once you go through something like this . . .

The first time he told me I was to have it done, it was like having my tonsils out, no big deal, no sweat, no problem. But the second time he told me, I got very nervous about it, I started worrying about it, I dreamed about it, I lost sleep. In fact, it got so bad, I wouldn't even check into the hospital the night before. I went to the hospital and got my blood work done and then told 'em I was coming home. And I stayed home until eleven o'clock on the day of my surgery.

I think it was knowing what I was getting into. It's kinda like getting married the second time. The first time you are happy and giddy and don't know any better. The second time, you know what you might be doing, so you are a little different about it.

I asked the doctor if my being so nervous and keyed-up could have caused any of the reaction I had following the surgery. He said, "Possibly," but he was more inclined to believe it was because he did so much more work, he was in there longer and he dug deeper and moved more bone than he did the last time.

V.
Broken Windows

A small hurt in the eye is a great one.

English Proverb

13. Glaucoma

Some people like to discuss their medical experiences over cocktails, and I had caught snatches of his story at a dinner party. During later conversation, I learned much about his leisure hours but little about his work.

He is a swimming enthusiast, a proponent of the healthful life. He is diet conscious, loves milk but also loves the harder beverages. He is in his middle 30's, slim and in excellent physique. Their children, a boy and a girl, are in their early teens. They swim in a pool in the backyard, which he refers to as a "play pool," but he does his workouts each morning in an olympic-size pool several miles away.

Their lifestyle is suburban casual. He drives a pickup with a gun rack in the back window. He also rides a motorcycle. It is apparent that he and his wife have frequent differences of opinion on many subjects.

●Eye Examination
●Increased Intraocular Pressure
●Glaucoma

There's quite a bit of incompetence in the medical profession. I've come in contact with so many doctors and I know of too many personal experiences of friends and other people that are just horrible, absolute gross incompetence, uncalled for. Just simple things like a recent study reported in the *Wall Street Journal.* Seventy percent, no, I believe it was 80 percent, of the doctors in this study on antibiotics didn't have any conception of what they prescribed and didn't know the contra-indications. The study would give the names of drugs and many of the doctors didn't know what they were. And they were prescribing them every day.

The fact of the matter is something has to happen to make me go to the doctor. This time I broke my glasses and I thought, "Well, it's been a long time and I ought to go to see if the prescription needs to be changed." Originally, when I got glasses, I'm not sure I really needed them. I thought they made me look older and some optometrist halfway convinced me that a little correction for reading wouldn't hurt. I wear them all of the time, for all intents and purposes. I really don't have to wear them all of the time, but I do.

Anyway, I went to see this eye doctor, and as a routine matter, he put the galvanometer on my eyeballs for glaucoma. I thought at the time he acted like something was up because he took the pressure, the readings, several times.

They were up, like 24, as near as I can remember. I think one eye was a little higher than the other. He made another appointment because he had some suspicions. I wasn't supposed to eat and I was supposed to come back and take the "water test." You drink all of this water and then they take the pressures again. He told me definitely that all indications were that I had glaucoma but he wanted me to go over to the University eye clinic to have some more extensive tests.

I was over at the University clinic a half a day. They had a real sophisticated tonometer-type thing where you sat in a chair and you put your head in this thing and they move the tonometer up against your eyeballs. They took color, Polaroid pictures and they gave me one. Then there was one where I laid on a table on my back and I had to lay without blinking. They had a butterfly on the ceiling to focus on — no, it was a red light. The butterfly was in the private doctor's office. I remember that it was kinda tough to stare at that light without blinking. Then, they did the peripheral vision test.

To make a long story short, my private doctor had me come back fairly regularly, once a week or every two weeks for a while. He gave me a book about glaucoma and said it was unusual for a person of my age, early 30's, to have it. He didn't say how the tests at the University came out. But he said there was no sign of eye damage. I caught it early. He put me on Epi one-percent solution and told me I'd be taking medication for the rest of my life. He also said you can build up immunities for one medication but said we're lucky now because there are so many different ones that we can keep changing off. There must be, because my pharmacist gets it in for me. He didn't have a single other person on Epi Number One.

He explained to me all of the things I wasn't supposed to do: see double feature movies, get excited, watch television in the dark and all of the things which would tend to increase intraocular pressure.

Do you know what the big change in my life style was? When he first said "glaucoma," gee, I thought that was just something old people got. I didn't know what it was, and, boy, I was plenty shook up. You can go blind. He flat told me, in so many words, and the book made it plain. You follow what they tell you to do or you can go blind. That scared the hell out of me.

But the biggest step, the hardest thing of all was the limit on drinking liquids. He said I couldn't drink more than six ounces of any liquid at any one time. I liked to stop and drink a glass of beer with my buddies, shoot some pool, that sort of thing and six ounces of beer isn't very much. In fact, it was because of this that I cultivated a taste for Scotch over ice so I could drink something while I was shootin' pool. I stayed with the program for a while but then I really began cheating on the drinks.

Anyway, I got to where I was going back to the eye doctor every three months. And I was putting in the drops every 12 hours, morning and night. It was really an inconvenient thing because I've never been able to put the drops in myself. But I was really super careful and stuck to the schedule. I kinda got over being all scared about it.

Every time I got a checkup, my pressures were well within normal, but I knew it was the medication that was keeping the pressure there. I asked him over and over again, but he assured me that there is no cure, that glaucoma doesn't get better. You can keep it from getting worse, but it doesn't get any better.

I started thinking, "Should I have gone and seen what another doctor said?" I just had little doubts poppin' around in my mind. Not that I didn't think he was a good doctor because I had quite a bit of confidence in what he said. But I didn't want this glaucoma and I must have asked him enough times because after I'd been on the drops two or three years he finally agreed to try it without the drops to see what would happen.

I went off the drops and my pressures didn't go up. I think he was expecting them to, but they never did go up. The doctor didn't say much, just told me to make another appointment at the University eye clinic.

They didn't order that whole battery of tests this time. The tests at the eye clinic came out normal and now I'm in my third year without the drops.

No one has ever said to me, "Gee, Mr. Johnson, you had glaucoma but now you don't have it." I can only assume that something screwy happened. I had high pressures, I was on the drops for over two years, I was diagnosed as having had it and now it's a complete turnaround. So I don't know. I really don't.

Since I found out my pressures were normal, I haven't followed any of the rules. I just went on livin'. Now, I'll probably go back to the doctor, this same guy, once a year.

I've heard nothing but good about this doctor and I feel very comfortable with him. I can talk with him. He seems to be interested in getting little details, even things in a far-out way, which might help him with a diagnosis. Of course, he's never said, "You don't have glaucoma now." I'm just assuming that I don't. I don't know. I'm not a doctor. I'm not pointing any fingers at this stage of the game but you have to wonder.

I've had so many experiences with doctors, being in the insurance business. I'm not real good at recall, but I think it's pretty sad. I think if I really got started down that avenue, we could use up 20 tapes.

There's this doctor I used to visit with. This guy is about 75 to 80 pounds overweight, really a slob. I've been up there when — he's too lazy to go to the bathroom down the hall — he'd pee in his sink. Honest to God. I've heard him talk about his personal experiences with patients and he's so far out of it. I remember there was this one doctor who was woefully inadequate, just terrible. It got to be a joke. I never went to him but if you heard that somebody was having trouble with their kid, you knew it must have been this guy they went to.

When I select a doctor, I call the county medical society. People don't realize. My pediatrician gave me the names of three ENT men when we needed somebody for our kid. I called the county medical society and they'll tell you where they went to school and everything about them. But more importantly, of the three she recommended, only one was board-certified in his specialty. I figure, hell, if they don't have enough pride to get certified in their chosen specialty, I don't want 'em messin' around with my kids.

> *No man values the best medicine if administered by a physician whose person he hates or despises.*
>
> Jonathan Swift (1667–1745)

> *The sweet road to health, say what they will,*
> *Is never to suppose we shall be ill.*
> *Most of the evils we poor mortals know*
> *From doctors and imagination flow.*
>
> Charles Churchill (1731–1764)
> *Night*

> *That physician will hardly be thought very careful of the health of others who neglects his own.*
>
> Galen (fl. 2nd century)
> *Of Protecting the Health*, Book V

14. Cataract

Until recently, he piloted his own airplane, but he has been grounded because of cardiac and vision problems. A private entrepreneur in the building game, he is personable, sharp, assertive in a way which is fair and commands respect. He is just past the middle of his fifth decade, but looks 10 years younger. He appears to have the ability to evaluate professional medical services more objectively than most people can. He senses when things aren't going right and gives credit freely when they do.

- **Clouded Vision**
- **Cataract**
- **Cataract Surgery**
- **Epithelial Edema**
- **Postoperative Glaucoma**
- **Iritis**

Let's start with the cataract surgery which I had known for some time was going to have to happen sooner or later. Last year, on October 7, which was the date established for the surgery, I went in to the Medical Center which was my old home away from home. (*He'd had surgery there twice before in a period of two years.*)

It was the simplest thing imaginable. I went in on a Monday night; Tuesday morning the thing was done. I had the phaco-emulsification procedure which, originally, didn't start out to be that way. I advised the ophthalmologist that I'd had bleeding problems during another surgical procedure and he thought that phaco-emulsification might be a better way to go. It was all over and I was out of the hospital by noon Wednesday.

I can't even remember any pain and the care, for the brief time I was in there, was great. No problem whatsoever.

After an interval of about 30 days, he put a soft contact lens on me, prescribed supplementary framed lenses and I was back in business. After another 30 days, I found that, little by little, either my lens or the cornea was clouding over. It probably took me four or five days to realize that no amount of cleaning was going to deal with the problem. So I made an appointment with the ophthalmologist and he peered in there with his lamp, raised off his seat almost a foot and called an assistant in to look at the worst case of epithelial edema he had ever seen. Then, he put a pressure instrument on and that too brought him up off seat because the pressure was 40, which was about as high as it could get. And scary. He didn't put a name on that condition immediately. He just said that the pressure was at an intolerable level and that I would have to stop wearing the lens. Also, I'd have to go on two different types of medication. Right now. Which I did.

After two or three visits to his office, the pressure did not seem to diminish greatly, just two or three points; he characterized it as a postoperative glaucoma. As far as I know, this is a by-product of cataract surgery, not the phaco-emulsification, and happens in four or five percent of the cases, according to him. He said that it was self-limiting, that in time the pressure would diminish and it would be okay. But it took four or five months to get the pressure down to tolerable limits to where I could resume wearing the soft contact lens.

"How did you see in the meantime?"

Not very well, because my right eye is really not that good. I had to function, in effect, with one mediocre eye. This was frustrating and probably a little bit dangerous from the standpoint of driving a car in, let's say, western

Arkansas with dusk coming on. But I finally was able to resume wearing the soft contact lens.

About a month after that situation was dealt with, something happened so that I couldn't tolerate the soft contact lens. I couldn't see with it in. So I went back to the ophthalmologist, and he finally diagnoses this condition as something called iritis, a condition I'd never heard of but which is in fact a legitimate kind of eye problem. It is, in some way that I don't understand, related to rheumatoid arthritis. I had to take a medication for this and during that time I wasn't able to wear the contact lens. This condition lasted about 10 days and then it was done away with.

"I notice that you are wearing a copper bracelet. Is this for arthritis?"

No, as a matter of fact I began to wear that a long time ago because of a condition known as tendonitis, which may or may not be related to arthritis. The next obvious question is, "Well, did it work?" and the answer to that is, it doesn't work for everybody. You've got to be a believer. I bought it on the spur of the moment in some remote town in New Mexico and my tendonitis disappeared. But the joker is that about the same time I began to wear the copper bracelet, I also began to utilize the whirlpool bath at the health club extensively. So I'm really not in a position to say that one, or even both, got me squared away. But, however it happened, I'm not about to relinquish the copper bracelet.

I resumed wearing the soft contact lens but I finally realized that it wasn't ever going to be satisfactory. You can only get so close in fit and in prescription with a soft contact lens; you can't get precise in either. The doggone lens would slide off the focal point, I guess, and I just didn't see very well.

"Why was the soft contact lens recommended to you in the first place?"

Well, I'm a little chagrined when you lay that question on me. He just sort of did it automatically, and it never occurred to me to question him on it. I just assumed that he knew what he was doing and this was the way it ought to be. But when it became apparent that my vision with it wasn't satisfactory and wasn't going to be satisfactory, that's when I began to think, "Maybe I should see another doctor." So I discussed it with my general practitioner who takes care of my little hurts and in whom I have infinite confidence, and he said, "Yeah, why don't you see another doctor. In fact, I just happen to know one and I'll call him and set it up." Which he did.

So I went to see ophthalmologist number two at the appointed hour and he examined me thoroughly. He said I had a good piece of surgery, that I was in good shape and there was no evidence of glaucoma or anything else. But, he said, "You're never going to see well with a soft contact. You can only see well with a hard contact lens." So I explained to him that a few years earlier I had tried hard contact lenses unsuccessfully. He pointed out that this is a whole new ball game. First of all, the eye has been greatly desensitized because of the surgical procedure, and secondly, he said, the impetus to make a go of it is far greater. So I said, "Okay, measure me up and get the lens." Which was done.

In due time, I got the lens and wore it within the framework of the break-in sequence that he had prescribed for about four weeks. At the end of the four weeks, all of a sudden, for no apparent reason, the lens clouded over. I presumed it was the lens, although I wasn't sure, based on my previous experience with epithelial edema, I thought maybe it was the cornea. So I called the ophthalmologist's office and told them about my problem, and I really didn't get the reception that I think I should have gotten. The girls who function as the doctor's assistants pointed out that you have to be very careful about having your hands completely clean, completely free of any grease or oil or anything like that. So I said okay and tried it for another couple of days. I was extremely careful about the way I cleaned the lens, the way that I handled it. I developed a technique that was close to what a surgeon would go through scrubbing in.

But it didn't work. I finally called the ophthalmologist's office again and demanded to talk to him. It was kind of a grudging reception that I got, but I finally did manage to talk with him. After we had talked about cleaning instructions to make sure I was doing that right, he set an appointment for me four or five days from that day. I got into see him, and he looked at my eye with the lens in. He told his assistant then to take the lens and clean it with lighter fluid. This was effective for what was left of that day; it was about four o'clock in the afternoon. My vision was good but the next morning when I cleaned the lens and put it in, I was right back in the same fix. It clouded over almost immediately. The clouding became manifest almost as soon as I put the damn lens in.

I put up with this for, oh, another two or three days. It finally reached the point that one morning I had removed and cleaned the lens 13 times. My wife made the observation that this didn't really make any kind of sense.

I called the ophthalmologist's office once more and said, "I'm in trouble. I can't see. Someone needs to look at my eye." They said, "Well, your next scheduled appointment is . . ." and they named a date which was almost a month from that time. "We'll see you then." And I said, "I won't have it. I demand to see the physician." In about an hour, the same girl called back and said, "The physician says there is nothing more he can do for you. He said that next Thursday Joe Smith is going to conduct a symposium on contact lenses at the eye institute, and why don't you go down there and see what he has to say." Well, I thought this response was monstrous. I decided then and there that I would indeed go to the eye institute for total eye care from that point on, and I would have nothing further to do with that ophthalmologist.

I would have to say that in all my dealings with physicians, this is the first time, at least the first time I was aware that I was being treated shabbily. I can't categorize his actions as anything but shabby. He simply wouldn't see me. To this day, I can't believe that that son-of-a-bitch would treat any patient, not just me but any patient, so cavalierly. I can't get it through my little marble mind why he would do this.

On December 14, I went to the eye institute, conferred with Dr. Nicholson, ophthalmologist number three, and at this point in time, I have to believe that I am in good hands. I feel very comfortable with him.

As it turned out, the lens which was giving me all of the trouble was not only warped but it had acquired some kind of a film that caused the natural tear fluid to bead rather than be partially absorbed into the surface of the lens, which is what is supposed to happen. It would bead up and there was no way that it could not film over. Now if ophthalmologist number two had taken that lens and put it under a microscope, he would have discerned this immediately. But he simply wouldn't do it.

I arranged to order a replacement lens which in due time came in and I began the break-in cycle all over again. At this point in time, this is my twenty-second day with this new lens and it's working just fine.

While all of this was going on with my left eye, I was also greatly concerned with the condition of my right eye which has a cataract in the formative stage, and it was my impression that my vision in that eye was diminishing at a very rapid rate. If I didn't get the left eye straightened out, I was going to be blind in short order.

But my visit to the doctor at the eye institute, Dr. Nicholson, convinced me that my right eye was not in as bad a shape as I'd thought. The testing he did indicated I had 20/30 vision in a room with normal lighting. True enough, in bright sunlight, the vision in my right eye diminished to perhaps 20/100. But with good sunglasses, this can be brought back to the neighborhood of 20/40, so, on the whole, I was greatly reassured. This, of course, was my first visit. Time will tell.

There is no way to know at what rate the cataract in my right eye will ripen. I think a good indication of the doctor's lack of concern over my right eye was that he said to me, "Unless something really serious develops, I'll see you in a year."

"You are a pilot, and you don't have an airplane now because you are grounded as a result of a cardiac condition, but what effect will your cataract surgery and the fact that you wear a contact lens have on your application for reinstatement of your private pilot's license?"

Actually the existing regulations permit certification of private pilots who have had binocular cataract surgery and who wear contact lenses. There are many instances of pilots who have been recertified by the FAA after cataract surgery. So I'm pretty optimistic about that. Once I get all of this straightened out, I intend getting back in an airplane. That's a strong goal with me.

Private pilots can be categorized in groups, like the flying farmers, the flying attorneys, the flying physicians. The rate of accidents, indeed the rate of fatal accidents, is far higher amongst the flying physicians than any other

category, far and away higher. And it's no mystery. It's because of their goddamn intellectual arrogance. They think that they are smarter than the
weather, which no one ever is. They think they are smarter than their airplanes, which they almost never are. They make enough money so that they
can afford to buy very high-performance aircraft. They get into a tough weather situation and in no time at all, the weather's got 'em beat. But they're so
damned arrogant that they don't understand this. All you have to do is look at
the statistics. The FAA will be delighted to provide you with the statistics to
which I refer. There are no old, bold pilots, but physicians don't believe this.
By virtue of the fact that, going in, they're the brightest and the best, they
think they can do anything. As their training goes on, this is drummed into
them, I guess. So, in time, they come to believe that they are not like mere
mortals. They know that the weather is deadly but they also know that *they*
have the insights and the training and the intelligence to beat it. Well, they
don't. Neither does anybody else. They buy these high-powered machines and
they think they can manage them. Well, sometimes they do but not always.
Between the weather and the high-powered machines, it's a deadly combination. So statistically, flying physicians are way out in front when it comes to
accidents. That's a fact.

> *The Eye altering alters all.*
>
> William Blake (1757–1827)
> *The Mental Traveler*

15. Detached Retina

*He is the dean of one of the health professional schools in a Midwestern
university. Because of his personal relationship with many of the medical
college professors on the same campus, his access to medical care is easy and
immediate. He is physically active, about 50 years old, and expresses himself
clearly.*

*His previous experience with the health care system occurred quite a
number of years ago and involved a deadly cancer from which he miraculously
recovered. This time, according to his ophthalmologist, he was not very
meticulous in his effort to follow his doctor's instructions. But his recovery was
uneventful despite his casual attitude.*

• Floating Black Lines in the Eye
• Retinal Detachment and Tear
• Surgical Correction

My symptoms began on a Monday morning following a weekend of very vigorous physical activity — ten sets of tennis — and the symptoms essentially were impaired vision of my right eye with very noticeable black lines that floated through my right eye.

I didn't give it too much serious thought during the day on Monday, thinking perhaps it was only one of those strange things following extreme exhaustion. But that evening, when I went home and covered my good eye, it was quite apparent that my vision was severly impaired. The following morning I had the same symptoms and about noon decided someone should take a look at it.

I called an ophthalmologist and related to him the symptoms. He asked that I come to his office within the hour, which I did. I was worked up by his technician, and then seen by the doctor within 30 minutes of my arrival. He examined me and determined that I had a detachment of the retina plus a retinal tear, and said that this would require surgery within the next 48 hours. He said he was going to place me in the hospital this same afternoon for bed rest so that I wouldn't disturb the injury any further. The tear was at the one o'clock position, but I'm not exactly sure where the detachment was; I presume it was in the general area, but it didn't seem to make that much difference so I really didn't worry about the location of the detachment. In the testing by the technician, it was apparent that I had some impairment of my visual field in the lower left quadrant of my right eye.

At any rate, the doctor called the hospital to make sure he could get a bed, which he was able to do. He also called for an anesthesiologist to make sure he could schedule surgery for the day following my admission.

Within an hour or two, I was able to sort of organize things and get myself home. I was driven home by one of my friends because the doctor had asked me not to drive any further. I went home, packed my little bag, and, in fact, my wife drove me from home to the hospital.

About 4:30 p.m., I went to the admitting desk, and they had my room assigned. One of the aides escorted me to my room — this all took probably no more than 60 seconds — and when I got to my nice, private room and it was a nice, private room, I got ready to go to bed.

Shortly thereafter, the resident who was on call during this period came in — it was within 30 minutes or so — and gave me a complete physical examination, took a history, et cetera, et cetera, and told me to take it easy. I think I got some Valium to tranquilize me, which was very pleasant.

On the following day, which was Wednesday, much of the morning was spent in laboratory testing, x-rays, et cetera, to make certain that I was in such shape that surgery was appropriate for the following day. Following the tests on Wednesday, the rest of that day was spent on bed rest — a very pleasant day.

Surgery was scheduled for fairly early on Thursday. They prepped me about seven that morning, went to surgery about 8:30 or so and operated. I understood that the surgery took about an hour. I'd had no preoperative pain or distress whatsoever; it was simply the impairment of sight and the black lines floating through my eye but no distress at all. Perhaps I should point out that I essentially have a fairly high pain threshold, so this lack of symptoms may not be common for all people, but this has sort of been my history when I've had previous problems.

"Could you read and watch television?"

Yes, I think I could, as I recall. I really didn't feel much like reading, but I did watch television, and I had no restrictions placed on me for that, so I could do just about what I wanted to do.

The preparation for surgery was very simple. The pre-medication made me completely relaxed, and the anesthesiologist and I saw each other no more than five seconds until I was completely dead to the world. To be perfectly honest about it, it was a very pleasant experience all the way.

I got back to my room sometime in the early afternoon after getting out of recovery. I was pretty groggy for much of the afternoon, but again, it wasn't unpleasant or difficult at all. In fact, I had no postoperative distress at any time following surgery. A patch was placed over the right eye, not the left eye, and I was able to watch television. I don't believe I read.

Each morning the nurse would come in, take the patch off, put the dilating drops in my eye, and within an hour or so the physician or the resident would come in and examine my eye. At some point in the morning a physician always came in to look at me.

I remained in the hospital for two days after surgery, went home on the third day. The operating physician examined me, I think, twice during the first week at home, removed the patch after the first week at home. The second week, I just took it easy, enjoyed life at home, went back to work the third week on a somewhat reduced schedule during that period.

That's really just about the story. I had follow-up examinations on two occasions, the last one being about six weeks after the surgery. Had examination for new glasses, which I now have and other than being kept off the tennis court for a period of three months, I had no restrictions placed on me.

I didn't know whether the tennis I played the day before my retinal detachment had anything to do with it or not. And the physician didn't even try to identify it. He said there's no real way to identify the cause of a detachment. He's known patients who, in fact, were in the hospital for some other problem and were resting totally and developed a detachment. So it's pretty hard to know. The only time you can really nail it down is when there's been a direct injury to the eye, and I had not had that.

Following the surgery, the doctor indicated to me that nine times out of 10 he can think of something he might have done just a little bit different, but this time, he'd done it just perfectly.

I have Blue Cross-Blue Shield plus major medical insurance. Although Blue Cross doesn't pay totally for the private room, I didn't have to pay anything more because I was given "courtesy" from the hospital.

Frankly, I had absolutely no complaints about my hospitalization whatsoever. The admission was very efficient. After I'd been in my room for an hour, the admitting desk called simply to get some information for my record, but that was all the interviewing the hospital did. Food was good, the nursing service was good; I had no needs that weren't cared for. Frankly, I had a very pleasant rest for a couple of days and enjoyed it thoroughly.

I was discharged with a note from the hospital saying I'd be billed later for any charges, so I didn't even visit the cashier when I left the hospital. I haven't been billed, and won't be.

I had a couple other hospital experiences, which go back 20 years now, for a problem which was considerably more significant than this one, and here again, the hospital experience itself was satisfactory, but there were significant postoperative stresses, and I was hospitalized for a longer period. I don't look back on that experience as one that, you know, I'd like to go through too many times. No fault of the hospital.

It's pretty hard to compare the two experiences insofar as the state-of-the-art of hospital care is concerned. They were two totally different types of hospitals and two totally different types of surgical procedures. The first one was in a 1000-bed university hospital and this last time in a 600-bed private hospital. You know, it's hard to compare. I'd say my earlier experience was perfectly fine, but again, the circumstances were so totally different it's hard to compare.

I certainly have no complaints, either about the medical care I received or the services in the hospital or the results.

"Then you are one satisfied customer?"

Perfectly. In fact, I'm a very strong advocate of the system through which I went.

> *Certainly physicians cannot prolong our lives by a single day; we live as long as God wills; but it makes a great difference whether we live miserably, like poor dogs, or keep well and fresh, and here a wise physician can do much for us.*

Johann Wolfgang von Goethe (1749–1832)

16. Congenital Cataracts

The story of this partially-sighted child was told to me by her mother who is the wife of the president of a small, private, church-affiliated college in the Midwest. There is one other daughter, and the four of them live in a huge, modern home on a corner of the campus. The child is petite, blonde, wears thick glasses but doesn't seem to let her limited sight inhibit her. Her mother works with organizations concerned with handicapped children and is involved with myriad campus functions. She spends much of her time and effort to assure that her visually handicapped child will have the special care and education she needs.

- **Visual Impairment**
- **Congenital Cataracts**

Maria was born in Phoenix, normal delivery, and as far as we could tell, normal pregnancy. I was in school, three months along in my pregnancy, and I fell pretty hard on the sidewalk after an English class. Later, the doctors I talked to seemed to think this stage of her eye development should have been passed. By three months, her eyes should have been pretty normally formed

I went into labor at a big hospital, was in labor 10 to 12 hours and had Maria, my first child. The pediatrician I had chosen came to the hospital, checked her out and told me I had a perfectly healthy, normal baby girl.

During the first month at home, since it was my first child, I guess I just didn't even think about anything being wrong, except I did see a lot of eye movement. Her eyes would roll if she became alarmed or frightened when I was changing her. I kind of questioned that and asked my mother about it. I don't know if my friends and parents didn't say anything because they were afraid to alarm me, but no one said anything.

When Maria was a month old, I took her to the pediatrician who said, "Something is wrong. She isn't following the light." He was trying to get her to follow a small instrument that had a little light on it and she wasn't following it. He said, "She's either severely visually impaired or blind. I have an ophthalmologist friend in town and I'll call him and get you right in."

So I got my husband and we took her right on over that afternoon. The ophthalmologist checked her very thoroughly and said she had congenital cataracts. He said that was a lay term for a lack of a better description of the real medical term for whatever it was.

At that time, we were thoroughly confused. I thought, "Well, this must happen a lot. She seems so normal, so healthy." I guess from that point on I first started discovering that the doctors, although they were very interested in any medical problems concerned, couldn't really tell me a lot about what she could see or what she would be able to see or to do with this condition. They said it was more a matter of me finding out, as her mother, what her capacity would be.

Looking back now, I do wish that physician had suggested that I get a consultation. If I had been more adept, I would probably have seen two or three more physicians. I wasn't asked to do that and now I think maybe I could have done more, seen more doctors or gotten a different kind of perspective on Maria's problem.

She was so young then that the ophthalmologist really couldn't check her thoroughly, that is, the back of her eye, the optical nerve. But at that time he did tell me that a sphincter muscle in the back here was not properly working, that her pupils were permanently dilated and that the condition could not be made 100 percent correct but we could probably keep it from regressing any.

Then we moved here and a doctor here in the city was recommended to me. I guess I was totally in his hands at that time. I was 24 then and I guess I didn't ever question what he said. I guess as you get older maybe you become a little bit more . . . uh . . . I don't know what the right word would be, not antagonistic, but you search into things a little bit more. But then I did exactly what he said.

Maria was six months old then. I almost became afraid to take her back each time because I was afraid something else would be discovered, or maybe the optical nerve did deteriorate or maybe the condition had regressed or the general health of her eyes had gone down. During this time, I tried to find someone who had the same problem but I didn't find anyone for a long time. When I did find some parents whose chldren had a visual problem, it was never exactly the same. Each time I went to the doctor, I was always very timid and very scared of finding out something was worse. And, too, I guess parents always have a sense of guilt, that things went wrong because of something they did. I'd always be afraid I'd come back from the doctor's office feeling worse but he would always encourage me about what Maria could do. I remember him telling me, when she was two, maybe three, that Maria was very bright. I had always sensed that her mind was very good.

The first doctor told me that sometimes these problems run in syndromes, that in addition to an eye problem, she might have a hearing problem or she might have some mental retardation or brain problem or heart lesion. This worried me constantly. I was always afraid I would find out the next problem. I guess my most encouragement came from sensing and knowing that things were okay mentally.

I worked with her a lot educationally when she was very young, kind of had my own nursery school with her and taught her a lot of things. I just kept going back to the doctor but I kept wondering, "There's got to be something I'm not finding out which will suddenly make Maria a hundred percent normal or okay." But eventually, you realize more and more that this just won't happen but that you can work with what you have. For me, it took four years to finally decide to be thankful for what I have and what state she is in.

The doctor did put her in the hospital when she was a year or two old, put her to sleep so he could look at the optical nerve and assured us that it was okay. We began finding out how important that was and we were told we had to check very carefully for glaucoma or any other eye condition that might set in because of a weakness there. I was always very relieved to find that her pressure was where it ought to be.

As a matter of fact, I've always wanted to let some other eye doctors look at her, at the risk of hurting my doctor's feelings. You always have the feeling that if there is any doctor on the face of the earth who knows anything extra special about this problem, you certainly want to know that doctor. So I recently asked another doctor to look at her file but he hasn't told me what he thinks yet.

I guess the most frustrating thing about the whole situation has been, as a parent, not only are you worried about the medical aspect of the eye — you want that to be good, you want that to be taken care of — but you've got to deal with the social and educational aspect of the child's development. That is kind of isolated from the medical field and I guess rightly so, but it is so hard to coordinate all three. There are very few people who can help you coordinate the child's total development.

The sphincter muscle is, I understand, what's keeping the pupil dilated. This is another thing, though. Reading medical books when there is a problem like this can be very, very upsetting. It can be both confusing and upsetting because you don't understand. You take things out of context. And really, I'm not medically oriented by any means. I am, if anything, artistically oriented, but I've always had the feeling that I wanted the doctor to understand that. "I can understand if you'll go ahead and really explain to me. Go deeper. Don't stay on the surface because I know there is more and my mind can comprehend."

You love to run into a doctor who is not condescending. If you feel like your mind is good too, you want your doctor to understand that. I talked to my husband about really getting involved and finding out all I could medically but we both decided against putting our time in that way. We decided to put that more in the hands of our ophthalmologist, but keeping abreast as much as we could without getting thoroughly confused or upset about it.

The problem of the dilated pupils is one of the main difficulties, as I understand it. In the formation of the eye, there are several veins which develop and hers stopped developing when the veins were enmeshed across the lens of the eye. One of the first things that we noticed were the little white spots, one white spot in the middle of each eye which, I understand, are blood veins running across the middle of her eye, making them more opaque.

Where in an adult, a cataract, if that is the proper name for this mass, can just be slipped out, in a child these blood vessels are all enmeshed and can't be removed. The doctor has drained these little spots. I don't know if this is true in other eye areas, but I have never run across another case exactly like Maria's.

As she became old enough that I could determine that she was seeing large objects, bright colors and large print, I knew that she could see enough to read. She wears cataract glasses at the ultimate strength which they can be. Bifocal in one lens only; if the bifocal were in both lenses it would be too strong and make her nauseated and dizzy.

Without these glasses, she cannot read. She reads regular print, goes to a regular school. When the print size drops in the higher grades, it will become harder for her. I think she can just about read newspaper print.

She does not seem overly alarmed about the problem. At times, she brings it up.

At one time, when she was two or three years old, a counselor suggested that she go to the school for the blind. I have great respect for that school but we decided to send her to a regular school where she has made outstanding grades. She reads very well and does well in math. She'll be in the third grade this fall. She shouldn't take the regular achievement tests but have them administered on a one-to-one basis, but accidentally she did take it. She placed in the ninety-second percentile on the California Achievement Test. I don't know how long that can last but it is saying something. Sometimes we can categorize these children too fast.

The movement in the eye was very bad at first but they said it would improve with muscle control until the age of six. If she can get in the right position, she can keep her eyes more steady. I've noticed that as she has gotten older, she's found out what this position of her head is.

She has no distance vision, but a child learns to fake this and a lot of people don't even realize this. I don't think Maria really comprehends that she doesn't have it, since she has never been able to see things at a distance. This morning we were at the zoo and there was a white leopard in a cage way off and the children with her said, "Look at that white leopard." And Maria said, "Oh, yeah." But she was looking the other way. Children are very resilient people.

The first inspirational contact I had with another mother was with a person whose daughter is albino. This child also had a movement in her eyes, so the mother faced the same problem so many parents have with visually-impaired children: Do we go to print or braille? This is one of the very most important questions these parents ask. So, meeting her, I soon found that she didn't realize either whether her child would be using braille or print, going to regular school or the school for the blind. Honestly, there is a certain point where you don't know what to do with the child. This is about the time they're ready to enter school and the doctor doesn't know either because this isn't his field. But you keep having this feeling, because I think most Americans have this feeling, that regardless of what goes wrong, someone's going to pick you up and take care of you. That's the feeling I lived with for two or three years. I felt, "They haven't discovered me yet. When they do, they'll come and they'll say, 'Oh yes, we know what to do about this.'" I think that Americans are raised being told what to do, where everything is, black and white, or objective. Then when something comes along which is non-understandable or hazy, you just kind of lose your wits.

Somehow, when Maria got to the age of six or seven, I kind of lost some of that helpless feeling. She is so independent, so spirited, that I realize she is going to barrel on through and work it out. I don't know if all children are this way or not.

There are many obstacles which a visually-impaired child must face, like driving. Americans think that everyone must drive and in America, about everybody does. There are different things which will have to be worked out with her each year, but those are things you just take as they come.

The doctor talks about two or three patients he has had who are similar to Maria. He talks about one very specifically who is now a schoolteacher and all. Maybe at a later date, Maria can wear contacts and normal size glasses along with the contacts. But now her glasses are the ultimate thickness.

There have been times when we have gone to the doctor and, not knowing how to relate to him about a particular problem, have come out feeling worse than when we went in. But with our ophthalmologist, somehow we, my husband and I, always come out feeling better. I have seen him get short with other people, nurses and others, but not to his patients. At one point, that scared me. I thought, "He's really protecting me about something very bad." For a short period, I got a mistrust, but after I overcame that, everything was all right. And we also had to overcome an age thing. We were afraid that he would be retiring soon or his health would be bad, but it has been seven years now. Of course, some day we'll face this with him, the day he will no longer be there to support us.

It did surprise me that he was unable to give me any direction about any other realm of the problem. In fact, he would come to me for information. I'd try to keep him informed about what we'd done about things like her education. But he had no answers. He didn't know where to send me. I guess that was the biggest breakdown: from the doctor's office to reality to the world. It is a very frightening feeling when there is nobody there to tell you what to do.

People are treated differently according to who they are. This was made very obvious to me in one instance when our doctor asked me to go to another ophthalmologist to help fit Maria with some special glasses. This other eye doctor is very good at this, has the real knowledge of fitting people, but evidently has no knowledge of working with children. His nurse was so kind but I've never encountered a ruder man. I don't know whether it was the day or if he was in a bad mood. I tried to explain to him that Maria has no distance vision. He put up some letters for her to see. Maria was old enough that she had a certain sense of dignity herself. Right away, after he had been very rude to her two or three times, she decided she wanted to go home. I showed him she could read because I had brought some books with large print. Maria read several words for him but then he would put up things too far away for her to see and she would try to fake them and he would get very angry. He told me to get her to cooperate and I explained that she was trying to, but he slammed the chair down and said, "You just bring her back when she is going to behave." I thought she had been very good so I said, "No, I'm not leaving." I'd waited a long time for this appointment and I didn't want to wait again so I said, "I'll call my husband; he'll come and he'll help." The doctor was a little surprised when I called my husband on the telephone and he said he'd be there.

When Greg walked in the door and saw the doctor, he said, "Hi, John." I had no idea they knew each other and he didn't know I was Greg's wife.

The doctor did a hundred percent turnaround. He was the kindest man and treated Maria so beautifully that I was sick, literally sick, thinking that other children were going to go through this and not be able to call someone the doctor knew. I was really kind of nauseated when it was over, and I really think I have a capacity for accepting people's behavior when I feel like they are being unfair. But to me, it was the rudest thing that I've ever had happen.

Come to find out, Greg and the doctor were in Rotary together, downtown. Greg believed me and he wasn't embarrassed and since that time we've been with the doctor on occasions when we have been very sociable, but it is very frightening to me to know that if some poor, ragged little child comes in there, he'll get a different treatment. Unless I just hit the doctor on a very bad day.

Maria needed those glasses desperately for school, and had we left and had to make another appointment, it could have been another two months and it could have gone badly again. To me, it was such an injustice to her.

But people are timid around doctors. It is either in *The Greening of America* or *Future Shock,* one of those books, I read them both and I don't remember which one, that talks about doctors, how human they are and yet, you don't want to say, egotistical. In a way, in a medical way, they are egotistical. They become superhuman because of the way people treat them. Until you've been around doctors as friends you don't realize that they have fears, too. But in the doctor-patient relationship, they sense how timid you are and that makes them more overpowering. They've got the edge on you. I think it is the hardest thing in the world for a doctor to stay human, in the sense that blue-collar workers are human. And lawyers and other professionals have the same difficulty.

I had a friend call me, a person I dated when we were in college. He is now a pediatric heart doctor. I could not believe the change, just on the phone. First, he identified himself as Dr. William Johnson and I said, "Bill. This is Janie." Then he told me how he had bawled out a mother that day and I said, "Bill, that's so cruel. That's doesn't sound like you." We talked about an hour and I said to him, "Don't treat that mother that way. She's at home, depressed, right now because you bawled her out." Somehow, if doctors could just sense how much hold they have over a person's feelings. Of course, some, a few, stay human and touchable.

Greg and I have talked about doctors and lawyers. Their vision is narrow, all medicine or all legal. It is very seldom that they branch out into other areas, read fiction, lead another kind of life. They are just a hundred percent doctors. They sacrifice their life to be a hundred percent medicine when they could be a little bit less doctor and a little more human.

All those, therefore, who have cataract see the light more or less, and by this we distinguish cataract from amaurosis and glaucoma; for persons affected with these complaints do not perceive the light at all.

Paul of Aegina (ca. 615–690)
Works, Book 6, "On Cataracts"
(translated by Francis Adams)

VI.
Sexual Systems

*The natural man has only two primal
passions, to get and beget.*

Sir William Osler (1849–1919)
Science and Immorality

*Venus found herself a goddess
In a world controlled by gods,
So she opened up her bodice
And evened up the odds.*

Harvey Graham (1912–   )
A Doctor's London, Ch. 7

17. Vasectomy

This slight, gray-haired man, possibly 45, is a clergyman who once served as an Army chaplain in Vietnam. The two children of his first marriage are grown; his current marriage is his third. He obviously plans to avoid venturing into fatherhood again.

He is soft-spoken, a liberal thinker and an experienced counselor. He doesn't believe in the immortality of the soul, life after death. He has a remarkable ability to present abstractions, but he also has a firm grasp on the reality of the here and now.

- **Sterilization**
- **Vasectomy**

The experience I had in seeking and achieving a vasectomy made me feel that the doctor was very uncomfortable regarding the whole matter. I don't know whether it was because I was a clergyman or what the problem was.

He had the interview with me in which he was considerably lacking in personal easiness. Then he had the interview with my wife and me in which the papers were signed, absolving him of all responsibility.

I was interested in having this done in the clinic, as an outpatient, but he told me I didn't want to do that because it was very, very painful. He insisted that I be admitted to the hospital because he didn't want to do it on an outpatient basis, but, of course, this procedure is very commonly done on an outpatient basis.

So I did enter the hospital, stayed overnight, had the surgery the next morning under a general anesthetic and went on home that afternoon. This may have been a painful process for the doctor but I had only very minor pain. There was a certain amount of soreness which you might expect from a surgical procedure, but I continued my normal activities immediately, both with my wife, as far as intimacies were concerned, and with my work. I found it to be what I had expected. From other sources, I had learned about the procedure. Here, locally, the Planned Parenthood people send patients in to the clinic on Friday afternoon where they get the procedure and then have the weekend to rest. I'm sure that approaching it that casually is a lot better for most people, but I suppose the doctor was protecting himself more than he was really protecting me. Anyhow, he discharged me in the afternoon, so I left the hospital, got on the bus and went home.

I had an appointment with him a week later and went in to his office. He said, "Well, I want you to come back. There's something I want to do but I don't feel like you're up to it yet."

So I came back in a week. He went through, trying to say that he wanted some procedures and then finally handed me a specimen bottle and said, "Take this home and bring me back a semen specimen so I can test your sperm." He was very uncomfortable about the whole thing. He previously didn't identify the procedure so I didn't know what in the world he had in mind. I supposed he had in mind a sperm test but it was so mysterious and it sounded like such a painful problem but it was only his own embarrassment.

I thought, well, heck, there's no sense in my going all the way home, getting this sample and then taking all the time to come back here for another appointment. So I closed the door, got the specimen — he was in another room — and then asked the nurse if she would give the doctor the specimen. She said, "Oh, no, no. You give it to him." So I found the doctor and gave it to him and he looked surprised to get it immediately, ran the test and said it was all right. I never saw him again.

I felt about this whole thing that where a man generally should be receiving support and comfort and strength of a doctor who feels comfortable about what he is doing, this experience, the hesitancy about doing the surgery, the talk about the pain of the procedure, the inability to deal with telling about getting the specimen, left me with a sense of incomplete relationship and inadequate knowledge of what was going on.

18. Sterilization

Laboratory technicians in hospitals are called technologists, and if appropriately educated, may be certified by the American Society of Clinical Pathologists, the physicians who supervise them. She was one of these ASCP technologists before she retired to become a full-time mother. Her children are 10 and 13 years of age; her husband is in charge of a large metropolitan library system. She is interested in human affairs, active in a liberal church which is a leader in community concerns. She hopes to return to graduate school to become a social worker.

- **Band-Aid Surgery**
- **Sterilization**
- **Cauterization of Fallopian Tubes**
- **Ileocecal Perforation**
- **Ruptured Intestines**
- **Abdominal Surgery**
- **Keloid Scars**
- **Intestinal Blockage**

To begin with, my surgery was elective. I felt that I was through having children and I'd read about the new band-aid surgery.

It's for sterilization. It was supposed to be a very simple procedure. The way it was described to me was that there would be a small incision made at your navel, a laparoscope inserted where they could see the tubes and make one small incision on your right side and cauterize both fallopian tubes, tie them off that way, for sterilization.

So, I wrote a doctor in the town where we used to live. I had checked into having it done here but there was no one doing it here at that time that I could determine, especially anyone that I knew. That's why I wrote to the doctor I had had there before. His response to me was "Certainly. We've done lots of those procedures. Come on down. It'll be fine." So the arrangements were made.

I'd asked him several questions about the surgery, but generally, he'd said nothing, just that you go in one day, have the surgery the following day and go home the next. Nowhere in his letter did he mention the risks involved and I had not read there was *any* risk except that I do know that anytime you undergo surgery there is a risk — the anesthesia; that's all I knew.

So we went down when the arrangements were made. Prior to my going into the hospital, I had met a friend who had just had the same surgery and she told me, bit by bit, what to expect.

"Had she been operated on by the same doctor?"

No, his partner. She told me what to expect in terms of discomfort. She went in expecting to have all of the bad things go wrong and nothing happened. She just felt great. She went in one day, had the surgery and went out the next.

"Did you seek out that person? How did you come by a person who just happened to have that particular surgical procedure?"

Well, she was a friend of mine when we lived there and I knew that she'd had the surgery done. We were at a party together and I was glad that she was there so we could talk about it. If she hadn't been there, I think I would have called her and asked her about it. She went to the same hospital I did which, incidentally, I had worked in as a laboratory technologist, oh, I guess, three years, so I was familiar with the personnel.

There was a little bit of a problem because my husband was going to be out of town during the surgery and he had to go sign the sterilization papers at the hospital early but we took care of all that.

My friend at whose home we were visiting took me by the hospital in the evening and let me out. At that point, I was a little bit worried about going in. I almost had second thoughts; what am I doing this for? After I'd worked at the hospital three years . . . . She let me out and I felt really very much alone at that time.

I was admitted and then tried to contact my doctor but they couldn't find him; he wasn't on duty that weekend. We had arrived in town Friday evening and I tried to call him on Saturday and on Sunday. When I was in the hospital I thought, well, surely he'll come by as I had not seen him for a whole year. I thought we'd be able to talk. He did not come by on Sunday. I thought that was a little odd.

Monday morning when they came by to give me my pre-op shot, I had decided that I was going to stay awake until I got up in that operating room so that I could talk to him before he started cutting on me. There were a few things I still had to ask him about. Sure enough, I did manage to stay awake after I had my shot, and boy, that's tough to do. I was thinking of everything I could imagine to keep awake. But it was obvious to me that he was not going to come by before surgery, so it was necessary for me to keep awake.

When we got in the operating room, I asked him about this and about that and he sort of explained what he was going to do. They pump CO_2 into you through a tube, and if they don't get all of the CO_2 out, he said that I would have some shoulder pain, but that was probably all of the discomfort I would experience. I guess the CO_2 sort of inflates your abdominal region so they can see better; I don't know.

But anyway, they performed the surgery and when they took me back to my room I was feeling okay. But after I got up to my room, I knew I wasn't going to go home that same day. I did not feel so good. I slept most of the day and the pain in the shoulder was there. He was right.

In the night, I felt a bladder infection. I knew it was a bladder infection because I'd had them before. And I mean it just came on me — powie! The nurse who was on duty was extremely nice, thoughtful and considerate, moreso than I would have expected. She called my doctor; they ran a urinalysis; it was a bladder infection and I got relief. They gave me some medication, pain shots and that sort of thing. The next day, he told me that, well, he was sorry but he'd forgotten to tell me that they had inserted a Foley catheter and that's why I'd gotten a bladder infection.

"You didn't know the catheter was there?"

No. They'd done it in surgery and removed it by the time I was in the recovery room. Of course, I would have known if it had still been in there but they had removed it before I was awake. It had come and gone. That was okay. I could understand that.

But he did say for me to make up my mind if I wanted to stay another day. Because I was feeling badly he thought I should stay in the hospital. Well, I was staying with friends, my husband was out of town, I didn't want to be a burden to my friends, so about ten o'clock that morning, the day after surgery, I decided that I really did feel pretty bad and that I wanted to stay another night.

By that time, the pain in my shoulder was really bad. I mean a lot more discomfort than the bladder infection was, and that's going a long way. I just thought, well, I just don't feel good in general but everything will be all right.

In the middle of the night that night I got terrible abdominal pains. This same nurse was on duty and I just can't tell you how kind she was to me. I had never experienced this before in a hospital but she was very busy that night and I was in intense pain and yet she found time to check on me and do what she could. She was in constant contact with my doctor, she kept giving me shots and more shots. Nothing relieved the pain.

The doctor came to the hospital finally, about five in the morning. He looked at my abdomen and said I had a "hot abdomen." He said that something had happened to cause my intestines to rupture. He called a surgeon, an internal surgeon — I don't know what his title was — and I did not know him but my doctor said he was good. At that point I didn't care. They could have cut my head off and I wouldn't have cared, I hurt so bad.

He said first we've got to take you to x-ray. While they were wheeling me down to x-ray, the woman who was in charge of nursing service for the whole hospital happened to be walking by. She knew me because I had worked there before so she went right to x-ray with me. She was a big, portly woman, reminds you of a Marine, but, boy, she was a tower of strength in that x-ray. They had to hold me up, I couldn't stand by myself. Here again, I really felt the strength from her. She's the kind you remember.

Anyway, they took the pictures. My doctor said, "Do you want me to call your husband?" And I said yes. He said, "We're going to have to take you back to surgery and repair whatever has happened to you."

They had to take me back to my room first and I could not understand why I couldn't go directly to surgery because I was in such pain. I just argued and argued with them and they said, "No, we have to take you back to your room first." But I didn't understand that.

When we got back to the room, the surgeon said, "Well, I want you to know, you'll probably have to have a colostomy." Of course, your feelings about that sort of thing are pretty powerful. I said, "You just do what you have to do." So I went to surgery thinking that was what they would probably do. The surgeon didn't think it would have to be a permanent one, probably a temporary.

My good friends didn't know any of this was happening to me. It didn't occur to me to have them called. I was staying with them and they felt responsible for me.

They took me to surgery and the anesthesiologist, I remember him, too. I no sooner hit that door than he was there with a needle to put me to sleep. He said to me, "I know that you are in a lot of pain." I didn't have to wait to get on that operating table; I was asleep when I was inside that door. And that was a fantastic feeling. The relief. I can remember thinking when he put that needle in my arm, "What a relief to just go to sleep." I remember his kindness, too. I thought, "How could he know that I felt this bad?"

I woke up in the recovery room with a tube going from my nose to my stomach, oxygen mask on, I.V.'s going. I did not know the worst, or what had happened, so I asked the nurse if I had had a colostomy because that was the most important thing I wanted to know and she said, no, that hadn't been necessary. That was really a relief. Plus the pain. The difference between how bad you felt when you went in and when you came out was so stark that I just couldn't believe it. I felt so good, even with all of this other stuff on.

I got good care during the rest of my stay in the hospital which was 12 days. I remember one morning feeling particularly bad. I had a pain in my left flank and kept asking, "Why do I have this pain that makes me feel so bad?" They said, "Oh, don't worry about it. We'll give you a little pain medicine." But by that time I developed a reaction to pain medicine. They finally found some stuff called Laratime, a narcotic they used during World War II, that would take care of it. Codeine and some of the others would make me so sick I just couldn't take any more.

One day when I was feeling so bad, they wanted me to walk but I just couldn't get up out of that bed. By this time the Foley I'd had and all of the tubes were gone, but I just couldn't get up. The chief of nursing service came by my room again that morning. She seemed to sense when I needed her. Florence Nightingale herself. She looked at me and said, "Now, you cannot look that way for the rest of our patients. You've got to think of our other patients." I was on the ob-gyn floor, you know. "I want you to get up out of this bed right now." So she put her arms around me, helped me up and literally drug me down the hall. "Now this is what I want you to do," she said. "You'll feel better." That was another instance of care above and beyond.

The doctor told me what had happened. When he went in to use the laparoscope, he usually has a 180-degree field, but that laparoscope wasn't working well, so they had to go to the 135-degree laparoscope. But he thought "Well, that's okay. I can see well enough." Then he picked up the cautery — by that time he had me cut open — and the cautery wasn't working well. He said he had to hold the wire kinda funny, up against the instrument. He said he guessed it just slipped during the surgery. Of course, he wouldn't know this until things happened. He really was sorry that it happened. I honestly, genuinely know that he was sorry. He was in my room two times, sometimes three times a day. Everytime he was in the hospital to deliver a baby, he'd stop by my room. If he was up there for any kind of emergency surgery, he would stop by, which would not be the normal times for him to be there, especially the first few days, when things were bad.

There were times that I was so glad I had worked in the lab, because my I.V. kept infiltrating. Nobody could find the veins any more. One Saturday morning, the doctor got it started again. Finally, I asked for the girls in the lab to come up because I knew they were better stickers than the nurses. And they were. They could finally get it started but they hated to come up because here I was, their friend, and they did not want to do that. No. It was pretty terrible. We were all relieved when I could stop that.

The instrument burned a hole in my intestine, right at the ileum and the cecum, an ileocecal perforation, they called it. I was fortunate because it involved mostly the small intestine. I hadn't had that much to eat since my surgery so that my bowels were still fairly clean. I don't think I had peritonitis afterward, which was lucky. I received heavy antibiotics.

Everything else went pretty well. They patched me up and said it would grow back just fine.

I had a giant, midline scar. It was as though they opened me up with a zipper, that's what it looked like.

This whole thing was pretty hard to get over, emotionally and physically. I was normally an active person and suddenly I became inactive and that was hard. I didn't feel like doing anything. I built up a lot of resentment against my husband about my being sterilized. Things were pretty tense for quite a while. It would have been easier to take the pill but the pill had really bad side effects for me so I couldn't take it. The other alternative, an IUD; our minister's wife had just had a baby with an IUD. All of these circumstances led me to think there was only one way. A vasectomy would have been a good answer, I guess, but we both decided it would be better for me to have band-aid surgery. It sounded so simple. Who would have thought?

As I said, the recovery period was a long time but everything was going along fine and then I started receiving all of the bills for all this stuff. I had asked the doctor before I left about paying for all of this because I knew it was going to cost quite a bit. He said not to worry about it because he was sure my insurance would cover it and if we needed any help filing the claims to be sure and let his office know and they would help me.

So I started receiving my bills and I began to see that it was going to cost us quite a bit. My doctor sent me his bill for doing the band-aid surgery. I got the surgeon's bill for the repair work. Until we went into major medical, there were quite a few out-of-pocket expenses. The deductible on our major medical was $100. I just felt like that after my insurance paid what it would, this doctor should pick up the rest of the tab, or even offer to, which he did not. Maybe I should have written to him and asked him to, I don't know.

The people we were staying with, the husband is an attorney and he had wanted me to file suit before I left. He felt that "this was a bad deal," but I said, "No, I really don't want to do that."

When we got home, I had to have a maid every week to clean my house. The medical bills came. After the $100 deductible, we had to pay 20 percent of the bills, which really wasn't a great deal. Then there were doctor visits here, because I was having more trouble, quite a bit of pain in my right side under where they had gone in to cauterize the tubes. I had to have a G.I. series, upper and lower, gall bladder series, the whole bit, proctoscope. The doctor here wanted to do all of that to see what was the matter. He said that the only thing he could see was the adhesions from the surgery that was causing my problem, from the repair.

When I got their bills, I decided maybe my friend was right, so I went ahead with the suit. My friend's law partner handled the case. There was still some doubt about what the future would hold, and in addition to that, I was still having back pain, too. This was about five months after the surgery.

The doctor where I had the surgery suggested that I have a three-month checkup here by an O.B. doctor, in addition to seeing an internist, and he, too, said that the pains were likely due to adhesions.

The lawyers contacted the doctor's insurance company, of course. The period from that point to the time of the settlement was a year. We settled out of court. It was $15,000. I didn't know how to put a dollar figure on what they were talking about. No one would tell me what type of future complications I might expect, which subsequently I have had.

The settlement came early in May, almost two years after the surgery, and the very last day of May I had to be readmitted to the hospital. Those adhesions had wrapped around my intestines and caused a blockage.

After the suit was settled, I had no further recourse. You sign away the right to sue again for the same problem.

Between the time I decided to sue the doctor and the final settlement, my state of health was kind of up and down. Eventually, I got to an orthopedist who told me my back pain was caused by muscle spasm. He gave me some muscle relaxers which did help that. The abdominal pain was there almost all of the time; sometimes it came and went. My emotional state was pretty rocky. The spring following surgery I came pretty close to a breakdown. I spend one whole week crying. Then I sought professional help for my emotional state.

As I said, approximately 30 days after the settlement, late one night, I started having bad abdominal pain. I recognized it as a different kind of pain and wondered why I had not had that kind of pain before. My doctor said for me to go to the emergency room of the hospital and they diagnosed it within an hour or so. It was an intestinal obstruction which they felt sure was from the adhesions.

I form keloid scars and this is something else which was very painful about the other surgery. That midline scar became a very bad keloid. I went to a dermatologist who treated it with x-ray as much as he could and then injected it with cortisone. Still it was very itchy, very painful, very bad looking, this sort of thing.

By having the tendency to keloid, they assumed that the inside scar would keloid, too, form that same kind of abnormal scar.

"Does anyone know why this happens?"

No. It's just heredity. And I have one child that does that, too.

There were two adhesions that had wrapped around a loop of the intestine, apparently, and caused them to block. They tried all night long by just a nose tube to relieve the pressure and could not. They decided I would have to go to surgery again and have those adhesions removed.

Of course, I was not looking forward to that because I knew what a mess it had been to recover from the last time around.

This is, I guess, the dumb thing I did. I told the surgeon I had a tendency to form keloid scars and would he please be careful sewing me up. "Do whatever you do to keep from forming keloid." It didn't work. I should have had a plastic surgeon come in. I got another bad keloid scar and I'm not willing to go back and have all of those cortisone injections again. It's just too painful. I'm talking about the skin incision. They can't do anythng about the inside scars.

The doctor says that if a person has more than two of those kinds of operations, to remove adhesions, they recommend removal of some of the intestines and stretch them out so that there is no place for adhesions to wrap around. And that, to me, is very frightening. Having had an accident in surgery before, I am not about to undertake a kind of volunteer surgery where they remove a part of my intestines.

I never saw the first physician again so I don't know what his reaction was to being sued. Previously, when we lived there, he knew me because I worked at the hospital but our relationship was not social. I was his patient while we lived there but I only went to see him once a year, for a Pap smear, if that often. Oh, I had had a D and C done and he had done that. So it wasn't a matter of having to confront him. If we had taken it to court, I would have had to. I don't know how that would have worked out. That was pretty frightening, too. Each step of the way, as far as the suit was concerned, I had to make a decision: did I want to go further? My lawyers prepared me for the worst. They said, "Are you willing to come down here and go to court and testify?" And I had to think a long time before I could think I was willing to do that.

In retrospect, especially since the added complications of the adhesions occurred, I do feel that he probably did not use his best judgment during surgery. If the instruments were faulty, I think he probably should have postponed the procedure. He told me right before I was dismissed that he had thought long and hard about it and this was not going to keep him from doing more of those procedures. But he did say they had become much too complacent about that surgery and that shock really rocked the whole town. A lot of my friends were doctors down there and they would come to visit me. People knew. I was not worried about his reputation being ruined by the suit because people already knew what had happened.

I think what motivated him to settle out of court was that he knew he had made a mistake. I really do. He sat right in my room and said he had gone over and over the procedure in his mind, reliving it to find out what had happened. He said there was a possibility that I could have moved during the surgery inadvertently, I guess a muscle reaction or something under anesthesia, but I find that a little farfetched.

The settlement paid for all of my expenses. The attorney worked on a percentage. I had no idea what the procedure was. His percentage was 30 percent but first they deducted from the settlement figure my out-of-pocket expenses for the surgery, telephone calls, maid service, all that kind of thing. They got 30 percent of what was left and I thought that was fair.

I'm real interested in the current controversy about malpractice insurance. I feel the double bind because I've been there. I do feel the physician has to be responsible to his patient. I feel that if there is blatant wrongdoing that a patient has to have recourse. You're dealing with something you have only one of, and that's your life. On the other hand, I think that there is a point where people become, maybe, sue-happy and ask exorbitant amounts. The percentage fee for lawyers? I feel my attorney did a great deal of work. There was a great deal of paperwork and record keeping and contacting that had to be done.

I'll be very curious to see what happens about malpractice insurance, having felt the bind of being a patient in that position and also having worked in the medical field where I am in contact with the doctors and can understand what their dilemma is, too. Believe me, I thought of all these things before I decided to sue. I know there are risks involved.

Before the surgery, I was not informed of any danger at all. After the surgery, the doctor went out of his way to communicate his concern, to try to think through the procedure and be as honest with me as he could. I feel he did what he could. And the surgeon I had here was really good, too. He was concerned about me; he went about his work very matter of factly but he checked in with me twice a day and whenever else he was on the floor.

Subsequently, I saw a magazine article which listed the odds of having this kind of complication as one in 500, where they burn the intestine by mistake. If I had it to do over, I would not have the surgery, because I know that the risks of surgery are greater than the risks of pregnancy.

> Mala Praxis *is a great misdemeanor and of-*
> *fence at common law, whether it be for*
> *curiosity and experiment, or by neglect;*
> *because it breaks the trust which the party had*
> *placed in his physician, and tends to the*
> *patient's destruction.*
>
> Sir William Blackstone (1723–1780)
> *Commentaries on the Laws of England,*
> Bk. III, Ch. 8

19. Fertility Test

This attractive, dark-haired teacher is 26 or 27 years old. She has been married two or three years, teaches fourth graders in a private school. Her husband works and goes to school at night, perhaps so that he may catch up with his college-educated wife, maybe just to escape a lifetime in the barbering trade.

• Inability to Have a Baby
• Fertility Testing and Treatment

When we went to our doctor because we thought one of us was sterile, he really didn't want to mess with us because he said, "Aw, you haven't been married that long. You don't need to be considering fertility tests." Well, that teed me off because it was not his place to make that judgment. If we'd been married only minutes, it wasn't any of his business when we decided to get help.

He said for me to stop taking the pill but he wasn't going to run any fertility tests until a year and a half after I'd been off the pill. This was our family doctor.

Just by asking around, we got onto another doctor. Fertility tests, of course, are really big ego tests, too. How much can you tolerate mentally? You are setting yourself up for the doctor to say, "You are not capable of childbearing." That's got to be a lot to take because very few people ever consider they won't be able to have a baby or father a child.

The doctor who treated us, as husband and wife, was very cold about it. He told us — I'll never forget this as long as I live — he said he had this one particular test he wanted to run, but it required examination 30 minutes following "spontaneous intercourse." That was so funny. He stressed the spontaneity. "Has to be," he said, "otherwise it changes the chemical balance completely." If you start planning, your anxieties and adrenalin and all sorts of things start clicking and it throws off the whole bit. This is what he said.

My husband has a good friend who is a gynecologist and he told him I was being treated by this doctor and, after hee-hawing for about 10 minutes, he said, "I can't believe you'd send your wife to that clown." But on the other hand, this doctor was recommended by a friend of my father, who is also a doctor. There's no way you can shop for a doctor.

Well, anyway, he did the tests and told us he couldn't find anything wrong. He did the tests between November and January; cost us $50 a whack.

"How did you manage the spontaneous situation?"

Well, he said any time between ten and two, Tuesday, Wednesday or Thursday. Of course, we both work; so finally, one day, I just stayed home from work. I told my husband that I'd be "spontaneously at home" between ten and two. It was a joke, a complete joke.

Then we changed doctors again. This time we went to the gynecologist who had laughed about us going to the first man. We went to him; well, I was there once a month for eight months. I don't know. It's sort of like, in this case, he didn't tell me what the deal was. He said, "Oh, I can't find anything." But I really like this guy; he's extremely personable and he helped us get Virginia *(their newly adopted daughter, age three weeks)*, so we for sure like him now, a lot.

He said to my husband, "Now don't think, just because you haven't got your wife pregnant, that you can go out and play around and think you're safe, like you've had a vasectomy. You might be with 10 women, one every night, and get 10 babies. You could leave a trail of kids because you are extremely fertile. It just might be the acidity of the cervical mucus."

He told my husband that my cervical acidity could be the problem but he didn't mention any of that to me. He never said that was a possibility. I like this guy and have no intention of changing doctors, but how come he didn't tell me that?

There were other things. Like taking Clomid, a fertility drug. He said, "Now, you can only take this four times, once a period." So for four months I took it and at the end of that time he told me to get the prescription refilled. And I reminded him that he had said I could take it only four months and he said, "Oh, it won't hurt you. You'll be okay." So I ended up taking it six months. But, I was having to make a judgment there. Was he right the first time and I shouldn't have taken it the extra two months? Or was he just buttin' me around then and it was okay to take it for an extra two months. You're really put in a position where you have to trust so much.

But my worst experience with health care has not been with professionals, it's been with the receptionist in the doctor's office. "Well, I'm sorry, he can't see you," she'll say. Some girl who has taken a typing and shorthand course in some business school will say, "What seems to be the symptoms?" She's not going to know anything about them if you tell her.

When that happens to my husband, he'll really gross 'em out. When he telephones and they ask him about his symptoms, he'll say, "Well, I've got this oozing, pusy sore on my butt!" and the girl gets all flustered and he gets attention that way. He usually gets to talk to the doctor then.

I used to be really enthralled by "knights in white coats" up until the time I was a senior in college, and then I worked at the university hospital in the emergency room. We had an inhalation therapist who was out in the parking lot playing cards and missed a "Code Blue" (hospital signal for emergency situation) and the patient died. He heard the call but he was in the middle of a poker hand and didn't respond. And then there was the medical student who was attending a patient who died. When this happened, he asked me to tell the daughter who was waiting there. He said, "You tell her. I don't know how to talk to kids that age." Just like that.

Of course, that wasn't the prize situation to work in because I worked weekends when the "gun and blade crowd" was brought in to the emergency room.

20. Sterilization

She is a young married woman plagued by a chronic health problem which is currently in remission, but which can become acute at any time. This circumstance put her life at risk during her pregnancy and the delivery of their only child. She thought she would never have a baby because sterilization surgery had been performed before she conceived. She sued the doctor for malpractice. The newspaper described her as a "sterile mom."

She and her husband, a blue collar worker, live in a modest home in a bedroom town adjacent to a large midwestern city. Their "miracle baby" is a beautiful, curly-headed girl, now kindergarten age.

- **Kidney Trouble**
- **Proliferative Glomerulonephritis**
- **Sterilization**
- **Childbirth**
- **Tubal Occlusion with Femoral Burial**
- **Laparoscopy**
- **Band-Aid Surgery**

The thing the doctors told me is you have these filters inside the kidney called glomeruli. The disease is a deterioration of these filters, the glomeruli. You go through an acute phase and once the filters are gone, they're gone. They can't be replaced. But you can go into remission.

"Is there a way to measure how much of this filtering system you have lost?"

No. As far as I know, all they can do is run tests to see how many casts are being cast out, B.U.N., creatinine, I don't know exactly what those are. It gives you an idea of the function of the kidneys at that time; it doesn't tell you how far the disease has progressed. I assume the only way you can do that is with a biopsy.

I was in college when I first started having a lot of problems. I had real bad protein, albumin, in my urine. That was five years ago. I was 18, a freshman in college. I'm 23 now. My family doctor thought it might be a case of virus nephritis, bacterial nephritis, whatever you call it, that could be treated with antibiotics. He treated me for three weeks — I was on complete bedrest at home — and when there was no improvement, he sent me to a specialist. The specialist, Dr. Larison, put me in the hospital, did a renal biopsy and found out what it was.

The biopsy procedure was very painful. They gave me a shot of Demerol — I don't think it was very much — and did everything in my hospital bed. They rolled up and stacked two pillows, end to end, and had me lay on them on my stomach. He gave me a local anesthetic, in the skin area. It was a needle biopsy; he stuck a needle through my back into my kidney.

It was very painful. He told me that they can put you under and cut you open, but this way you're awake and it's not as dangerous. When you're awake you can let him know when he hits the spot. It took around 20 minutes. I had never had that much pain.

On my first visit, Dr. Larison told me that birth control pills have an adverse effect on the kidneys. He also said, when the time came that I wanted to get married, to please talk with him first. He stressed that.

I was going in for routine tests all along, and when James and I decided to get married, I told the doctor. He told me again that I couldn't take birth control pills but I could use any other method I cared to choose. He said that childbirth put a lot of stress on the kidneys and getting pregnant could be dangerous. He even said that if I did get pregnant, I'd have to have an abortion. He said, "I'll tell you how strong I feel about this. If you were my daughter, I would have to do an abortion."

I studied about IUD's when I was in nursing school — I had a little bit of nurse's training — and I had heard about cases of children born with IUD's in the placenta. It's risky. Besides, an IUD is not a preventive. You can go ahead and conceive and then the fertilized egg is lost.

Dr. Larison suggested that I be sterilized and recommended that I go to a Gyn man. I worked on OB at the hospital as a unit clerk and know some of the specialists but I really can't tell you why I settled on Dr. Smith. I mentioned to him that I had to be sterilized and he mentioned this procedure. I asked another OB-Gyn man, Dr. Bedford, to be in the operating room with Dr. Smith.

Dr. Smith said they would bury the Fallopian tubes in a uterine muscle. I looked up in a medical dictionary what occlusion means which is a blockage or "to stop up." He called the procedure tubal occlusion with femoral burial. I just assumed that "femoral" was the muscle he buried them in. He never did really explain it to me. He said he had never done this procedure before but he would research it beforehand.

I had a Fanstill incision which is crosswise on the hairline. It was about six inches long. I asked to be put on OB because I worked there, I knew the people who would take care of me. But they put me across from the baby nursery. That was rather depressing.

When Dr. Smith came to take the sutures out, I don't know how they do it but somehow he did the stitches underneath the skin and brought up both ends on each side of the incision on the outside. You are then supposed to clip the ends and take the suture out. Well, he couldn't get it out so he just cut it off and left it. I didn't think much about it at the time but it was just another one of those things.

He did this early in March and I was married in the middle of April, the following month. I made sure that I had enough time to recover from the surgery. The reason why he picked this surgery was because I was interested in a possible repair or reversal of the sterilization process five or six years later. My kidney doctor had told me that sometimes when the kidney disease has been in remission for that length of time, it is safe enough to go ahead and bear a child. Naturally, if I could have a child later, I was interested.

"So the Fallopian tubes are merely collapsed and buried in the muscle tissue?"

And secured. He told me that if this procedure was ever reversed, if I were lucky, I would have a 20-percent chance then of becoming pregnant. He didn't give me any figures to indicate how safe I was before the procedure was reversed. He led me to believe, though, that I'd be lucky if I ever had a child after the procedure was reversed.

I had my last period on April 25, two weeks after I was married. I remember the day because I've always been bothered with (menstrual) cramps, real bad. Dr. Smith said that the next time I had my period to come in and he'd give me something for it. The bottle of pills he gave me was dated April 24, so that was the correct, true date. My baby was born on February 1, nine months and two weeks later.

Not long after the sterilization surgery, when I went back in for a checkup, Dr. Smith said that the hospital was going to receive a laparoscope soon and he wanted to perform a laparoscopy to see how everything was. He would make a very, very small incision, insert this scope and see how everything was in my abdomen. I didn't think anything about it, but when I told Dr. Larison about it, he was outraged. He was so mad. He said, "What the hell does he want to do that for? Why would he want to do it unless he was unsure of his work?" That didn't hit me until later; I was too dense to realize what was going on at first. He, Dr. Smith, wanted to put me under, put me in danger again, to check on his own work. Besides, I'd have had to take off work again.

After the operation, I was talking to Dr. Bedford who assisted Dr. Smith with the surgery and had seen me when I was open. Just out of curiosity, and almost jokingly, I asked him, "Well, how was everything inside?" He turned around and almost snapped my head off. He said, "I didn't do anything. Dr. Smith did it all." And then he turned away and walked off. Ordinarily, he was very friendly to me.

When I began having symptoms of being pregnant, I had a pregnancy test run at the hospital. They ran two tests, a short and a long one, and they were both positive. Then I went in to see Dr. Smith who also gave me a test which was positive. He gave me a shot of progesterone, which is a hormone to make you start your period if you are late but it won't make you start if you are pregnant, only if you have some other difficulty. I didn't start.

The next time I went in he could really tell I was pregnant and I told him I thought I deserved a free delivery. It was a mistake of his. We didn't have any insurance. I knew my kidney doctor would want me to have an abortion but I also knew I wouldn't.

"Is the biggest risk to the kidneys during pregnancy or at the time of delivery?"

Really a combination. Dr. Larison said that it could affect my kidneys adversely, even two or three years after the birth. How, I don't know. With nephritis, I have trouble with swelling and pregnancy just complicated that. But as far as any great difficulties, no. My albumin was up. My obstetrician said there were no complications but they don't always know. I have a heart murmur and I had some tachycardia *(rapid heart beat)* while I was pregnant. Also, I had a tumor on my ovary which I understand is not uncommon. It didn't have to be removed or anything. But kidney-related, I didn't have excessive trouble.

My labor pains started early in the morning but I wasn't dilated very much. They put me in the hospital. I was going to try to have natural childbirth, but for the week before my daughter was born, I had bronchitis real bad and I couldn't do my breathing exercises or anything.

In the afternoon, the doctor broke my bag of waters to see if that would make me deliver faster. I was mad because everybody was talkin' but nobody was telling me anything. The nurse asked me if, when they prepped me, they had prepped my stomach, so I knew something was going on. Later on, the doctor . . . .

Backtracking again, Dr. Smith told me before he did the sterilization surgery that he wouldn't charge me except what my Blue Cross-Blue Shield I had through the hospital would pay. After he found out I was pregnant, he charged me $135 extra. When I pointed out to him what he had said earlier, he deducted $100 of it, leaving me $35 to pay. It was the principle of the thing. And besides, I didn't have any money anyway. After that, I changed doctors, went to Dr. McKinsey.

Back to the delivery. Dr. McKinsey said that labor would be hard on my kidneys and he didn't want to push it too much. He said he wanted to do a section.

I never did get into hard labor. It was painful and I'd been at it all day and by that time, I was so tired that I was ready to agree to anything, just to get it over with. Because of my bronchitis, I had to have a spinal, couldn't have gas. The doctor had a very difficult time administering the spinal anesthetic. He shot me time after time after time. He kept moving up, moving up and I'd have a contraction and it was very painful. He asked me what it felt like and the only way I could describe it was like electricity going all through my body 'cause I guess all of my nerves were jumping, I don't know. He did comment that I was so swollen, so . . .

"Edematous?"

Yes, that he was having a difficult time and had to move higher and higher. He did it so high that it really felt funny breathing, almost. He didn't get that high, but it was close.

Judy, the baby, was healthy. My pediatrician was in there; he was a little bit concerned about her health due to my kidneys. In fact, she was so healthy, her Apgar test was 10, which is as high as it goes. That's good for a section, really is.

But that stupid anesthesiologist. He put a mask on me so I could breathe oxygen and it would let me breathe in but I couldn't exhale. I shook my head and told him to get it off me, it wasn't working. But he put it back on again, snuck it over my head. The second time I told him to keep it off, he did. I was pretty mad.

There were a few jokes in there. The doctor said he was going to put his initials in my belly because I had so many scars now.

The next days were bad, painful. I have a real bad problem with gas. With that kind of surgery — he cut clear from my umbilicus to the pubis — you get air in your intestines from handling them.

I had Judy on Friday night, and the following Friday morning he came in, took the sutures out and discharged me. As soon as he discharged me I got up and went to the bathroom to clean up and get ready to go home. I bent over and picked up Judy's diaper bag, which didn't even weigh a pound, and started feeling some liquid running down. It was blood. My incision had split open, almost the entire length. I was pretty scared. Another doctor came in to see if the inner layers had split open, too, which is what's dangerous. All during the week, I had noticed a serous discharge on my bandage but when I mentioned it to the nurse, she said it was normal. What it boiled down to, they just left the incision open and I went home like that.

"Gaping open?"

Well, I did have a couple of four-by-fours over it, but I was open. The abdominal cavity layer was closed, though. What happened was that I'd had so much edema in my tissues that it just didn't heal. Too much fluid retention. It took at least four weeks, maybe six. It seemed like forever before I could take a bath. The incision finally closed by itself. It took a little while before I could feel secure about not dropping my innards out.

After the last visit to Dr. Smith, when I found out for sure that I was pregnant and I asked him for a free delivery and he offered me a 20-percent discount, that's when I went to his receptionist and found out that he had charged me $135 extra for the sterilization. I started crying because I was very upset and frustrated. I didn't know what to do. It was unfair. I went home to my parents' house and was bawling to them. My father advised me to seek the advice of a lawyer.

I didn't know what lawyer to see, so my father went to the senior partner of a law firm he knew and told him the story. He said, "Yes, there is a very good chance. We'll take the case." When we all went in for an appointment, my father, my husband and I, they shuffled us down to the junior partner. He talked to Dr. Larison, my kidney doctor, who wrote what I thought was a very supportive letter. After that, the lawyer turned the case down.

Then we got another lawyer, who kinda gave us the shuffle, too. I told him the whole story and gave him a list of expenses we had paid. From that time on, for a period of at least three years, I didn't see him again. In the meantime, this lawyer died, his partner took over the case, changed firms and took the case with him. They just now wrote me a letter telling me they wouldn't continue the case. They didn't tell me why. They had filed suit and did what they called "dismissal without prejudice." I have one year to refile the suit if I want to.

I went to a lawyer friend of our family who talked to this lawyer who had my case for the three years. He said I had a 60-40 chance of winning the case but said that juries in this state are not very sympathetic with the plaintiffs. They are usually sympathetic with the doctors. He thought the most settlement I could get would be from $10,000 to $15,000.

I didn't know how much the lawyer was suing for until the day it came out in the paper. It was $86,000, to cover medical expenses, loss of wages, physical and psychological injuries and support, care and education of the child.

Several times I had asked him how much he planned to sue for. I told him many times I did not want to break the man. I just felt that retribution was due us; all of the expenses we were out, everything. I still think that I should have been consulted about how much to sue for.

Fifty percent of any settlement would go to the lawyer and any expenses or court costs would come out of my half. He thought that expenses might be $2,000 or $3,000. If the settlement was $10,000 I'd get only $2,000 after expenses and that wouldn't even cover my medical and hospital bills. Besides, it was a risk. We don't have $3,000 to put up in case we lost. We don't have a penny in the bank. We'd still be out court costs. For that reason, I can't continue. I have no choice.

I can see how it might look to a jury. They might say, "What kind of mother is that who wouldn't want her child?" I feel like Judy is a miracle child but, my gosh, I went through a lot to get her. I love my daughter and I wouldn't take a million dollars for her. But no matter. For me, it was a big risk, one which I was led to believe I wouldn't have to take. I could have died.

When I recovered from my section, I discussed with Dr. McKinsey what was going to happen now. He is a Catholic. He explained that he will do hysterectomies for women who need them. In my case, he felt like I needed a hysterectomy because there is no way I can have another baby or take the risk. A second child would be even doubly risky. For this reason, he was willing to do it.

But he didn't want to do major surgery on me again right after my section, which is when it would have to be done, right away, rather than take the risk of becoming pregnant again. He thought another operation right away would be too hard on my kidneys.

So he sent me to another doctor who does a lot of sterilization procedures; asked me, if nothing else, to talk to him because he knew my hesitation on going through it again. The procedure he does, you use a laparoscope to do it. He makes a very, very small incision in the umbilicus and then a lower one, farther down the abdomen. They are so small they don't even require sutures. Then he goes in, cuts the tubes and cauterizes both ends.

"Band-aid surgery."

That's right. I asked him how much of the tube he cuts off and he said an inch. That kinda scared me because I'd heard about them growing back.

Cauterization is pretty safe, or I thought it was, in my limited knowledge. He said it was a very, very, very low risk surgery-type thing.

I had to do it. I didn't want a hysterectomy but I was scared of another ligation procedure. So we went ahead and I made him promise he'd cut off more than an inch. He cut off four inches.

Before the surgery, he told me he might have trouble because of scar tissue inside. He'd have to just wait and see. But it wasn't bad at all. It healed up real nicely.

It was a fantastic procedure, outpatient surgery. I went into the hospital at eight in the morning, got in surgery about 9:30 and got out at noon. I've recommended this procedure to a lot of people since then.

In August, after Judy was born, I started having very severe headaches. As a student in high school, I had trouble with hypertension which resulted in headaches. This time, I noticed a big lump at the base of my head. The doctor said to get that kind of a lump, you either have to have a sore on your head or have been bitten. He couldn't find anything, but he gave me some medication.

One night it got so bad, I had to go to the emergency room and get a shot. I don't know if you call it a migraine, but it was a very severe headache. The next day the doctor put me in the hospital. In the meantime, the lumps had spread to five or six at the base of my head. Strangest thing I'd ever heard of. He told me it was an accumulation of poison that my kidneys wouldn't get rid of. He gave me medication, strict diet and kept me on bedrest for a week. That's all he could do.

Since that time, all I can say is, I've been very lucky. It's been in remission.

I have a battle with my weight, always have, probably always will. Dr. Larison is a very outspoken man and he really gets down on me when I weigh too much because it is detrimental to my kidney health. The less weight you have, the less work your kidneys have to do. This is the kind of man Dr. Larison is. He as much as told me not to bother coming back until I decided I was going to get the weight off. He can't help me if I can't help myself.

"What method of weight loss do you use?"

I go to a doctor, another doctor, and he knows all about my problem. He is a "weight doctor" and he has me on a diet pill; it's an appetite control pill. He keeps real close watch. I have to go in once a week. I lost 55 pounds and then gained some back. Of course, I diet, too, foodwise.

Getting back to Dr. Smith and the lawsuit, I would like to take some action. We've recovered, it's been a battle and we've lost a lot along the way. But I would still like to make a complaint to somebody, not to get the money, but to let people know what's going on. Since this happened, I've heard that a lot of people complain about Dr. Smith. I remember one girl's baby died; it was something the doctor had done wrong. And another girl was in labor over 36 hours and he wouldn't do a section. He finally had to but he let her go that long.

Maybe there's more to it than people know because a lay person doesn't know all of the things a doctor does. They just don't tell you.

My family doctor told my kidney doctor that they'd had a lot of complaints about Dr. Smith, the hospital, that is. It's unethical for one doctor to say something against another one, I think, so it's always done under the table. You'd think something could be done. And Dr. Smith is smug, he's so smug!

Like my kidney doctor says; we sat and talked one day. He said, "Look, Brenda, doctors are only human. It's a practice. They are practicing on people every day. Doctors can make mistakes. I've made mistakes, but all I can do is go to the person and say, 'This is what I've done wrong and this is what I want' to do to fix it.'"

I had not even thought of suing Dr. Smith except for his attitude. It wasn't until his attitude changed, after he charged me for the surgery when he said he wouldn't, that I saw a lawyer.

VII .

Baby Production

Parturition is a physiological process — the same in the countess and in the cow.

W. W. Chapman (1866–1950)

21. Childbirth

A curly-haired blonde, 17 years old, she is the mother of a one-year-old boy. She is exceptionally bright, possesses more street learning than book learning, the result of a very early independence from her adoptive parents. She adores her son although she gets exasperated with him often. She is raising him by herself because she declined to marry the child's father. She says she will raise her son to be a famous person, perhaps to carry the title which is now his nickname, "The Senator."

She is a person whom you cannot avoid liking although she describes herself as "a selfish bitch." She smokes incessantly and when she is in that kind of a mood or the situation provokes her, cusses like a sailor. Although she did not finish high school, she passed the G.E.D. (general education degree) examination and is a freshman in college. She wants to become an accountant.

• Childbirth

Cause and effect, cause and effect. You go to bed with someone and you get pregnant. You get pregnant and you have a baby. You have a baby and you get old, fast.

Can you believe it, I'm almost old enough to vote. I'm old enough to go to an x-rated movie. I'll be 18 in August.

When I was pregnant, I could see the baby's whole foot against my tummy and a whole hand print, his little fingers outlined against my tummy. And you could tell his head which was a larger round lump, bigger than an elbow or a heel. It was so neat.

The first time I ever saw Mike move I was getting into the bathtub. I saw my stomach jump and I almost freaked out, it was so neat. I'd lie there in the bed with almost all of my clothes off and watch my stomach bouncing around. And the cat just loved it. She'd crawl up on top of my tummy and just purr while the baby was kicking her.

I was in labor for 26 hours. I asked Pat, this lady I worked for in the flower shop, what it felt like when you go into labor and she said it was like having gas pains. Well, I'd been having this horrible case of gas all day long so we giggled. We both knew I was in labor but nobody wanted to say it. Mike was supposed to be born on the twenty-fourth and here it was the twenty-fourth and I was in labor.

She timed my gas pains and they were 10 minutes apart then. She took me home with her and we had dinner: pizza, strawberries and ice cream and iced tea. I'll never forget the iced tea because that's what I threw up when I was in labor.

All of a sudden my gas pains were two minutes apart and we went to the hospital. They couldn't believe I was in labor because they couldn't feel any contractions. Thought it was false labor or something. The reason they couldn't find any contractions was because I was all baby. I lost 20 pounds in the first four months and then I gained back 21, so actually I only gained one pound. So finally one of the nurses felt a contraction and they took me to the labor room.

Ann Johnson. She's the one who gave me a hard time when I was in labor.

I remember her name because afterwards she tried to be my buddy-buddy and give me the *Living Bible* and the whole damn stuff. I hated her. She gave me a harder time than Mike did, by God. I can't stand pain at all. I have a very low pain threshold. You stick a pin in me and I hit the ceiling. Some people can stand pain and some people can't. Well, here I am in labor, I was in labor for 26 hours, and at the time I was in my deepest labor, it was the middle of the night. I wanted to get some sleep. I didn't want to go through this damn havin' a baby until the next day. I was tired. I'd have a pain and right away, God, I'd have another one. I was going, "God, I can't believe this is happening." I started making a couple of grunts here and there, I didn't holler or nothin', but you've got to grunt, at least. And, damn her, she came in and she goes, "Would you mind keeping the noise down. There are other patients in this hospital trying to sleep." I said, "Damn it, I wish I was one of them."

She kept saying, "Be quiet, be quiet," and finally I said, "You fuckin' bitch. You shut your goddam mouth!" Here I'm the patient and she's the nurse and she's giving me a hard time. I really couldn't believe that. In fact, I was doing okay with my breathing and everything, had everything going pretty well. They told me how to breathe when I came in and I was doing okay until she gave me that hassle and then I started crying, I couldn't breathe right. I couldn't catch my breath and the pains started getting worse. I couldn't control them at all. She really messed up my labor for me.

When I was in labor, I kept having this feeling, "They're all out to get me." I felt like the nurses were going to take my baby away, because they were so weird and so mean. I'd had two hypodermics, I was in labor and in pain. It wasn't logical thinking. It was a "fuzzy think." It was from having watched *Rosemary's Baby* two months earlier, I assume. We went to see it when I was seven months pregnant, which was real smart, but you know how weird teenagers are.

My labor was so slow. It maybe took four hours to dilate from one to two. I got to seven centimeters about eleven o'clock the next morning, the twenty-fifth. At 11:15 I was dilated to 10, bang. I skipped over eight and nine and went straight to 10, zip, like that. And I was so tired and kind of out of it from fighting and all. I don't even remember going from the labor room to the delivery room. All of a sudden, I was there.

When I was having Mike and I was in there in the delivery room, I was popped wide awake. Nothing could have put me to sleep. You could have knocked me up the side of the head with a boulder and I wouldn't have fallen asleep. The nurse told me to sit up and she came out with this needle and I thought, "My God, what is she doing?" I didn't know anything about having a baby. I hadn't taken any course on it and nobody told me anything about it. My mother's never had a baby. *(She's an adopted child.)* I said, "What is that?" and she said, "It's a saddle block." I'd heard of that so I thought, "That's cool," and then she stuck the needle in my spine and, yow, it hurt so bad.

They told me to put my feet up in the stirrups, sit up and bear down. I didn't know what she meant by "bear down" so she said, "Just pretend you're going to shit your britches." So I said, "Is that why you gave me that enema while I was in labor?" Apparently they do that so when you bear down, you won't shit all over the doctor.

So I sat and grunted and the doctor grinned at me and when I asked him why he was grinning he said, "You're so red." They kept telling me to bear down while I was in labor and I didn't know what that meant but when they finally told me what that meant, I said to myself, "I'm going to do it right, by God." *(Laughs and gives a grunt to demonstrate.)*

The baby was just starting to come out and his head was out and nothing else and the doctor told me to sit up and I got to see his head. It was really gross. Covered with slime and everything. But it was so neat, seeing your kid's head before anything else.

Then he pulled him all the rest of the way out, and I'm telling you, this is what really impressed me. You're going to die, everybody thinks it's so gross. When he took Mike out and held him up, that fuckin' umbilical cord was beautiful, it was purple. It was all twisted, it was beautiful, it was gorgeous, I couldn't believe it. I thought, "God, what a pretty cord. Who cares about the baby, that cord is gorgeous." A pastel violet. Boy, you ought to have a baby, you'd love that cord. It was really neat.

"Were you in pain at that time?"

Oh, no, heavens no, are you kidding? I'd had six hypos; I'd had an I.V. and a saddle block and I was feeling pretty good then. Elevil and Valium are nothing compared to having a baby. That's a real trip. Plus the added effect of seeing this slimy, gross-lookin' baby. But it's mine and nobody can do anything about it. It's my kid. The doctor held Mike up. How do you describe something that's so ugly it's beautiful? He was the ugliest, ickiest, most horrible mess, yellow and purple and red and green and black. The whole shot. At the same time he was the most beautiful thing I had ever seen in my whole life. Amazing how I'm the only person in the whole world who has ever thought that.

When I was in labor, though, for about 15 hours, maybe one o'clock that morning, I figured I was going to die. I didn't know whether the baby was going to live or not but I knew I was dead. I had it all mapped out. I knew that nobody could live through that much pain. I don't know whether it was a real thought or the hypodermics they gave me, the hassle, the fighting. It was a pretty scary thing.

It was kind of weird, though. I only gained at the most three or four inches while I was pregnant and to see that whole baby, that gigantic creature, come out of my little tiny tummy was really weird.

After I got back to my room, Pat came to see me and I wanted to sit up and talk to her. I wanted to tell her all about the most terrific thing that had ever happened. This nurse came in and told me, "Don't sit up. If you sit up after having a saddle block, you'll throw up." And I was just going crazy. I can't stand to stay still when something exciting is happening. I want to jump, I want to leap, I want to throw myself against the wall. But they wouldn't let me.

When Mike was three days old, I dropped him on the floor. Mike is like I am, he's a sleeper. I love to sleep. In fact, I'd like to be a mattress tester, do that for a living. Anyhow, they treated Mike like they treat every baby. "You are going to do this because you are just born and you're under our care and we have routines and schedules and you're going to do what we tell you to do." At two o'clock in the morning they would wake Mike up, change his diaper and bring him into the room to be fed. He was breast-fed. By the time they got him in the room, he was asleep again. He didn't want to wake up. I practically had to force feed him, tickle his feet to keep him awake.

I'm also a sleeper, and who in the hell is up at two o'clock in the morning? No idiot in the world is going to be up at that time of night, 'specially this idiot. So there we were, all cuddled up together; he was nursing and I was stroking his hair — he had such long, pretty hair when he was born — and smelling him. Babies smell like babies, you know. And we fell asleep together.

We'd been asleep about 45 minutes. The nurses hadn't checked or anything. All of a sudden I heard this horrible scream. I jumped up, sat up and looked down and there's my baby, wrapped up in blankets, screamin' and kickin' on the floor. I liked to have had a heart attack. My first thought was, "My mother's going to kill me."

I rang for the nurse and she came sauntering in. They never paid any attention to me because I rang that buzzer all of the time, mostly because I was so bored and so lonely. I got down and picked up my baby. I was in hysterics because I thought he was dead, for sure. But he wasn't hurt, thank God.

Hospital beds are too high. My baby fell off of a high hospital bed, hit his head on a potentially dangerous bedside table that swings over the bed, and falls to a bare, uncarpeted, hard floor. It should be mandatory when the patient is breast-feeding her child that the rails should be up. They shut the barn door after the horse got out. Then they put the bed rails up, pillows along the thing, the whole shebang.

There are so many times I wish I was pregnant again, without having another baby, just to be pregnant again for a while. Except that it is uncomfortable when you have a full bladder and the baby bounces on it.

It is so weird to think about it when you are pregnant. You think, "God, there's going to be another person in this world because my stomach is bouncing around." It's a weird feeling, hard to describe.

When I first had Mike I looked at my tummy and thought, "God Almighty, I've got all these stretch marks on my tummy." I had one weird one which I loved. It was a beautiful brown one which went straight up and down my stomach. Right down the middle. And the weird thing about it is that every one of my stretch marks just up and walked away. They're all gone. And that's not always the case. My doctor said that he had only one patient who lost her stretch marks. I guess I was pretty lucky. I think it depends a lot on how well you take care of yourself. If you get fat and all, you're more apt to keep them. It has to do with your skin's elasticity. It may have something to do with being young, too. Anyhow, I don't have any stretch marks except on my boobs. I had those when I was 12 or 13 because I used to eat lots of candy when I was a kid and I got super, super fat. All of my stretch marks landed on top.

> *She grew round-womb'd and had indeed, sir,*
> *a son for her cradle ere she had a husband*
> *for her bed.*

William Shakespeare (1564-1616)
King Lear, I, i, 14

22. Septic Abortion

She is young, 25, but much more knowledgeable about the medical world than most consumers her age. Her acquaintance with matters of health care comes from her lifetime ambition to become a doctor as well as her work as a cancer research assistant in both laboratory and clinical procedures. She is animated, agile, bright-eyed. Her two girls, ages one and three, have very different personalities: The oldest is outgoing and full of talk; the youngest is quiet and unsmiling. Her husband is a senior in law school. They live close to a university medical center in the capital city of a midwestern state.

- **Miscarriage**
- **Septic Abortion**
- **Premature Delivery of the Foetus**

I think it probably started when I got pregnant the second time; and it was again with an IUD.

"The second time with an IUD? Wasn't that discouraging?"

The first time I thought it was pretty freaky, but no, it was rather exciting. I have to admit that making a baby is an awfully . . . . If you've ever thought about something from almost nothing, it is pretty miraculous.

I'd had some problems with this two-month pregnancy. All along I'd had slight, episodic bleeding, very slight, but still that's not normal. But I was riding to work every day with a friend who had had two pregnancies and both kids were old enough to be in junior high school and she had bled during both pregnancies so that made it seem to me less unusual that I had that problem, especially with an IUD which could easily cause it.

One Monday at work, I was good for nothing. I was unable to walk all of the way down the hall without feeling faint. I had to lean up against the wall or sit on the floor for a minute before I could make it the rest of the way. It was rather obvious to my boss that I was having problems. He knew I was pregnant and that things weren't really going right. In the middle of the afternoon, he called the doctor for me. I was working in the medical center for a research laboratory so it was very convenient for me to walk across the street to see the doctor. My white count was low so it looked like a viral infection to the doctor when he examined me and did a blood test. I did have a couple of symptoms of what could have been the flu.

"A viral infection does not elevate the white count?"

It lowers it in a lot of instances, in contrast to a bacterial infection, which increases it. The doctor gave me a prescription for Amphycillin, in capsule form, to take at home. I was to record my temperature a couple of times that night and let him know the next morning how I was feeling.

That night, I was not feeling up to going out to have the prescription filled and for some reason I didn't have my husband do it either. I just went to bed and I began bleeding more heavily, but, again, it was episodic. And I was chilling, which is also an accompaniment to fever. I finally remembered to get the thermometer out and record my temperature. Every hour and a half I would begin to have a high fever with chills. It would last a half hour. It was odd to have it cyclic which is more like a parasite or bacterial infection. My husband Steve didn't sleep with me that night because we thought I might be getting the flu.

I was so cold whenever I had chills that my back would contract in a violent arch. I had the electric blanket up to 10, which is the maximum, and I never sleep with it set over two or three. I was just freezing to death. I was literally chattering.

Close to morning, I recorded my temperature once more and it was 107 degrees. At that point I was hot, rather than cold.

My hair was dirty and it is very important to me to have clean hair in order to feel good, so I wanted to get up and wash my hair before going to the doctor. I knew I'd be calling the doctor and going to see him that morning, but I couldn't even sit up in the bed, let alone get out and wash my hair.

When I did call the doctor, and as soon as I told him my temperature, he asked for no more information, he just told me to get on in to see him right away. So I went, dirty hair and all. Things were so distorted to me, vision-wise, that even though Steven was driving carefully, things looked close. I thought he was driving too close to other cars and things. When he parked at the hospital, I said, "Watch out!" because I was scared that he was going to hit a car. Everything looked weird.

The doctor examined me again and told me to go have x-rays taken because he was sure by now that I was probably aborting.

Getting x-rays meant going downstairs and waiting. I was told to take off all my clothes, put on this white gown and go out and sit in a chair in the waiting room. To take off all of your clothes when you're a female and you're bleeding and sit in a white gown isn't exactly cool. So there I sat. I asked Steven to get me another white gown and I flipped it out, so nothing would get on it. So when I stood up I was going to try to be cool and keep my rear end covered as I went past people. Luckily, I was not bleeding badly at that point, so nothing embarrassing happened. That was one of my biggest fears at that time.

Finally, it was my turn for x-rays and they took a couple of quick films and I went back out to wait to make sure that the x-rays were okay. Well, we waited and waited and waited and, meanwhile, I felt myself bleeding again. So I asked Steven to go check and the girl said, "Oh, yes. They were fine, a long time ago."

I went back up to the doctor's office and he said, "We're going to put you in the hospital to watch things." And then he told me, as nicely as he could, that it was probably too late to save the baby. Well, I had a feeling all along, with the spotting I'd had from the beginning, that things weren't going to make it. But it was just the fact of accepting it.

The problem was that if I were contagious, I couldn't be put on the OB floor. I had to be put on the medicine floor and the medicine floor was full. The hospital was very, very full that day, but they found a room for me, gave me a nightgown and I crawled into bed.

After that, I remembered the history and physical. The interns and residents were most suspicious that I had tried to abort this baby myself, because I had the IUD, I was pregnant and was aborting. That was a high point in their questioning, "Did you really want this baby?"

They interrogated me along a lot of lines, this being one of them. I was afraid they would think that I had tried to cause this abortion and that wasn't the case at all, so I became very defensive. I said, "I was trying to plan my babies, not prevent them." It was not that I didn't want a baby. I thought that it wasn't time yet. My first baby was just barely over a year old.

The second suspicious thing was that my fever had been cyclic. Throughout the x-rays and the waiting and all, I could predict when my fever would start. I could tell the doctors and attendants that my fever and chills would start at 11:30 and at 11:30 they would start again.

The part I remember which I really didn't care for was the I.V. with the Amphycillin. I have never wanted to have an I.V. because I have seen an operation and what size intracath or venacath had gone into the person's arm. I just couldn't believe it. And to know that was going to go into me. But it did, and very easily, with no pain because they put xylocaine in. But as soon as they put the Amphycillin in, it irritated the vein and made my arm ache and ache and ache.

Before they put in the I.V., they took blood samples so they could culture it for sepsis. Everytime my fever spiked, they'd take more blood for cultures, so it wasn't too long before I'd had enough needles to take care of me for a lifetime. I was becoming very needle-shy and not a very nice patient.

The next problem was that the I.V. stopped up. My veins couldn't take the Amphycillin. The I.V. kept stopping and the nurses kept coming in and scolding me for stopping it. Apparently, something I didn't know, patients don't like it when it burns and they reach up and shut it off. But I was hurting more when it wasn't flowing so I was attempting to make it go again. Several times I restarted it by myself because I couldn't get a nurse to answer my call.

"How did you do that?"

I piddled. I stroked and I jiggled, I pressed and I bubbled and I squeezed.

"Where did you learn this technique?"

I didn't. I just messed around. I figured out that that's drippin' and that's stoppin' and that's going in and that's not making it and something had to be happening. Meanwhile, my veins started streaking red, clear up to my elbow. You could see what was being irritated. That was the biggest irritant of the whole hospital visit, the I.V. Nothing else. Just a simple I.V. That's what I hated about the whole hospital stay.

The next day, after bleeding quite a bit that first night in the hospital — the nurses confirmed that I had lost quite a bit of blood — I had still not eaten because I had been put on N.P.O., nothing by mouth, as soon as I came in. I was starving because I hadn't eaten anything because they wouldn't let me. By Wednesday morning I said, "Whatever you've gotta do, do it, just so I can get some food."

And I said, "And you're not going to put me out. It'll be done under local." So the doctor said okay and he sent in a soft diet. It was so horrible I couldn't eat it. I couldn't even look at it.

I was told I was "on call." We decided Wednesday morning to do the surgery, complete the abortion. The operating rooms were scheduled for that day, so they had to wait until one was empty and it was convenient for the doctor.

I believe it was close to one o'clock in the afternoon when the doctor came in and said, "This is going to be the easiest shot you've ever had in your life." I said, "I don't want it." And he said, "Don't worry, it's not going to hurt a bit because we'll just put it right in your I.V." I repeated, "I don't want it," but he went ahead anyhow and said, "It'll be all right." I found out later it was Demerol-Vistaril which stung like hell.

Vistaril is put with Demerol to keep you from vomiting. Demerol alone would make you vomit. Well, it burned even worse than the Amphycillin did. Within a minute or two, I felt drunk or rather high. The Demerol got to me very fast but my arm still hurt. It was still streaking red and the I.V. was not working well. They put me on the guerney and mobiled me to wherever they mobiled me. Then they transferred me to the operating table.

I had my hair, my dirty hair, back with a barrette so it would be out of the way. At least they let me do that. Instead of stirrups on the table they had canvas loops, up in the air, and that's where your heels hang. As they were scrubbing, I went into another chill and the nurse and I discussed how to get the I.V. working. We were busy bubbling and pinching and stroking and rubbing and squeezing.

The doctor did a suction currettage which is the way I wanted it. That means suction is used to take off the endometrium, which is being shed anyway by the abortion, and what had not already been expelled is sucked away into a container and saved for measuring, doing a pathological survey on the structure and whatever.

I was draped and cleaned and ready to go and the doctor did a para-cervical block, which is numbing around the cervix. Then he did a dilatation. He described it to me and it was kind of interesting. The cervix is kinda like styrofoam and when you insert this graduated cylinder, the cervix stays open for a while, as though you had molded styrofoam, while you work on the uterus.

Because I was a good patient and on good terms with him, the doctor promised he would not strap down my arms, which I did not want. Being half drunk on Demerol, even though they said, "Now remember, don't touch the green sheets," I did fine until he said, "I'm not hurting you, am I?" And I said, "A little bit right over . . . " and I started to touch where he was hurting me and somebody grabbed my arm and said, "No, no."

They finished the currettage, which took only a few minutes. I felt only pressure, no pain. There was no pain to it at all. When they were through, I said, "Now, let me see what you took out," and they handed me a Dixie cup of what looked like blood clots. That was all. It was a tiny Dixie cup and there wasn't much in it. That was it.

The doctor said he almost didn't get the IUD. A problem is that IUD's sometimes fall out and females don't know it. But I claimed mine was still in there. He said he didn't see the tail of it and I reminded him that he had cut it off for me. It was only through x-rays that they realized it was still there, because it is radiopaque. He worked and worked and worked and finally got the IUD out.

They were having so much trouble with the I.V. they decided to switch to the other arm, but I said I didn't want it. Despite my protest, they began working on the other arm and put the I.V. in it. I'll have to admit it didn't hurt any more. This was a new vein which wasn't irritated yet and it didn't hurt to put it in. It was a relief.

Meanwhile, my legs were up in these canvas loops and I said, "Okay guys, get my feet down." I could not get my feet down by myself and it was a great relief to have my legs down.

We made jokes and talked and they covered me up and wheeled me back to the elevator to take me up to my room. The elevator was stuck and we waited for 20 minutes. The electricity to the two elevators for patients had gone off.

No one had bothered, in fact, I had asked for it, and no one had given me a sanitary napkin for after surgery, so there I lay for 20 minutes on a stretcher. I never have cared for the guys who usually cart you around because they're just in it for the money. That's their job, but I've never cared for being naked under these weird sheets and being toted around by one of these guys. Well, there I lay, bleeding all over the guerney, waiting for the elevator to be fixed.

By the time I got back, my room had been loaded with flowers. It smelled like a funeral home. Steven was there. I was tired. Demerol depresses me, unlike what it does for a lot of people, so I was not in a good mood. I asked him to please leave. And he did. I was finally able to sleep for the first time.

Instead of eating hospital food that evening, Steven went out and got me a Wendy's hamburger and a malt and brought me chocolate chip cookies and cold milk from home.

By this time, I had made friends with a couple of the residents and they were borrowing my Playboy magazines and coming in and making jokes. The next morning the crew came in to see how I was and I said, "Fine, but will you please take out the damned I.V.?" By then my arm had swollen to three times its normal size. I looked like I had on a baseball glove. All of my fingers were big and fat, and my hand was big and fat and my arm was big and fat. The I.V. had infiltrated. The nurses had come by in the night to see that the I.V. was dripping but they didn't pay attention to where it was dripping to and I was asleep. I slept well.

The swelling in my arm gradually went down. It was just fluid and it went back down in a day or so, but it was rather astonishing to wake up and find my arm that big.

After the surgery the fever and the chills were gone, but the backache stayed on for a number of days.

The IUD was a particular kind which, about that time, was known to have caused 26 or 27 deaths throughout the country from sepsis. It has since been taken off the market.

I refused to have another IUD except the Copper Seven. This kind was still being tested and was not on the market. The basis for the Copper Seven is that the plastic is wrapped with copper wire and the copper somehow prevents implantation of the fertilized egg. And that's a form of IUD. It was the only kind I would have tried but I couldn't get it. So I went onto the pill for a month. But I've never been fond of the pill or trying to remember to take it every night at ten o'clock or every morning at six o'clock. I don't care to subject myself to possible problems in the future, either. So I quit it on my own and two months later I got pregnant, on purpose.

23. Childbirth

This young mother is single and lives alone. Her pregnancy was extremely difficult for her mother to accept. For a long time her mother didn't want her friends to know that her single daughter was going to have a baby. This idea didn't seem to bother the patient's father, however. He seemed to accommodate his thinking to the reality of the circumstances almost at once.
    She is tall, redheaded and in her late 20's.

• Childbirth

I went through prepared childbirth classes but I flunked my final exam.

My doctor recommended that I go and take these classes at a Lutheran church on the south side. The LeBoyer method was the one I wanted. LeBoyer is more concerned with what the child goes through during labor and delivery than he is with what the parents go through; the feelings of the child, the first things that the child sees and hears, the pressure on the baby's head as he comes out, all of that good stuff. He feels that you should make the baby comfortable as much as possible because birth is too traumatic an experience as it is.

"What is that supposed to do for the child later on?"

According to him, it makes for happier children. They are not so aggressive, not so unkind to other people and to animals during their growing-up years. They play different, they do their school work different than other children. He has done over a thousand babies and some of them are now eight or 10 years old. They run tests on them once a year to see how they react to different things. And they come out different, all of the time.

My doctor, and maybe one other in town, uses the LeBoyer method. The reason he didn't use it with me was because he was already angry with me for flunking my prepared childbirth.

You are supposed to be able to go through labor and delivery without any anesthesia but I had an epidural right before the baby was born. That's a form of anesthesia and there are only two anesthetists in town who can even do an epidural. It is similar to a spinal, but instead of going into your spine, they go around it to a certain place in your back and inject a medicine which partially numbs you, from your waist to your toes. But you can still wiggle your toes and it wears off in exactly two hours, so you've got to be really close to delivering the baby before they can even do it. All it does is shut off your labor pains when they get really hard.

I went into labor at one o'clock Saturday afternoon. The first six hours were easy; we stayed home. My sister was my coach and she came over. We ate, went through our contractions, went through our breathing exercises with each contraction and did everything just fine. We were very happy with it. You have to have a coach and my sister went through the classes with me. Most of the people have husbands as coaches but my sister was mine and that worked out fine. The daddy didn't want to be a coach, said he was scared to be in the delivery room.

We called the nurse at the birth center, which is next to the doctor's office, at about 4:30. We told her what kind of contractions I was having and how far apart they were. She told us to wait another couple of hours and meet her at the birth center after six o'clock. When we got there, she checked me and I was "fully effaced" but not dilated. So I had quite a ways to go yet. The thinning of the cervix had happened but I wasn't yet dilating to let the baby out. She told me to go back home, eat some food, drink some wine and have a comfortable evening because I was getting just a little bit uptight. That's when the trouble started, right there. I got separated from my coach for about 45 minutes, thanks to my other sister. She went home in one car and I went home in another. That got me all off track because she wasn't there to go through the breathing with me and keep me relaxed. You really need your coach, more than anybody else in the world right then.

When we got back home, my mother decides to pick a fight with me. By the time my coach came in, I was ready to leave. I didn't care if I didn't ever see any of those people again. My whole family could go jump in the lake. You see, they all showed up at the birth center the first time I went up there. They had a case of beer, three bottles of wine and a whole bunch of other stuff in the trunk of the car. They were going to the living room of the birth center and throw themselves a party while I was having my baby. And I would just as soon they would have stayed at home if they were going to have a party. They were driving me bananas, this whole troupe of people following me wherever I went.

Finally, my coach got back; she puts a glass of wine in my hand and a glass of wine in her hand and we went walking, all around the neighborhood. The nurse said this would get my mind off the contractions so we did; we went for a long walk. I bet we walked two miles.

When we got back about 9:30 the family was all sitting around eating hamburgers. So we sat down, too, and had a hamburger with them. It was awful, made me sick to my stomach. Made everybody sick so there must have been something wrong with the hamburger.

Well, we kept going through the contractions, watching television and things like that.

Everytime I had a contraction, my mother tightened up both her fists and sat there and watched me, with bug eyes. She was feeling left out because I could only relate to Becky, my sister who was coaching me. You really have to concentrate, you have to stay right with your breathing. If your coach gives you a suggestion, "You're getting too uptight, go to a higher level of breathing," you've got to go.

About midnight, when we called the nurse again and went back up to the birth center she said, "You're right where you were six hours ago." I hadn't dilated any at all in six whole hours with two-minute contractions every five minutes. I was so uptight, so upset that I couldn't have relaxed if I'd wanted to. My whole body was just one tight knot. I was angry at my folks, my little sister and the whole world.

I asked the nurse for a quarter dose of Valium, that's what they tell you to ask for at the birth classes. You start out with quarter doses and then you won't feel so bad if you have to have a little bit to keep you going.

The nurse pulled a Catch 22 on me. She said, "That's not enough to do you any good," and she didn't give me any. So, half an hour later, I asked for a half dose and she gave me the same answer, "That's not enough to do you any good." She kept fighting me all the way. By this time, I was crying and I didn't care if I lived or died. I was in very hard labor and really upset.

Finally, about 15 minutes later, I said, "Give me the whole shot." Then she said, "I don't feel like you're going to be able to do it. I think that if you need a whole shot of Valium, you ought to go to the hospital." This was about one o'clock in the morning. I was on the brink of complete madness by that time.

The nurse talked to my doctor then for the first time. He didn't even know I was in labor; she hadn't been able to get ahold of him.

My sister talked to the nurse, asked how much longer it might be, since I wasn't dilating. The nurse said it could be 12 to 14 more hours. Here I was going almost completely crazy. My sister and the nurse agreed that I needed some medication but the nurse wasn't going to give me any.

Then my sister and I talked a minute and she said, "Let's get out of here." The nurse at the birth center called Memorial Hospital and told them we were on the way.

The nurse at the birth center had Valium there and she had authorization from the doctor to use it. She runs the birth center, does everything but deliver the babies, and yet she wouldn't give me any medication. It didn't make any sense to me. As soon as I got to the hospital and got a shot of Valium in me, I started dilating. Beautiful. I was still in very hard labor. I was not quite in control of my breathing but I was working on it. The shot of Valium helped me and an hour later they gave me some Demerol. I got Valium in one hip and the Demerol in the other.

Demerol is not a good thing to have. It is plenty strong enough but my sister said I started talking funny. For about 10 minutes, I was out of it completely. I was doing my breathing exercises all right but I was saying things that didn't make any sense. I was goofy. And the Demerol made the baby sleepy which is one of its side effects. And that's not a good thing for the kid.

They called the anesthetist about the time they gave me the Demerol. He lives 45 minutes away from the hospital and I was dilating all of this time. I must have been somewhere around three or four centimeters. When he got there, I was five centimeters. The anesthetist was a neat doctor. I'm going to send him a thank-you note. He was spectacular, the whole trip. He was just an exceptional person to have there.

He came in and did the epidural, which takes approximately 10 minutes. They give you eight little shots up and down your spine and then put a catheter in around your spine, a tube, a big tube, as a matter of fact, around your spine close to your waistline into a thing called your dura or something on the other side of your spine right down there. They put the catheter into that part of your body and then bring a tube around to the front of your body and tape it down. They shoot the medicine in from the front so you can lay back down on your back again.

When he got that done, he checked me again and said, "Holy, my God, she's at nine and a half centimeters. Let's go." And we were on our way to the delivery room. It took just 10 minutes to go from five centimeters to nine and a half.

My sister said that it was as much the psychological effect of having the epidural as having the epidural itself. It was just knowing that the pain was going to stop. I knew that when I got through with what he was doing, it was all going to shut off and I wasn't going to have to put up with looking forward to a two-minute contraction every five minutes for the rest of my life. It relaxed me and the baby decided she wanted out.

It didn't take them 30 seconds to get me into the delivery room because they knew that baby was comin' quick.

"Where was the obstetrician all of this time?"

God must know because I don't. He walked in one and a half minutes before that baby's head came out and that's no joke. He got there just in time to catch her. He did not say, hi, bye or nothing to anybody except the nurse. I don't know if he didn't like the anesthetist or he was mad at me for having to have an epidural after I'd gone through all of this prepared childbirth or what it was, but he didn't say a word to anybody except the nurse the whole time he was in the delivery room.

Just to show you what a far-out guy the anesthetist was, we were all muckin' around in there while they were putting this sterile stuff on my legs, getting me up on the delivery table, saying don't touch this, put this arm here, grab this over here if you need to push; you know, the little handles on the side of the delivery table. We were doing all this as fast as we possibly could because everybody knows this baby's on her way, right this minute. The anesthetist walks around, cool as a cucumber, sticks his finger in where the baby is, pulls out a little lock of dark hair and then stands back in the mirror and says, "Can you see that?" And I said, "Yeah, I can see that." And he says, "That's your baby's hair, not yours." And I said, "Far out," and sat there and watched my baby's hair for a few minutes. It was just a really neat thing for him to do.

About that time, my doctor walked in and doesn't say anything to anybody, including the mother, which made the mother very angry. He did talk to the nurse for half a second, sat down and popped the baby's head out. That quick. While the doctor was aspirating the baby, the anesthetist stood off to one side and said, "Wow, look at those ears. I'll bet it's going to be a boy."

The doctor reached up and pushed down on my stomach to help the baby out and it took only a minute and a half between the time the baby's head came out and the baby was all the way out. He plopped the baby up on my stomach and he didn't even tell me boy or girl. The anesthetist reaches over, lifts up her leg and says, "It's a girl. I'm wrong again."

From the minute she was born, which was 4:21 in the morning, until they took her out of the delivery room, he kept up a running commentary, "What a pretty little baby she is." "What dark hair she has." All of this good stuff.

They thought she was not very alert, that she was breathing rather sluggishly so they only kept her on my stomach for a minute or two, long enough for me to look her over and count her fingers and toes.

The doctor told me in advance that he has cut out the warm bath even in his LeBoyer deliveries. To him, that is changing the baby's body temperature three times in 15 minutes and he thinks it is harder on the baby to do that than to keep a baby warm on the mother's tummy the whole way. For a baby to go from 98 degrees to a 70-degree room into a 98-degree bath and then back out of that into a 70-degree delivery room again is harder on it than to keep it very warm on the mother's tummy after delivery.

After two or three minutes, they cut the cord and put my baby in the bassinet, which the doctor wouldn't have done at all under the LeBoyer method where they leave the baby on your stomach the whole time. But she was breathing kinda slow, so they put her in the bassinet on oxygen for a few minutes.

The whole time she was in the bassinet, the anesthetist stood right there and said, "Oh, look, she's got her finger in her mouth." "Oh, look, she's got both eyes open." "Oh, this one's a keeper. She sure is pretty." And on and on and on. He told me every single move she made because I couldn't see her when she was in the bassinet.

The doctor sat down there and stitched me up for 20 minutes. I don't think he had time to do an episiotomy so I guess I tore. And in the back of my mind, I believe that he was angry enough that he wasn't going to do one anyway. "By God, if she wants to be that way, we'll just let it happen the way it happens." But he did put in a bunch of stitches, I know that much.

After that, they took the baby away. That just about devastated me, right there. If I'd had the baby at the birth center, she would never have left my side. That's another one of the doctor's "rules to live by." The baby never leaves momma. But my kid did. They wanted to watch her and I went along with whatever was best for the baby. They said I could have her back in an hour and a half if she was doin' all right.

They took me back to my labor room, which they also use for a recovery room. I was there for three hours.

Right after the baby was born, I started shaking, really bad. I had started shaking earlier, about midnight, having these weird, weird muscle contractions. My legs and arms were doing this (*demonstrates vigorous shaking*).

When I got to the hospital and they gave me medication, it stopped and then after the baby was born, it started again, almost immediately. The nurse told me that was normal, but I've never heard any other mother talk about it. I guess I shook for 45 minutes before I calmed down out of it.

I felt kind of let down because I wanted my baby and they wouldn't bring her back. I kept saying, "I want my kid. I want my kid." They kept changing my little pads, coming in to ask me questions, checking my blood pressure every 15 minutes. I had to have some kind of special I.V. in my arm because of the epidural. They told me it was some kind of medication, yukky-looking stuff, a yellow, jelly-looking stuff in a bag. Every now and then, they'd come along and squeeze the bag.

At quarter 'til seven in the morning, the nurses are getting ready to go off shift. This is the only thing in the hospital that drove me buggy. I hadn't gone to the bathroom yet but being numb from the waist down from the epidural, I can't go to the bathroom. I have very little muscle control. The nurse kept saying, "You have to go to the bathroom." And I told her when this thing wears off, I'll go to the bathroom, no problem." She said, "Yeah, you probably could, but I'm going off shift; we'd better catheterize you." So they did. She wanted everything to be perfect when she went off shift even if it meant catheterizing me when 20 minutes later I could get up and go to the bathroom.

I laid there until 7:30 and even I knew that was longer than the hour and a half they said my baby would be gone. So I started screaming again, "I want my kid." Also I kept saying, "Take the I.V. out. It only has to be in for two hours and it's already been over three. I'm fine." But they kept squeezing the little bag saying, "Oh, there's only a little bit more medicine. You're going to have to pay for it, so you might as well have it in your body." This is kinda backheaded logic.

Breakfast wasn't served until after 8:30 but I wasn't hungry, not for hospital food. If someone had offered to take me out for Eggs Benedict, I would have gone, but cold eggs and cold cream of rice cereal? I ate almost half of it and gave the rest of my breakfast to whichever my brothers and sisters were sitting around. They all gathered around in the hospital as soon as they knew I was going to be there. My mother stayed home. She was still angry and she'd be damned if she was going to come to the hospital.

She has been angry during my whole pregnancy. It was such an easy pregnancy and my sister was doing so well as my coach. Of course, my mother never had prepared childbirth. She went through labor the hard way and they gave her a saddle block and then knocked her out with gas right before each one of her babies were born, so she never has seen a baby born. I think it bothered her. It made her a little bit jealous.

So I ate this dumb breakfast and they picked up the tray and I kept saying, "I want my baby, I want my baby." And everybody else around in all four rooms that I could see through the door, got their babies. One lady said she wasn't ready yet and had them wheel her baby back to the nursery. And here I was, jumping up and down, wanting my kid. I couldn't believe this lady didn't want to see her own baby.

I got out of bed, walked to the door and said to the first lady I saw in a pink uniform, "I want my baby and I want her now. If you're not going to go down and get her, I'm going to go to the nursery and get her." She said, "Yes ma'am. What's the last name?"

When the baby was brought to my room, they gave me all of the stuff to try nursing the first time, which is a dumb thing to do. They give you this alcohol to put on your breasts and it tastes awful. A baby doesn't want anything to do with a nipple that tastes awful. So after the nurse left, I got up and washed the alcohol off my breasts and then nursed the baby. She did great then.

Twenty-two minutes later they came in and wanted to take my baby away again.

The girl who brought my baby in had timed it. She said, "You've had her for 22 minutes. And I said, "Yeah, and I'm going to keep her, too." "But all of the babies go back to the nursery after they've seen their mothers." I said, "This one is 'rooming-in.'"

The hospital had rooming-in but it turns out that at night they take the babies back to the nursery unless you scream and jump up and down.

Fifteen minutes later, they came to get the baby because the pediatrician was there to examine her. Well, why can't he examine the baby in my room where I can watch? That wasn't the way they did things so they took my baby away again and it was an hour and a half before they brought her back.

"Were you feeling all right by this time?"

Good God, yes. I was feeling great. I had my clothes on by then. When they told me that rooming-in meant that the baby would spend the night in the nursery, right then I said, "I'm not going to be here by nightfall." My doctor zipped through my recovery room about 7:30 to see if I was still alive — he didn't talk to me, he just whizzed through — and I asked him, "When can I go home?" He said, "You may go home if the pediatrician says the baby is all right." He left and I haven't spoken to him since; and I may not, either.

The pediatrician said she was all right but that she was awfully tiny. She weighed six pounds, three ounces. He told me she was a 10-month baby. That's the reason she's peeling all of her skin off. He said that all 10-month babies will peel their whole body off.

The coating which covers the baby, the vernix that the baby wears while it's floating around in the bag of waters, wears off in exactly nine months. If the baby stays in longer than that, it's just bare skin against the water. It gets her all wrinkled, like doing dishes too much. There was another whole month of that, in the water with just bare skin. So it dried that whole top layer of skin out, which comes off. Her face has already peeled off pretty much — she's five days old — but her whole body looks like her fingers.

I cried for a couple of days after she was born because it didn't go the way I wanted it to. Every time I thought about it, I got so mad, and so discouraged and so disgusted. I feel like I had flunked out of school. I was upset with myself because I should have suspected, way in advance, that my mother was going to pull something like that.

My mother didn't speak to me the first two months after I told her I was pregnant. She likes the baby's father; he is married. She doesn't like that very much because my father was quite an alley cat while they were married. There's no other word for it. He was and he admits it. The only side she can see is the father's wife's side. That's the only side she relates to because that's where she was when she was having her babies. The fact that I would have a baby out of wedlock gladly and do it because I wanted to, she just couldn't handle it. The biggest hangup she has, they are going up to Minnesota this weekend to see her brothers and sisters and her parents and she is not going to tell them that I've had a baby. But the funny thing is, I can name at least three of my cousins who got pregnant before they got married or got their girl friend pregnant and had to marry her. I can name seven or eight of my aunts who have skeletons in their closet which are atrocious. A lot worse than having a baby out of wedlock. And still she doesn't want to tell them; she's embarrassed to tell them.

Later, when I was six or seven months along, I began bringing up the subject more often and she began to open up. What happened to you during your pregnancies? How did you feel about your babies? We went out shopping together once and she drifted slowly past the little-girl dresses in the infant department and that did it, right there.

I've got an easy baby to take care of; some mothers don't. This one is no problem.

I think that mothers who are uptight about motherhood have a rough time with their babies. It is as much the mother being uptight as it is the kid being a problem. But we don't have those problems. When she's hungry I stick a nipple in her mouth. Every time she eats she goes to the bathroom, so right after she nurses, I change her diaper. She nurses every three hours, sometimes every two, whenever she is hungry. I have been giving her one ounce of formula as well as breast-feeding her because she was so dehydrated but the doctor says I don't have to do that any more. I wanted very much to breast-feed my baby. It is very important to me, a proud thing. It is like passing a test in school.

(She gives the baby a bottle but the child does not seem to want it so the mother pulls up the right side of her T-shirt, opens the flap of her nursing bra and exposes a full, brown nipple which the baby takes eagerly.)

That's very painful for the first second or two. She's got both of my nipples cracked pretty badly. Until she gets the nipple far enough back that she's not chewing on it any more, it hurts. But the doctor says we'll get over that. She'll get better at it.

She doesn't like my shirt at all. It gets in the way of her nose and her breathing, makes wrinkles on her cheek. The biggest trouble we had was me learning to put a finger in there *(pressing down on her breast right above the nipple)* to keep my breast out of her nose. And nobody ever bothers to tell you that. It took me a while to figure that one out.

> *Where did you come from, baby dear?*
> *Out of the everywhere into here.*
>
> George Macdonald (1824–1905)
> *At the Back of the North Wind,* Ch. 23

> *Here we have a baby. It is composed*
> *of a Bald Head and a Pair of Lungs.*
>
> Eugene Field (1850–1895)
> *The Tribune Primer,* "The Baby"

24. Miscarriage

The description of this event is only fragmentary because the woman's story is told by her neighbor, a concerned 30-year-old mother. She is like an older sister to the patient, empathic and experienced, but she was powerless to get the emergency room people to pay attention to what she perceived to be an urgent problem. Having borne several babies herself, she knows how anxious a girl who is pregnant for the first time can become.

• Premature Delivery of Foetus
• Miscarriage

We had come home from church and I was just preparing dinner when my neighbor's husband called and said, "Could you come over? Ann needs you."

I went over and Ann was in pain. She said she was cramping, explained what had been going on. What it was, she was having a miscarriage.

I'd never been through a miscarriage, you know, threatened, but I hadn't, so I just didn't know too much about it so I just tried to reassure both of them.

While I was there, the doctor called back and they decided she'd better go on to the hospital. Her water had broken, she was passing bloody mucus and had this severe cramping. She was four or maybe four and a half months along.

To my knowledge, she had never been in a hospital since she was born. This was her first pregnancy and she and her husband were totally bewildered and frightened.

They went in. She just had her robe on—I don't think she had anything on under her robe—and they put one of these little, attractive gowns on her and put her on one of those little, narrow, emergency room tables. Her husband stayed in the waiting room and I stayed with Ann in the emergency room.

A nurse's aide came in and took her blood pressure and temperature, I believe, probably pulse, and left. No one came. They had called her doctor and they said he was on his way.

And no one came and no one came and no one came.

She was bleeding rather profusely and she was shaking. Never did a nurse come in that room once since they got her in there. Ann said, "Susan, I feel like I'm just laying in a pool of blood. Would you look?" I lifted the covers and she was. She was laying in a pool of blood. I'd never seen so much blood. I said, "Yes, Ann, you are bleeding a lot. Just a minute and I'll go ask somebody."

I don't think they were particularly busy. Her husband was the only one in the waiting room. He was sitting there by himself, you know.

I contacted a nurse and said, "She's really bleeding a lot. Shouldn't you come in?" She didn't respond so I said, "Well, is there something I can pack around her to absorb some of that blood. She's just laying in a pool of blood."

And the nurse said, "There's a cabinet in there. Reach in and get some towels and pack around her." I went back in, found the towels to pack around her to soak up the blood.

Never did a health worker come in before the doctor came. I estimate that was an hour. I left when the doctor came and she went ahead and expelled the baby there in the emergency room.

The doctor explained that they were going to do a D and C and she'd be in the hospital for a day or so. But before that, she was almost to the point of hysteria.

Of course, I know that when someone's bleeding like that, it looks like more than it is, and I couldn't say how many quarts or liters Ann lost, but the nurse should have at least taken a look. For all she knew from my description, the girl could have been bleeding to death.

To this day, Ann wouldn't go back to that hospital. If she were dying across the street from there, she wouldn't go to that hospital. I don't know whether she ever discussed the incident with her doctor but I was going to write a letter. I thought my view would be more objective than hers. She and I talked about it later. She was very upset about it and we decided that I should write a letter. We felt there was no excuse for this kind of treatment.

But I never did write the letter. I'm not very good at writing.

VIII.
Water Works

As men draw near the common goal
Can anything be sadder
Than he who, master of his soul,
Is servant to his bladder?

The Speculum, Melbourne, No. 140 (1938)

25. Enlarged Prostate

He is near retirement. He is a graduate-level social worker who heads an agency which deals with family problems. He did not learn about children from personal parenting because he and his wife are childless. The agency he heads counsels people with family crises and takes temporary care of the children.

He is bald, medium height, with a tendency to carry a few more pounds than he would like. His habit is to work at the office on Sunday morning while his wife attends church and then go by for the after-service coffee hour and the socializing.

- **Difficulty in Urinating**
- **Enlarged Prostate Gland**
- **Prostatectomy**

The realization that I would have to have surgery on my prostate came after a routine physical checkup examination by my family doctor. He said I had an enlarged prostate and that I'd have to have surgery eventually but this was not imminent.

At the point I began to notice symptoms, difficulty in urinating, my physician referred me to a urologist who agreed that I'd have to have surgery sometime. We didn't set up a date because at the time there was no reason to. We talked about the mortality rate from the prostatectomy operation; I was naturally interested in that, and he assured me it was well under one percent and that age didn't make any difference as far as that risk was concerned.

Not too long after that, it became increasingly difficult for me to urinate and I became worried and uncomfortable so I called him and we arranged a time that was convenient for both of us. He got me a bed in the hospital for several days later.

The hospital sent me a form to fill out so that when I arrived there for admission they wouldn't have to ask me all those questions. I filled it out and mailed it back in but it didn't do what it was supposed to. I don't think they even had the form because they asked me the same questions I had already put down and mailed in. It certainly didn't save any time because, not only did I have to answer the same questions all over again, I had to wait about two hours until they could get me a "number." This was a new hospital, that is an old hospital which had just moved into a new building, and apparently, they had new procedures which didn't work too well. That's what the administrative intern told me when he came around and I talked with him about it. The hospital had just opened on the first day of the previous month and I was admitted on the fourteenth, about 45 days later. There were a lot of other people waiting around to get admitted, too, so it wasn't just a problem with my admission. This number they were waiting to get apparently had to do with identifying my medical record. Well, I'd say there was something wrong with middle management because you got the impression the people in admissions didn't quite know how to get things going. And there were other instances which I'll mention later.

This hospital has all private rooms and my room was certainly adequate. It had everything I needed, bathroom, shower, TV, all of that. But there was something wrong with the heating system. All of the air comes out of one vent and blows right on you and it's either too hot or too cold and always too strong. The maintenance people who came to see about it when I complained said that there was still debris in the lines of this new heating system and gave that as the reason you couldn't adjust it. All that sounded a little dubious to me. I had to put extra pillows and blankets on top of the unit so that just a little of the air would come out. But you'd think that wouldn't be necessary in a new building with a brand new system.

Then the faucets kept dripping and there wasn't any way to shut them off completely. They have these long blade handles, but they were put on backwards so the ends of the handles touched together before the water was completely cut off. I told the maintenance man that the noise of the dripping faucets didn't bother me. I just hated to see all of that water go to waste. Well, he turned the handles around, said they'd have to do that all over the hospital.

The bed was lousy. It was so hard and uncomfortable that I woke up with a pain in my neck that was worse than the pain from the surgery. I slept the first night because they had me doped up, but the next two nights I slept in the chair because I just couldn't stand to lie in that bed. I even had abraded heels because the sheets were so rough and had to put lotion on them to relieve the irritation.

The nurses said they'd had complaints from other patients about the beds. I asked for a different mattress and after two nights sleeping in the chair, they got me one but it wasn't a bit better. I could tolerate being in the bed part of the time but for the rest of my 11-day stay, I was up and down, getting a goodly proportion of my sleep in the chair. Oh yes, the nurses said they thought it was something used in the laundry that made the sheets so rough. You got the impression that the mattress was selected for its durability rather than how it felt to the patient. I sleep on a hard mattress at home — I don't use a bed board — but that bed in the hospital was the hardest I'd ever tried to sleep on.

The food was almost inedible, not because it started out bad, but because it wasn't cooked right. The system in this new hospital was to make up the trays, freeze the food and then cook it in a microwave oven just before it is served. The problem was, though, that the people didn't know how to work the microwave ovens and the food came in about half-cooked. Therefore, I didn't eat much and all in all, I lost eight pounds. Now for me, that was therapeutic because I needed to lose weight anyhow but the next guy might not think so. And, of course, I'd like to have the privilege of selecting poor food, not have that the only alternative.

The whole food service system seemed to be inadequate. I tried for four days to get dry cereal for breakfast but they kept sending up hot cereal. And the little individual salt containers that you break open, like the ones the airlines use, had been frozen. This makes the plastic brittle and when you try to open the end, the whole thing fractures and the salt dumps on your food. Little, irritating things like that.

Fortunately, they had a well-stocked refrigerator at the nurses' station filled with soft drinks, fruit juices and the like. Since they wanted me to drink a lot of fluids anyway, I got all of that I wanted. In the evening, when I'd get hungry after being unable to stomach the food they brought to me on the tray, I'd go to the nurses' station and get what I wanted so I didn't starve. The nurses were well aware of the situation. In fact, one night one of them asked me if I wanted her to send out to McDonald's for a hamburger.

I had no complaints about the professional care except for the anesthesiologist. I didn't even see him until five minutes before he put me under in the operating room so I didn't have a chance to find out what kind of anesthetic he planned to use. And then they had given me a sedative before I was taken to surgery so I was already half out of it. I wanted a general anesthetic and that's what he gave me but I didn't have an opportunity to say so. He should have come 'round to my room the night before so we could discuss it and I could get my questions answered.

Another thing, I woke up after the surgery with a really sore throat as a result of an instrument, I think they call it an airway, which the anesthesiologist used. Now, whether or not it could have been lubricated some way I don't know, but this is what I think is wrong. He didn't tell me about any of this beforehand and I believe he should have. I called his office later and asked him to telephone me but he never did. I thought he should have explained some of this to me.

When I came back from the surgery, I had a catheter in my penis so my bladder would empty and I also had a drain in my abdomen half way between my belly button and my penis. I never could understand why the drain didn't hurt. Here was a hole in my abdomen with a tube sticking out of it but it never did hurt.

The catheter makes you feel like you need to urinate all of the time and that is uncomfortable, but after awhile you get used to that. And then there is the fear of losing the catheter during the process of defecation. I won't go into the gory details but you feel like you must be very careful or the catheter will be expelled. At one time, there was a little blood around the catheter but that didn't bother me as much as the thought of losing the catheter and having to have it reinserted. They put it in while I was still in surgery. Well, it stayed in okay and the doctor removed it the day before I went home.

While we were talking about this operation before the surgery, the doctor had said that I would probably drip for a few days after the catheter was removed but that this condition would clear up. He also said that there were cases in which patients were left permanently incontinent after having a prostatectomy. Well, that had me worried and I was concerned until after about five days at home when I regained control. I could visualize myself going around wearing a bag the rest of my life.

When I mentioned this later to the doctor he said, "Oh, that only happens to maybe one man in a million." He hadn't told me the odds before. Had I known it was a million to one shot, I'd have saved myself a week of worrying.

Later, I saw an article in the *New York Times* which explained all about this condition, the enlarged prostate and the surgery and all. It had diagrams which showed what happens and how the situation is corrected by surgery, what the mortality statistics are and all of that. I sent him a copy with the suggestion that he ought to get reprints and distribute them to his patients who have this problem. Then the men who face surgery would have a better understanding of their condition. He seemed interested in my suggestion but I don't know whether he'll actually follow through with it or not.

I had some pain after the surgery. The doctor said I could expect an occasional bellyache due to adhesions but these went away. I stayed off work for two or two and a half weeks and gradually felt better. The weight I lost, eight pounds, was a side benefit and I'm trying to watch what I eat so I can keep it off.

Because the Blue Cross-Blue Shield coverage I have at work paid most of the bills, this surgery wasn't any financial problem. There are things about the bills that I'd change, though, if I were doing it. For example, the drugs are not specified, it just gives the date and says "Drugs" and tells the amount on the bill. If I were the insurance company, I would want to know what drugs were provided because it's too easy for the hospital to make a mistake and overcharge.

The other bills are confusing. There is a charge for blood and one for administration of the blood. X-rays are the same way. There is a charge for taking the x-ray and another one for interpreting it. Just a simple explanation of things like this on the statement itself would relieve the minds of lots of people who try to understand their hospital bills.

I think hospitals try to do a good job but I can't say that they, or any other health institution for that matter, are really planned or seen with the patient as the number one consideration. I suspect that most of them are run for the convenience and benefit of the people who run them.

First need in the reform of hospital management? That's easy! The death of all dietitians and the resurrection of a French chef.

Martin H. Fischer (1879–1962)
Quoted by Howard Fabing and Ray Marr in *Fischerisms*

26. Kidney Shutdown

He is a tall, dark-haired sinewy man in his late 20's. He was one of the town's firefighters before the attack of nephritis changed his life.

I sat by his bed in the tiny bedroom of a modest home in a small Southwestern town. It was a high, hospital-type bed, and on the opposite side of it was the kidney machine with its plastic tubes hooked up to a permanent shunt in his left forearm. The bright-red blood flowed out of his arm, circulated through the washing cycle of the dialysis equipment and back into his body. His short, chunky wife operated the kidney machine, which seemed to dominate the small room. Two toddler-aged children wandered in and out of the bedroom as we talked.

When the appointment was set up for this visit, he made a point of scheduling it at a time he would be on the kidney machine, so I could see the dialysis process in action while we discussed his illness.

- **Nausea and Vomiting**
- **Kidney Shutdown**
- **Glomerulonephritis**

First of all, I didn't know anything was going on. I got sick at work one day and they forced me to go to the hospital.

"Where do you work?"

At the lumber company and the fire department. I was working at the lumber company when I got sick. They took me out to the County Memorial Hospital and took a blood test and run a bunch of other tests on me. The doctor come in and said that I had some kind of kidney problem.

"What kind of symptoms did you have?"

I just got sick, just vomited. All of a sudden, I got hot and had to go to the bathroom and vomit. We didn't know what caused it. I thought I was all right but they said I looked bad and made me go to the hospital.

The doctor took the tests and said I had a kidney problem; he didn't know what it was and that I'd have to go into the hospital. So at two o'clock in the afternoon on the day I got sick, I was put in the hospital.

They ran urine specimens and ran dye into my veins and into my kidneys. I stayed in the hospital three days and that's all they did, urine specimens and this dye stuff. He told me he didn't know exactly what it was and he wanted to send me to the city, up there to a hospital to see if they could find out exactly what it was. He said he had a pretty good idea but he wasn't sure. This was my family doctor, a general practitioner.

Three days later, I went into a hospital up in the city. That was a great hospital. All they did was take urine specimens, 24-hour urine specimens. Then they did a biopsy the third day I was there and sent me home. They never did tell me anything, they didn't give me a diet, they didn't tell me what to do or nothin' about it except that I had something wrong with my kidneys.

This was an internal medicine man up there and they had a kidney specialist come in and do the biopsy. But after the biopsy, they just sent me home, told me I had some kind of kidney disease. They were waitin' on the tests on the biopsy to come back.

So in the meantime, I'm at home and my feet start swellin'. So I called my family doctor and he said I have sinus trouble and he gives me medicine for my sinuses. Course I couldn't breathe. I'd get tired walkin' across the room. I'd get literally exhausted.

Well, at this time I couldn't work, of course, so I'd stay at home and I was afraid of losing my job because you just can't do that around here.

I'd call the doctor and tell him, "Hey, my feet are swelling," and he'd say, "Don't worry about it. That's part of the disease." And I call him back and say, "Hey, my face is swelling." "Don't worry about it. That's part of the disease."

Well, I got to where I couldn't breathe at all, so I went out there. I went to the emergency room and my doctor came in and said I was hyperventilating. "Breathe into a sack," he told me. At the time, my lungs were full of liquid; he didn't know it and I didn't know it but I wasn't hyperventilating.

So I came back home and three days later I had to teach a class at the fire department. I knew that I had to teach that class or lose my job, because I'd been off so much. So I forced myself down to the fire department and I stayed down there about an hour, I guess. I couldn't breathe, I couldn't walk, I couldn't move. And I couldn't see. When I walked out of the house, everything had "snow" on it. It was unbelievable. And I was more comfortable riding in a car than I was sittin' here at home. I could breathe better. I guess it was because of the fresh air comin' in through the windows. But I couldn't drive, I couldn't walk, I couldn't see, so finally I decided to go back out here to the hospital.

The doctor took a blood count and it was 2.9; the hemoglobin was 2.9. So they rushed me to the city and took me to a different hospital up there this time.

The first thing they did there was x-ray and I could hardly stand up for x-ray. They were great up there. Everything was just click, click, click. They were waiting on me when I got there. They put an I.V. in and started preparing me for the kidney machine, which I'd never heard of. I never thought I'd be a patient of this kidney machine, this dialysis machine.

Then they operated on my arm and put in tubes, sewed veins and arteries together so I could be on the machine. When I woke up, I was on the machine.

I was kinda surprised because all of my family was up there, you know, and when you see everybody you haven't seen for 10 or 11 years you think, "Well, this is it. I'm gone."

They had told my mother that there wasn't much of a chance but they were going to try. The blood count was so low that they didn't know if they could do anything or not.

Anyway, I woke up on the machine and they were all there, and that kind of scared me. They gave me two pints of blood, they couldn't give me blood before because if they did it would mess up the chemicals of my kidneys and therefore change the routine of a transplant, if I could get a transplant. So I had to be on the machine before they could give me blood. They could have given me blood at the County Memorial Hospital but it would have messed up my blood chemicals.

This time they kept me there for three days. He let me come home on the weekend because the weather was getting bad. He gave me instructions on what to do, gave me a strict diet. I can have 400 cc's of liquid a day which is about two cups, and I can have six and a half ounces of high protein which is anything from a living animal — meat, milk, cheese — and 16 ounces of low protein. That really gets me more than any of the rest of it because I always ate all the time. I can only have 87 points of sodium and 57 of potassium. They gave us a book that tells you everything about every food you eat and we have to sit down and figure out just exactly how much is in which foods that I eat and if I don't, I gain weight like crazy. When I gain 10 pounds or so they have to take it off with the machine.

Then I heard that the VA Hospital had dialysis machines so I asked the doctor in the city if he would transfer me from there to the VA Hospital. He didn't like the idea but still he said yes, he would do it. He told me I'd have a better chance of getting a transplant staying with him but with him, I was having to pay the bills. At least 80 percent of the bills; the government was paying the rest, so he said. But I felt like I needed to go to the VA because everything was paid for there.

They taught my wife how to run the dialysis machine at the VA Hospital, from the first day we got there 'til the day we left. They put a permanent fistula in my left arm so I could get on the machine with needles instead of these tubes that were in my right arm. Then they pulled the tubes out and that's about it.

I went back up there twice a week for eight weeks but now I have a machine here at home. The VA furnishes the machine, all of the equipment for it, furnishes all of my medicine. I dialyze three times a week here at home. We don't pay for a thing. They even pay for our trips to the city; we get travel pay for comin' up there.

"That solves your medical expense problem, but it doesn't get you a job."

Hallelujah! Social security takes so darn long to get started. I get disability from social security but it hasn't started yet. It's been months and months and months. They keep telling us it will come through. We called her the fifteenth of this month and she said there was no reason why it shouldn't be there and she'd put a "Critical" on it and get it here. I told her they were about to repossess everything we have, which they are. You can't blame them. It's been five months and if you can't make a payment, the people kinda want their money.

They won't let you work or stuff like that. I guess you could get some kind of job to do but really, when I do anything strenuous, I get out of breath. I can't walk four blocks without being completely exhausted. I get a small pension from the fire department, $46 a month, and then I get a VA disability which is $164, a non-service-connected disability. And then I'll get social security on top of that, if they ever get it started. If I get a job, they'll cut off the social security, which will be $65 apiece for my wife and two children and I'll get $250 a month. So I'd have to get a job which paid me $500 a month net to make it worthwhile. And it would have to be a job where I could go on the dialysis machine three times a week. I stay on it six hours each time. I guess I could do it at night but I do it now in the daytime.

"What is the outlook for a transplant?"

Well, they say it's good, but you gotta wait for just the right kidney. Everthing's gotta match up, you know. They say a car wreck victim is mainly where I'd get my kidney. I could get one from my brothers or sisters, but none of them are old enough to consent to giving one. Mom and Dad want to but they say it's better to have it from a brother or sister if it is donated. I'd rather not take it from them. I'll wait until I can get one from somebody else, someone that's had a car wreck or someone that's definitely going to die that would donate their kidneys.

Any kidney you get, well, they can't tell how long it will last. Most of them last about two years and then your body rejects it. Eventually, your body will reject any kidney that's put into it because it's a foreign body put into your body. But he said sometimes they last two years and sometimes they last twenty. What time you do have it, you don't have to have the dialysis machine, you don't have the diet and it's well worth the effort of having the kidney transplant. We're still hoping for one but it's just wait and see. But you can live on the dialysis machine forever. It does the same thing as the kidney.

Sometimes if she *(his wife)* is taking off a lot of weight with the machine, I really cramp. I just turn into a pretzel. She practically has to put me to sleep with Valium. But, otherwise, I have never had any pain. My kidneys didn't hurt me at all during all of this conflagration of events. The only time they hurt was right after the biopsy. I urinated blood then, but the doctor said that was normal. But never any pain. Nothin'. It just all came all of a sudden. Even when I started vomiting at first, I just thought it was one of those things. I wasn't hurtin' at the time, never did hurt.

The more weight you gain, the higher pressure you have to run the machine at. I've been gaining around 10 pounds every two days, which is really a no-no. They say you are supposed to gain between one and two pounds a day, which I cannot do. I can't stick to one or two cups of water a day, especially in the summertime. The food part of it, they say it's not so much the food you eat, though the potassium level and all that stuff counts, but it's mainly the liquid you drink because you retain all of your fluids. My kidneys still act some but they aren't functioning. I pass out water but it's not filtered. The kidneys haven't cleaned anything. All the garbage and stuff goes back into the blood stream.

The doctor here told me what he thought it was I had before I went to the city, and it did end up to be that, glomerulonephritis. But he didn't have all of the equipment and stuff to say for sure.

After I got back from the city, I went back to work with the tubes in my arm and got that infected and they made me quit working and now I haven't worked. I was in college at the time this happened. I'd enrolled in the last half of my second year in college and because this all happened in January, I never did make it back to school but I plan to go back, yes, definitely and get a degree. My interest was firefighting and I was going to major in fire technology. Now, I guess I'll major in music or English, one of the two, and teach. I'd like to teach. The VA will pay for school. I have plenty of schooling left. I was in the Army three years; spent one year in Vietnam.

A funny thing about a kidney patient. Everyone of them craves something. I craved gasoline. I would do anything in the world to get gasoline, to sniff it. I finally got off of it, thank God. I talked to several other kidney patients up there at the VA Hospital and people craved rocks. They would actually eat pebbles. Mine happened at a filling station. We were sittin' there, filling up with gas, and all of a sudden, I had to have that gas, had to have it on a Kleenex to sniff. There was one guy up there who had to have this blanket over his head or he wouldn't go, couldn't go. It was unbelievable to me. I didn't know what was going on.

Now, if I want to go on vacation somewhere, I can call any VA Hospital in the United States two weeks ahead of time and dialyze at that center when I get there. It takes two years to go to Hawaii.

The doctors have told me — you can't drink anything, you know — but he said if you want to go to a party and get drunk, go on the machine before you go, have your party, get drunk, but go back on the machine as soon as you get back. So really, the machine's not that confining. If I wanted to go get drunk, I could go get drunk.

The doctors can't tell you when you might get a kidney. They just run the tests and if they get a kidney in that fits you, they call you and you've got 48 hours to get up there and receive the kidney. They find you wherever you're at. I don't know how they match 'em up but they told me that there are so many numbers that have to match up and if it comes up that all of them match up but three, they're not going to do the transplant. They have to match up very close. It's sort of a lottery. I have to wait until something happens. It's not like getting in line. It's just like waitin' for your kidney. It's gotta match you. They might get 10 kidneys in today but if none of them match me, I won't get one.

They have to keep the kidney alive and they can keep it alive for 48 hours. Apparently, there are a lot of transplants happening and they say that in the future, they'll have a dialysis machine the size of a cigarette package that you can carry in your belt. As far as I know, it's not on the market yet, that's all hearsay. But they've come so far working on it that anytime they could come on the market with it. You see, it would be a 24-hour deal. You'd be dialyzed all the time. Just like having an outside kidney, sort of like a pacemaker. It would be on the outside and connected to the bloodstream. They're coming right along with it. They say that the kidney is the only organ in the body that can completely give way and you still can live. There isn't a machine for any other organ. That's amazing to me.

Eventually, they'll take my kidneys out and then I'll go on dialysis every other day. I have to watch that diet real close. For example, I went to Kentucky for two days and came home and I'd gained 18 pounds. It was really hard getting it off, hard on me and hard on the machine. They had to run 450 pounds pressure.

A lot of people, when they find out they've got this disease, they just give up. That's what the doctors told me. They won't try or do anything. But I want to go back to school and do a lot of things and I'm going to do them. But there's some people they wheel in up there in a wheeled chair, can't walk or anything, and they put 'em on the machine and take 'em off and wheel 'em out and they don't do anything. They are just a vegetable. Well, I'm not going to end up like that. It was a shock to both of us, my wife and I, when we didn't know what was going on. Her sister died of kidney disease several years ago and it scared the devil out of us when we found out I had one. But we've gotten used to it and we've decided, what the devil, if you can't live without it, you've gotta live with it.

We don't let it affect us in any way. The children are used to the machine, I'm used to it, she's used to it. But a lot of people come in here and see the blood going through the machine and go bananas. Her daddy won't even come here when I'm on the machine.

Another interesting fact. The first two hours you're on the machine, you can eat and drink anything you want. After that, the machine won't take it off. Everything I can't have, like watermelon and cantaloupe, I eat during the first two hours. I get three good meals a week that way.

The only thing that bothers me about being on the machine is cramps. When the machine is pulling off more than my body can take, I cramp. Leg cramps. Well, I have had some stomach cramps and when the pressure is real high, sometimes I cramp all over. But she gives me Valium through the blood stream and that relieves me. I go to sleep then.

When her sister died, they asked for her organs for study. At the time, her parents didn't feel that they should give my wife's sister's organs to science.

Right after she had died, it was a very complicated thing. But we've decided that when I die, whatever, I want my organs to go to science so it can help somebody else.

When I first found out about the dialysis machine, I thought, well, I'm one in a million but it's not like that. There are millions of people on dialysis in the United States, all over the place. It's unbelievable. There's hundreds and hundreds.

There's always someone a little worse off than what you are. We've got our problems but somebody else has got more than we have. But we've kinda got it down to a routine now.

You've gotta look at it that way. You can't feel sorry for yourself or you're going to kick the bucket.

Bones can break, muscles can atrophy, glands can loaf, even the brain can go to sleep, without immediately endangering our survival; but should the kidneys fail . . . neither bone, muscle, gland nor brain could carry on.

Homer W. Smith (1895–1962)
From Fish to Philosopher, Ch. 1

IX.
Hole in the Wall

He has a rupture,
hee has sprung a leake.

Ben Johnson (1573?–1637)
The Staple of News, Act I, Sc. ii

27. Hiatal Hernia

He is a combat veteran of World War II in which he piloted fighter planes. Now in his 50's, he is still associated with military aircraft, working as a civilian employee for the Air Force in a Midwestern air-materiel installation. In fact, he has been there ever since his discharge from the armed services and is now a supervisor in electronic data processing. His wife works there, too. Their children are grown and have moved out of their early post-war subdivision home.

- **Acid Stomach**
- **Hiatal Hernia**
- **Corrective Surgery**

I was introduced to my doctor by my sister, who felt like he was a good doctor and I feel like he is a good doctor, even to this day. He did at that time a lot of insurance cases and he was pretty important at the hospital. Anyway, I went to him with my problems and he gave me pills and the usual routine, come to find out, and kinda brushed me off. This was with my chest condition; I had pains in my chest. This was back right after I got out of the service and I don't know whether or not they were able to diagnose hiatal hernia at that time. I was a fighter pilot, you see, and I lived a pretty high life and flew P-51's and I was in the service about three years in World War II. I had this continuing condition after I came out and they gave me a 10-percent disability on a head injury. The doctor at that time felt within himself, well, it's mental and I really think the man was partially or mostly right. I put my head through a gun sight, three inches of plate glass, across my left eye. But as far as any recurring condition due to the head injury, I don't know of anything.

So I think he probably diagnosed my case about right, as a mental condition.

Since then I went to several doctors. I went to this family doctor up here who since has committed suicide, by the way. He said, "Well, maybe we'd better give you an upper G.I. series." That was just before my operation. So he sent me across the street from the hospital and they did it there. And they said, "Yes, your stomach is about a third through your diaphragm. And this could cause trouble."

I could have had this condition since birth or it may be that it was something that happened as a result of an injury. Nobody ever spoke to me about the cause but I can remember incidents in my life. We were playing soccer when I was a kid, and a big kid, twice as big as me, kicked a soccer ball full tilt and hit me right in the pit of the stomach. Whether this could cause it or not, I don't know, but I do know that I was bent over and I got me a good'un. I almost blacked out before I could get my breath. In fact, I really needed a little first aid then, and didn't get it. But how the condition came about, I don't know. I went back to the VA and told them that possibly the stick in the airplane caused the damage, jabbing me in the middle. But they wouldn't listen to me, for additional compensation.

The doctor diagnosed it through the x-rays as a hiatal hernia and told me I ought to have it repaired. He told me I should get it done before I got any older. It wasn't going to get any better, that was for sure. It was getting to the point that when I'd lie down at night the acid would come up my esophagus into my mouth.

"How old were you?"

Forty-seven. The family doctor asked who I wanted to do it and I asked him and he recommended one. I took his word and they performed the surgery.

You know, one thing has crossed my mind. The patient himself won't always give the doctor the true answers on things. He'd get better answers from the closest kin, the one the patient knows best. A short interview of the man's wife or sister or brother or mother or father might help a lot. Not that it should be extensive or anything. Such questions as "Say, what's troubling this patient?" Not that the doctor should do the interview himself but have it on record, to give him some idea of what's affecting the patient. I know if you go into a hospital, generally it's for a physical condition but we have a mental condition, a state of mind, too, and in many cases doctors tend to forget this mental condition until they come to the point of saying, "Well, this patient just doesn't have the will to live." Somebody that was thoughtful enough to ask and try to find out a few very simple things; maybe the man might have just got a divorce or maybe he just lost his mother or his brother. When I went to the hospital, I'd had some serious complications in my family. Course the doctor didn't know that and it might have helped him to know that during my stay.

During my stay there, I think I got proper treatment, but I don't think they had enough full-time registered nurses to take care of the work load. I really don't think so. The poor lady who was up there, I think she had the whole floor. Every time she came to wait on me it appeared to me that she was just trying to do things too fast. She didn't have any time to take personal attention and speak to you like an average human being, kinda like a knot in the wall.

After the operation, the doctor told me he had taken out my appendix. I was surprised but it just means to me that I won't have to have another operation for appendicitis. I really feel like it's a good thing. This is my attitude. He made the judgment, you know. He probably said, "That man's got a good chance of having appendicitis, so let's just get it now."

"Were you disturbed that they didn't tell you ahead of time?"

It never bothered me.

The surgery is difficult in itself. What it does is cause a lot of inflammation in your esophagus and that thing swells almost shut. Immediately after surgery and for days and for months, I had to chew my food until it was almost liquid. I don't know if you can visualize the feeling, but you swallow and it doesn't go down. You'll be sitting there, trying to eat your meal, and you've got a couple of bites that didn't get all the way to your stomach and you have to wait awhile until those muscles can take it on through that very small opening. He told me this before he ever did the surgery. He said, "You're going to have to chew up your food real good before you swallow it." And this is exactly the way it happened. Even now, if I'm a little bit upset and eat my food a little bit too fast, I'll notice these symptoms and slow down.

One thing while I was there at the hospital, you see, I have a bad back. Lower back, right down between the hips. Nobody's ever said it was a disk or anything. I got hurt while I was in the service. So while I was in for this hernia operation, believe it or not, my back hurt me as much as my front. I'd tell the nurse this when she'd come in and she'd try to help me as much as she could. They had to give me quite a bit of medication to get any rest at all. I'd lay there until two o'clock in the morning and they'd give me a hypo.

It was a lot worse in the hospital because of the immobility. People who don't have a bad back may not understand this, but if you've got a bad back and you're going to get laid up in bed, you ought to consider some special arrangements, special therapy or a way to lay in that bed or something.

I have hospitalization insurance, so the cost of the surgery wasn't a major problem. I have to pay the first $50 deductible and the insurance pays 80 percent of the rest. Something like that. I was off work over a month, closer to two months, and when I did go back to work, I had to creep around. You don't get over major surgery just like that. And all of that time, I had sick leave so I didn't lose anything.

Of course, I'm a little strong about insurance. As far as I'm concerned, we shouldn't have any insurance at all. I'd rather be self-insured. You start as a young man setting aside money and as you grow older and need it, then you use it rather than this myriad of insurance companies. Why, you've got as many insurance companies as you've got flavors of ice cream. And every time you turn around, here's another warning about cancer or spinal meningitis or something. This is not right. I think it is preying on the public.

"Why did you have insurance then, if you are so opposed to it?"

Well, a man has to line up with his community where he lives. If everybody else is buying insurance, he should get the best bargain he can get. It's either that or nothing at all. I work for the government but still we have to pay two-thirds of the premiums, I think it is.

"Even though you are philosophically opposed to insurance, you aren't sufficiently opposed to . . . ?"

No, I'm not that hard-headed. And I do try to take care of my family.

"Since you are a veteran and work for the government as a civilian employee in an air base, why didn't you go to the Veterans Administration Hospital to get your operation?"

Well, I could have. I have faith in the doctors at the Veterans Administration because I think that they can call in any specialist they might need for a particular problem. But, I also had this insurance and my doctor recommended a private surgeon. So, it didn't make any difference whether I went to the VA Hospital for free or had it done by a private doctor and had it covered by insurance. Also, there was the question of location. My doctor said they had good facilities in the hospital close to my home so I figured it was better to have it there than way across town at the VA Hospital, so my wife wouldn't have to drive so far.

I was in the hospital a week. I wanted out. You know, I don't like to stay in hospitals, even for major surgery. I don't want to stay any longer than it takes to do the job. I'm ready to go out. I don't care anything about laying up there in that electric bed you can move any way you want and watching color television. That's not my idea of a vacation, not when you've got your middle sliced open.

I was moved into a ward before surgery with a man who had a heart condition which worsened, but after surgery they put me in a private room at my wife's request. Personally, when a man has a severe condition, I think he should be alone but it's all right for two recuperating patients to be in the same room if they are well on their way to recovery. When you're laying there groaning and hurting, you don't want any company.

One other thing I noticed which was kind of peculiar. I had a lot of friends that sent me flowers. And the doctor gave me some kind of intravenous medication. Oh, you might say I wasn't all there after the operation, but anyway, they had these lines in my arms and up my nose and one in the back of my hand. I could smell what I thought was flowers and the heavy odor bothered me and so I asked my wife to get those flowers out of my room. But when she got them out, I realized it wasn't the flowers, it was the medication.

It's hard to remember how much pain I had. It's a good thing the good Lord blesses us with the ability to forget pain, or we'd be in trouble, wouldn't we?

28. Double Inguinal Hernia

Sometimes the complications of a hospital stay override the initial complaint. This young accountant went into the hospital to correct one problem, came out of the hospital with a problem he did not anticipate. He is of medium build, not small, not large. He is a college-educated city dweller with a forceful manner. He and his wife and their two-year-old adopted daughter live in a subdivision of sprawling, same-size houses which have no windows on either side because they are built so close together.

- **Double Inguinal Hernia**
- **Corrective Surgery**

Over the course of the years, I've had many physicals, for the armed services and that sort of thing, and every time the doctor informed me, "One of these days, you're going to have to have a hernia repair. You are subject to it. It's hereditary."

It's in the groin. The tubes, as they went through the stomach lining, slanted; instead of going straight through, they went in at an angle. That's why they had to be repaired and corrected. During the years, working at various kinds of jobs, I'd strained it, put a lot of stress on it. The outer wall had torn; the inner wall had not. When it started hurting about four months ago, I went to the doctor and he said, "Yeah, it's time to have it repaired."

I'd been doing some yard work and probably strained it more than usual. That brought it to the point that it was really noticeable and the pain did not subside. The pain was just on one side. The doctor said that side was real bad and needed to be repaired. He also said that probably within a year, I'd have to have the other side done. I'd already thought about it because my older brother had exactly the same problem and he'd had his hernias done at the same age I am now, 32.

The surgeon my doctor referred me to said, "Yeah, let's go ahead and do both sides because I'll be in there within a year to do the other side, if you don't have it done now. If we go ahead and do both sides now, you'll have one six-week recovery period and that's it." That made sense to me. I couldn't see going to the hospital twice because I didn't want to go to begin with. I'd never been a patient in a hospital and I didn't want to be.

More than anything, I didn't know what was going to happen. I didn't understand hospitals and even though I'd been with my wife when she had her hysterectomy, I didn't know what happened after she got in the operating room and that bothered me. Nobody can tell you what goes on and they can't explain the feeling you have as you go through all of the different procedures. I told the surgeon about it, the way I felt, and he kept me pretty doped up right before the operation. It didn't bother me any when I did go in; I was calm and relaxed and almost knocked out completely. I remember very little about it until I started waking up.

When I did wake up, I discovered that my front teeth were missing.

This happened after the operation as I was waking up. Apparently, I bit down on an airway. They had some blocks in there to keep me from biting down but I bit down anyway and snapped off two caps on my front teeth.

My teeth had been capped eight years prior to that time but it snapped the original teeth off, too, this time, broke them off so they were not cappable any more. My dentist had to pull the front two teeth and then cap two more beside them to hook the bridge to, to make a four-tooth set. That was all taken care of when I got out of the hospital.

During the hospital stay, the service was basically good. The nurses, about half of them were concerned enough to check on you and half of them could care less. I went to this hospital because my surgeon preferred going there. I figured that if the surgeon was going to cut on me and he preferred this hospital, I'd better go there. I didn't want him to be upset and make mistakes. What do I know? Also, I wanted a private room and that was the only place I'd be guaranteed a private room. That's all they have. My wife had been in semiprivate rooms before on three different occasions with rather elderly patients. One of the patients died, one was dying and we don't know what ever happened to the third one. It made my wife uneasy, nervous and very uncomfortable while she was there. I didn't care for that kind of environment. It's a shame those patients were in that shape and I really felt sorry for them, but at the same time, I didn't want to hamper my progress toward recovery because of some outside influence.

As I said, about half of the nurses were real nice, very courteous, efficient and concerned enough to come and check on you. The other 50 percent, well, you might ring for a drink of water and you might get it two or three hours later and you might not get it. I wouldn't rate the care highly at that hospital. The story was that the hospital was understaffed and the nurses were busy some place else but I was not very happy with the care, to say the least.

As far as my recovery was concerned, the doctor had issued orders for painkillers. I could have shots or pills and the first couple of days I took shots. If I called and told the nurses I was hurtin', they came immediately. If I called and told them I wanted a drink, that was another story.

I was in the hospital five days and went back to work two weeks later. I didn't have any more sick leave; I had to go back to work.

After the surgery, which was done at noon, I was knocked out most of the day. I woke up about seven o'clock, asked for a drink of water, and it was then that I discovered that my two front teeth were gone. The next morning, the anesthesiologist's nurse came in to see me, but before the operation, on Sunday, she asked me questions about allergies, past medical history, anything they might need to watch for. She asked me if I had any caps, bridges or plates or whatever in my mouth. When I told her about the caps on my two front teeth, she said, "That's important. We really want to watch and be extra careful." When she came back in Tuesday morning, she talked about my missing teeth and said, "Boy, I'm sorry that happened." And I said, "Me, too. Who's going to pay for it? That's a thousand dollars or more of dental work." She said, "Oh, don't worry about it. The anesthesiologist has insurance. It'll cover it."

It almost didn't. I had to hassle him to get everything settled. The anes thesiologist said he had done everything correct and he really shouldn't be paying for it, but seeing as how his nurse had said that somebody would take care of it, he was going to. Of course, I talked to my lawyer who said, "If you can get him to settle it at all, let him pay for whatever he'll pay for, because if you fight him, there's one doctor, somewhere, some place, who'll say he did everything correct. Consequently, you won't get nothing. Some place there is a doctor who'll take some money to get up in front of a jury and say that. Get whatever you can from the guy, just whatever he'll settle for. Don't take it to court, just settle it."

Anyway, he is paying the full bill but it did take two weeks to get it worked out.

"What would you have done if the anesthesiologist had not paid off?"

I would have fought it. I would have gone to court to try and get some restitution out of it. I didn't figure it was my responsibility after what his nurse told me before the operation. Somebody didn't do their job right. I don't know the exact definition of malpractice. My dentist called it "neglect."

I think a lot of doctors have taken bum raps from people claiming malpractice and that's not fair. I really don't want to hassle anybody. I just wanted somebody to take care of my teeth.

My dentist was rather upset by the situation. He said that through normal usage, I would never have broken my front teeth off, they were that strong. He couldn't imagine anything that hard being in my mouth. My dentist uses a rubber airway in his office when he anesthetizes somebody. He inferred that somebody at the hospital took the blocks out too soon and, through negligence, allowed me to bite down on something hard, probably a metal airway. He said someone was at fault because I was not awake enough to comprehend what I was doing. He said that when people come out from under an anesthetic, they do different things. Some try and fight and some bite and some do other things.

My dentist was upset because he's done a lot of work to save my teeth. I've got bad teeth and I've got a lot of dollars invested in my mouth. Then to lose my front teeth like that is rather disheartening.

It seems to be working out. I don't particularly like my new teeth but at least they are paid for. I couldn't have afforded the thousand dollars it cost to have them repaired.

But as far as everything else was concerned, the doctor who performed the surgery was a super gentleman. He explained everything he was going to do. The only thing he forgot to tell me was how much it was going to hurt. Even my brother didn't bother to tell me. He said he figured that if I didn't know, it wouldn't bother me as much. Probably he was right, but I said, "At least the doctor could have said something about it," and my brother said, "Well, what does he know about the pain? He's never had a hernia repair."

I was out of bed and walking by nine o'clock that night after the surgery. Of course, the nurse threatened to use a catheter on me and I decided to get up. I couldn't use the little pan laying in the bed and she said, "Look, you either go or I'm going to have to bring the catheter!" I said, "No, we're not doing that."

"Why couldn't you use the urinal in the bed?"

I don't know. There's something about it when you hit that cold metal. Even if you were dying to go, there's no way after hitting one of those cold things. I couldn't relax enough. The feeling's not right. You are in the wrong position. Of course, I was a little dopey at the time. But when she threatened me with the catheter, I said, "Just get me up out of this bed. I can walk to the bathroom."

I think there's a lot of room for improvement in the health care system. I don't know what it's going to take to change it. A few doctors and more than a few nurses seem to have the attitude, "I really don't want to hassle with you. Come back later, or don't come back." The nurses' attitude seems to be, "God, I don't want another patient. I don't want to have to take care of another one."

Every Tooth in a Man's Head is more
valuable than a Diamond.

Miguel de Cervantes (1547–1616)
Don Quixote, Pt. I, Bk. III
Ch. IV (translated by P.A. Motheux)

29. Hydrocele

This patient is "the Senator," now a year old. His health problem is discussed by his young mother, the 18 year old who described her experience in childbirth earlier. The child is a beautiful and well-behaved infant who apparently sailed through his encounter with the surgeon with great aplomb.

- **Hydrocele**
- **Hernia**
- **Corrective Surgery**

When Mike was born, I always thought he was — this sounds so gross — well-endowed. You know, some little boys are. Anyhow, little Jimmy across the hall is only eighteen months old and his is twice as long as David's and David is three. So I just assumed he had bigger, you know, down there.

What is the technical term for those little things, the ones that everyone else calls balls?

"Testicles?"

Yeah. So I always thought he was super potent, or something. One day, my mother and I wanted to go shopping so we left Mike at the day care center. I'd left him with three other people before and nobody had ever said anything about it. But when we went to pick him up, this girl who was taking care of him was almost hysterical. She says, "Your little boy has a hernia. He's going to die, he's going to die." She said his testicles were swollen and his abdomen was hard. But I thought, "Well, it can't be that bad." So I took him to the doctor who checked him and he said, "Yeah. He's got a hernia."

Only it wasn't a hernia, I think they call it a hydrocele. Okay, when a little boy is born, their testicles haven't descended yet and their intestines have to move apart a little to let the testicles descend into the scrotum. Right? And then they are supposed to go back together but sometimes they don't and so the bowels can slip into the scrotum. That's the way the doctor told me. I looked it up in the dictionary and hydrocele is supposedly a body cavity or something like that, which I assume is what it is. But everybody calls it a hernia, so I call it a hernia like everybody else does.

The doctor said Mike would have to go to the hospital to get it fixed but my mother, being the hysterical creature that she is, decided that we were going to get the very best for her grandson. I couldn't afford it and she wasn't going to pay for it.

Anyhow, we went to Dr. Brown; he's a specialist.

"This was at your mother's suggestion?"

Suggestion! Huh! I was under 18 at the time and I had no choice but to do what she said. She said, "This is it. The very best for my grandson come hell or high water."

"Aren't you happy now that she made you take Mike to a pediatric surgeon?"

No, because Dr. McCrory could have done the very same. Dr. Brown was okay, I guess, but I wasn't really impressed with him at first. He never once smiled and he acted real grumpy and everything. He really turned me off.

The hospital sent me a letter telling me when I was supposed to bring Mike in. It said, "Please get here before noon" and something about they wouldn't have a bed after that. Well, we got there and sat for three or four hours. It wasn't that long but it felt like it. It was about an hour and a half. Then we had to fill out all of the forms for insurance and all.

Then we took him up to his room and the nurse went to take his temperature. She lifted up his legs to stick the thermometer in and he had real bad diaper rash on his bottom which he hadn't had that morning. It just developed during the day and his bottom was bleeding, it was so bad. And it was scary. I didn't know that babies got diaper rash so bad it would bleed.

In a way, I was worried about Mike and in a way I wasn't. The thing is, my mom's melodramatic, always has been and she taught me to be melodramatic. I really wasn't worried about the surgery itself because everybody said a large percentage of little boys have to have this operation. It's really nothing, kinda like a tonsillectomy. I said I was worried about the surgery because it sounded a hell of a lot more logical than what I was really worried about. I was worried about how I was going to pick him up and take care of him. What if I bump the wrong place and the stitches bust open and he bleeds all over? That sounds stupid so it was easier to say, "God, I'm worried. What if he dies in the operating room?"

He went in the hospital on Monday, he was operated on Tuesday and I believe we went home Wednesday. It surprised me that it was such a short time. I thought that when people got operated on they stay in the hospital for months.

When I got him home, nothing I had been worried about happened. Mike didn't even seem to be bothered by any of it. I sat there and poked his stitches to see that they were all there and that didn't even bother him.

There was something I didn't understand about the operation. Dr. Brown said that he made the incision inside and the stitches were on the inside. There was some plastic sort of stuff over the outer wound. I don't know what in the world he was talking about, but I do know that the stitches were not visible.

"How did you know where to poke?"

Well, you could see where the incision had been made, there was the red mark and it was kinda puckered over. And there was this plastic seal stuff. I don't know what it was. Apparently it was there to keep the incision from getting infected. After a while it got dirty and worn from having diapers rubbing on it and it fell off. Apparently, they put that plastic on instead of a bandage. There was no bandage. I really don't understand it. It was weird.

After the operation, I suppose his scrotum was smaller but I really didn't pay that much attention. I was paying more attention to where they made the incision. I didn't care whether his testicles were big or little or what.

There was a little emotional upheaval after the operation. It is really hard to think of your little tiny baby, just a year old, having a scar. God creates a perfect creature; babies are perfect. When they are four years old, they may fall off their tricycle and skin their knee and then they are not perfect any more. But up until that time they are pretty well perfect. But Mike has this adult imperfection on his body. It upsets me. My perfect, wonderful, soft, smooth, bouncy little baby, and now he has this adult-type scar.

There was this one particular nurse who was nice. She was always telling me how pretty he was and what a good boy he was. I'd worry that he was going to cry the whole time I was gone and when I'd get back she'd say, "He stopped crying right after you left."

But they did make one mistake. They took his blanket away. Those idiots. Those jackasses. His Linus blanket! And he had fits the whole time until I got back and gave it to him.

One thing that freaked me out is those little jackets they put them in, with the straps, one attached to one side of the bed and one attached to the other. I know it is a good idea because it kept him from falling out of the bed. They did that to all the kids but it is freaky to have your kid tied down in a straight jacket. But they can't really take any chances of a kid falling out of a bed and killing himself.

The only time I had any feeling toward Dr. Brown that was the least bit nice was when he first came out of surgery to tell us everything was over with; that was the first and only time that he ever let loose a grin. It was a one-sided grin, sort of maniacal, like, "I cut the kid open and I did it right. Hah!" I don't know; when he came out with that shit-eating grin on his face, it freaked me out.

The hospital keeps sending me a bill for five dollars every month. I get the same bill and the same letter every time. And I don't have five dollars to send them. They have the same big red warning on the bill, "Please Remit Immediately." Welfare paid the rest of the bill, I hope. If they didn't, the hospital's not going to get paid.

I guess I'll keep on getting that bill until I finally scrape up the money to pay it. They'll probably turn it over for collection. Of course, it was welfare who paid most of the bill. My mother wouldn't pay it. She'd buy me a hundred-dollar dress but she wouldn't pay Mike's hospital bill.

X.
Sensitivity

It may seem a strange principle to enunciate as the very first requirement in a Hospital that it should do the sick no harm.

Florence Nightingale (1820–1910)
Notes on Hospitals, Preface

30. Penicillin Reaction

She lives in a comfortable ranch-style home on a tree-shaded suburban street. Cars and a pickup truck clog the gravel driveway. Teenage children come in and out of the living room and call on the telephone. A small poodle commands the sofa with shrill barking until he is banished to the kitchen.

She is plump and has black hair piled high. She works as a switchboard operator in a downtown office now but previously she managed a family-owned business. Her husband is employed at a military base after a career as an Air Force officer. She is affable and gracious.

- **Bee Sting**
- **Allergenic Reaction to Penicillin**

I don't remember whether it was a bee or a wasp that stung me. We had gone to a city about a hundred miles away for a weekend. We were out by the pool at our friend's house in our bathing suits, playing with the kids. I was sunbathing and a bee — they said it was a bee; I didn't see it — stung me on the breast. It hurt real bad and I started to swell where it had stung me but then I started having chills and getting dizzy. My friends thought I might be going into shock so they took me to a hospital where they gave me some kind of reactionary shot.

I started swelling up so they decided to admit me and keep me over night. The next morning a doctor came in and asked me if I was allergic to anything. I told him I had once had a penicillin shot for strep throat which had caused swelling and a rash that itched. He said, "Fine," and supposedly wrote this on my record.

Later on this nurse came in to give me a shot. If you've ever taken penicillin, you know what it looks like. It's milky looking. And I asked her if that was penicillin and she said, "We are not allowed to say." So I said, "If it is, I'm allergic to it." But she went ahead and gave me this shot.

Everything seemed to get all right. I was in the hospital two days, my swelling went down and the doctor gave me some medicine to take home with me. But after I got home, I started running a high fever; I got so I couldn't drink and things tasted funny. At that time I smoked, but I couldn't smoke. I thought I was just sick for some reason but the next day I got sicker. I could hardly breathe and was so sick I couldn't lift myself off the bed. My sister came out, took my temperature and said I had 105 degrees. We are military so she took me to the base hospital. In the meantime, she had called the doctor who had taken care of me in the hospital and when he heard of my symptoms, he said, "My God, we've given her enough penicillin to kill her. Get her a doctor quick!" The prescription they sent home with me was penicillin, plus the shot they had given me in the hospital. They gave me an ACTH shot at the base hospital.

I was in terrible pain and by this time, my breasts had started swelling. The guy who was in the emergency room at the base hospital gave me a shot and said, "If that doesn't work, I'll be back in a few minutes and give you something else." Then I began having these terrible cramps in my stomach. I told my sister, "Take me to the hospital where I was. That man up there messed me up and he's the one who's going to fix me. These people don't know what they're doing. This kid's going to come back and give me another shot and my stomach's hurting bad."

So she took me right back where I was at first and they started giving me different kinds of reactionary stuff for penicillin poisoning. My breasts kept swelling and swelling and swelling 'til they were stretched so far that I could see my face in them. You couldn't believe skin can be stretched like that but it was tighter than any drum I'd ever seen. They were so shiny I could actually see my reflection in them. They were huge.

They were filled up with fluid but whether it was from the penicillin or the bee sting, they never did tell me. I was practically delirious and this went on for two weeks. I thought I was getting better because I wanted out of the hospital so bad but I was terribly weak. The doctor said he thought he could release me and I came home. Although my breasts were still swollen, the doctor said he thought the swelling would go down. He told me to put packs on them and to rest.

Well, I wasn't home but a couple of days. I was so sick that I couldn't take it. My breasts got so tender that I couldn't even move. My sister took me back up there a hundred miles and they readmitted me to the hospital. This time, I ended up staying in there four months.

They started the never-ending process of trying to figure out what was causing all of these reactions. By that time, I was reacting to everything they gave me. They decided to pump the fluid out of my breasts, so they took me to the x-ray room to locate the fluid. But by the time they'd get me back to the room, it wouldn't be where the x-ray showed it was. And they didn't use a needle to pump it out. They cut and put in a hose, a siphon hose. Finally, at my suggestion, they took me to the x-ray room and drained the fluid out before it relocated. They took a half-gallon jar of fluid out of there two or three times a day.

They moved me to different rooms while I was in the hospital. They say cortisone has a reaction on you and you get sorta dingy after a while. I didn't sleep much and I'd hear things at night. So I asked this nurse's aide who used to hide in my room and watch television at night, "What is that noise I hear. Sounds like an elevator or something." And she said, "That's the elevator that takes cadavers downstairs." "Are you trying to tell me that my next step is downstairs?"

They put me in a room with an elderly lady who had blocked intestines. For some reason or other, they couldn't operate on her. She was in so much pain that they had to keep her doped up on drugs.

In the meantime, the doctors had put drainage tubes in each side, so the fluid would just run out of my breasts. It was horrible. It was just like acid and it burned and it smelled bad. It was really rank.

Well, one night I woke up to find this woman at the side of my bed and she jerked all of the tubes out of my sides. She was just clawing at me. I went into hysterics, screaming and nurses came in and this old lady took off running down the hall. Of course, she was so doped up, she didn't know what she was doing. I guess the nurses and attendants really thought I was crazy because I pointed down the hall and said, "She went thataway."

They tried everything to drain my breasts, even let an intern put this pumping machine on me. He would fasten this machine up to me and flush this fluid through my breasts and back out. It was pure clorox; I know, it smelled like it. Talk about nerve-wracking. If you can think about pouring clorox water on a raw sore and flushing it around. Usually he left the machine on there an hour but this one night he didn't come back so I rang for the nurse and asked, "When's he going to come back and take this off?" And she said, "He's gone to an intern party." I said, "You've got to be kidding me." And she said, "No, he won't be back until tomorrow." I asked her if she knew how to take that machine off of me and she said, "I don't know anything about it. That's one of his inventions." They were actually allowing him to experiment on me. That's what it amounted to. I had seen him put it on often enough so that I shut the thing off and got it off of me.

By this time I weighed 83 pounds and nothing would grow except my fingernails which were out to here. My husband was overseas all this time but I kept thinking I'd get all right. But I'd lost so much weight and I shook all of the time. They had me so jumpy because I never knew what was going to happen next. And I didn't have anybody to come see me except on weekends. My mother was taking care of my children and my business and, of course, I was a hundred miles from home.

The doctor told my mother that one of the drugs he had me on caused reactions and not all of them were good. Now, I know, if anyone takes cortisone unless it's a matter of life or death, they are out of their mind because it's really a dangerous drug. It has too many side effects. I asked him to take me off of it and he said he couldn't. And do you know how I got off of it? I started palming a pill a day. Each time they would bring me pills, I'd palm one and if that didn't change the way I felt, I'd throw it back in the pot and palm another. And finally I had a whole jar of these pills I'd palmed and that's the way I took myself off of it.

One time when I called the doctor, he came in, sat on the side of my bed and cried, absolutely cried, and said, "I tell you, I don't know what to do for you." I begged him, "Please let me live. I've got a purpose in life. I've got three children who need me." He said, "You are going to have to get up out of that bed in order to get your strength back. I want you to get up in a wheelchair at least twice a day."

By this time, they had moved this woman with the blocked intestines out of my room and I was quite concerned for her. She had told me several times, "They're killing us both." And I kinda believed her. So I went down to her room to check on her. She'd been operated on in the meantime and I wanted to see how she was getting along. I wheeled down there and had just gotten in the room when this head nurse came in and grabbed my wheelchair and flew me out into the hall and back to my room. "You know you're not supposed to be in there." Well, I was crying and mortified and couldn't understand why they'd treat me like that. Then this girl came in and I said, "What's wrong with me? Why can't I go down there?" She said, "Don't you know what you have?" "Oh, my God, what do I have?" And she said, "You have staph infection."

All of my life, I never had one blemish on my face, even when growing up. I thought it was caused from being in bed so much but I was getting sores on me. But I didn't know anything about staph infection.

"Hospital acquired?"

Yes. And I thought, "My God, how long does it take to get over that." This was toward the end of my hospital stay, the four months. But I still had sores on my face when I came out.

And, believe it or not, they let me out of that hospital, scott free. They were so glad to get me out of that hospital, they didn't charge me one dime.

They decided the only way to cure my breasts, they had destroyed so much tissue and, actually, I think the clorox water did it, was to go in and take out all that tissue. So they operated and here I am, flat-chested. Nothing. They just lifted my breasts and took everything out and that was it. I was in the hospital about two and a half months before they decided to do that.

They had started giving me hormone pills, too. There was a girl in the hospital who collected for an anesthesiologist and she came in everyday to see me. She and the nurse's aide who watched television at night in my room were the only regular visitors I had. One day she came in and, you see there were no mirrors and I couldn't see how I looked. The only one I had was in an overnight case and I very seldom had the strength to get it out and look at myself. She said, "My God, look at your face! Have you looked at yourself?" "What's the matter?" So many things had gone wrong that I would panic when someone would say there was something different about me. "You have a mustache and a beard." And I did. I'd started growing black hair on my face. The doctor said whatever he was giving me was causing a male reaction and I said to him, "Forget it. I don't need it. And I'd lost all my hair, too. So there I was, flat-chested, no hair, growing a beard and had real long fingernails. I looked like some kind of an animal. So they stopped the male hormones. I never did know why they gave 'em to me in the first place.

Then they did breast implants, but they took them right out. I kept them a month but my body rejected them. You see, I had so many things wrong with me by then that my body just wouldn't take care of anything else, I guess. The doctor said it was better to take them out. He said maybe I could have them later.

One of my breasts grew back to a substantial size. But this side, I never could get it to release. I'm telling you, I pulled on them whenever I could to get them to release. Adhesions grew them to the wall of my chest and it took a long time before they came loose from my chest. He told me that if I got heavy and stayed heavy, maybe they would come back because that's what breasts are, fat tissue. But the one never grew back.

After I'd been in the hospital some time, I knew I needed some kind of help so I called this friend of my husband's who worked with military dependents at the base and asked him what to do. I knew I could never pay for all of this. When your husband is overseas, you can get medical assistance other places. So when I saw I was going to be in there, and in there, and in there, I called my husband's friend and told him everything that was happening to me. I think he went up there to the hospital and investigated and that's why the hospital settled without charging me anything. I never did hear from them about the bill and I know the military didn't pay for it because I asked. It was probably because of the staph infection I got while I was there. While my husband's friend didn't tell me how they handled it, he did tell me not to worry about getting a bill.

The doctor said if I'd never been given the penicillin, I would probably have been all right and none of these things would have happened to me.

XI.
Save the Bones

The human body . . . indeed is like a ship;
its bones being the still standing-rigging,
and the sinews the small running ropes, that
manage all the motions.

Herman Melville (1819–1891)
Redburn, Chapter XIII

31. Fractured Vertebrae

This 56-year-old black man wears a brace to support his back. He is an aircraft maintenance worker, medium build, a high school graduate, married.

He was almost ready to be discharged from the hospital, spent his time walking the corridors. After being in one room for a week and a half, he was told he had to go to another room and he wasn't pleased.

- **Injured Back**
- **Fractured Vertebrae**
- **Fusion Operation**

When I found out I was going to change, they'd got the bed all cleaned up and the lady that had been working in my room, she came down and told me, "You're going to move," and I said, "Why move? Where?" "Down the hall," she said and I said,"Why do I have to move? I was thinking about goin' home tomorrow or the next day." She said, "I don't know why." In fact they just told her I was going to move.

I finally kept waiting for someone else to tell me I had to move and nobody told me. I went up to the desk, the admitting office up there and talked to the head nurse down there and said, "How come they're pickin' on me, want me to move?"

"Aw, no," she said, "You don't have to if you don't want to."

"Well, you know, with double rooms like these they have to match up the sexes and they even have to match up the diseases sometimes. It creates a problem. And another thing, this hospital empties out on the weekend."

I noticed that. That's the reason I started to raise Cain. I was really going to balk on that. My doctor was gone on vacation 'til next week and he said next Monday he'd probably let me go home. That's what I was depending on. The other doctor came by, see'd how I was doin', checked my records back up, said everything was goin' along pretty good, see. I don't know which doctor this were. Then this big doctor came along. He had all my books, all the books of everybody he wanted to see. And he moved me.

"This won't make any difference as far as whether you go home on Monday or not, will it?"

No, but it was just the idea, you know? You get in the room and you kinda get used to it and you don't want to leave until you get ready to go home. And then you turn around and you gotta move. I moved down here. I had my television up there in the other room; course the boy, he wasn't able to pay for television. He could look at it if he wanted to, but the TV's mine, you understand. When I come down here now, I don't know whether this TV belongs to him (*motions to the other bed, then empty*) or not. I didn't think it was on but I got to messin' with it and it's on.

What I gotta do now is go through all that transfer paperwork changin' this and that, and bring everything I had down there to this room and get set up again.

The reason I'm here, I fell and hurt my back. I was working under Boeings out at the air base. I'm a sheet metal mechanic. We replace skins, ducts and skins, anything that's necessary on one of those planes when they come in. Tear 'em down and redo 'em all over and all that.

I fell off a stool about four and a half, five foot high, flat on my back. I hurt three vertebraes. This was a month and a half ago. It messed me all up.

There might have been something in there before; don't never know about your back. But it sure messed it up this time.

I'm a civilian employee and we get workmen's comp. Uncle Sam'll pay the bill. I have another insurance, same as Blue Cross-Blue Shield, but it's Aetna, see. We have it and I tried to find out if they'd pay anything on it and they said no. As long as we had federal workmen's comp their insurance wouldn't pay a thing on it. You couldn't claim a thing on it at all. They wouldn't pay a thing on it even if workmen's comp didn't pay at all.

I've been here about a week and a half, come in Monday, had surgery on Tuesday. Doctor told me I'd be in two weeks.

When I got hurt out at the field, they got a bunch of doctors there but they couldn't determine what my relations was on everything so they just told me, "You got nerve problems in your back." So I picked out one doctor and went to him and he sent me on up to town, up here to the hospital. I stayed one night, took x-rays that day. Next day, they take x-rays and then release me. I ended up with another doctor who picked me up from there, see. He's a surgeon. He gave me a few days to come back and then I took a cardiogram. I took that cardiogram and was in the hospital from Wednesday to Friday. They sent me home, said stay home, don't do nothin'. You've got one vertebrae sitting there, the last one, ready to pop off any minute.

They fused everything. I feel pretty good but I don't know how long it will be afterwards, after I get home, get through with this other. See, they haven't taken the stitches out of it.

I'm going to have to wear a brace from now on. That's bad news. It'll wipe out my sheet metal work. In sheet metal, you have to climb up on ladders, get up on a stool, be where you walk up on those planes, out on the wings, stoop and bend and twist and everything else. Sometimes you gotta get down on your hands and knees and crawl in places, and then you gotta make those points and that's where I won't be able to do any of that.

I'm set for retirement. I'm 56 and I can retire on a medical workman's comp.

I worked 16 years with the railroad, the Santa Fe. A car inspector. I went and checked up and found out how much I could draw. I'll have retirement from the railroad and the government and I've worked a lot of social security so I can still retire from them. I figured I'd just go ahead and retire. I can see I ain't gonna be able to do no work. It's going to be hard for me to stoop. I'm going to have to be wearin' this brace from now on. I figured I'd be better off takin' those retirements and settin' down, takin' it easy. Set around the house and enjoy the rest of my days.

"Has your friend taken pretty good care of you in the hospital?" (An L.P.N. had just entered the room.)

She's taken care of me. She's really nice. I've been in the hospital before, in '60 and '71. Had a gall bladder. Only one thing about it, in '71 when I was here, after the first night, this nurse went home and they figured I was all right and they shut the door, pulled the door to, and I liked to died that night. I ain't kiddin' nobody.

I had needles in both hands and one down my throat. I couldn't do nothin'. I was hurtin' so bad. I needed something to stop me from hurtin'. I started screamin' and hollerin' and I don't know how long I did that. Finally, the little boy that was workin' orderly that night, he finally, he said he just happened to come out in the hall and he could just barely hear me. He told me the next couple of days, he said, "I could just barely hear you sayin', 'I'm dyin', I'm dyin'.'" When he heard that, he said, "Well, I'd better see who this is." When he came in there, he said I was just tumblin' and so he run and got two doctors and two or three nurses.

The light was off, couldn't get to the light, couldn't do nothin'. Had just come back from the recovery room. They'd given me some medicine so I'd go on back to sleep and I woke up way in the night. That's when I thought I was gonna die.

That was in this hospital and my family doctor and all of the doctors I've had take people to this hospital.

I've never had any money problems on account of bein' in the hospital but I'm lookin' to have some financial problems. I've begin to think about it because they's so many people that has retirement and not too much money. I've been thinkin' I'll have trouble down the road. I'm wondering whether you take Medicare or try to hold the insurance you have. I'm wonderin' what Aetna would have. I'll ask the Aetna man. I was up there not long ago so I know where to go to see the company about it. I been thinkin' about it pretty hard. You gotta think about your future.

32. Fallen Arch

He is a barber. He dropped out of college earlier, but now at age 30, he has decided to return to school and complete his undergraduate work. Extroverted and talkative, he obviously loves to be with people, to exercise his sense of humor.

- **Leg Pain**
- **Difficulty Walking**
- **Fallen Metatarsal Arch**

Starting about two years ago I went into the family physician because I thought at the time I had prostate trouble. I had no idea I had a foot problem because when your rear end hurts you don't think of your foot.

I went in at great expense — to me at that time it was a great expense — took the drugs for prostate infection. The doctor gave me the examination and tested my urine but he said he couldn't find anything. Evidently, the tests hadn't picked it up so he told me to take the drugs anyhow.

I think he was treating the "hypochondriac." First of all, the doctor is a close family friend. I think it's bad to go to any physician who knows you personally. If they're too involved with you personally, they may think you're a little neurotic or under pressure at the time. I was taking finals at school and he probably thought I had a psychosomatic disorder and the drugs would suffice to clear it up.

At class, sitting on those hard chairs, I would have to sit on my right hip. This was traumatic to say the least because you have internal pain and you don't know why. I took the drugs for a couple of weeks but I didn't get any particular relief at the time. I just kept on with the drugs and the cranberry juice and this bit they treat prostate trouble with. I finally did get to feeling better where I could walk but in the upper part of my leg there it was extremely painful. There was no pain in my foot at all.

Two or three months later the internal pain became so intense, it became a mental trauma. My physician says it's this or that but he's not finding anything. I'd have pain every waking moment. The only time I'd have relief was when I'd go to bed.

So I went in again to see the same doctor and he said, "Oh, you've got a hemorrhoid." You know, take a hot bath, Preparation-H, this bit. So I went along with this. It wasn't as bad this time, but it was a periodic-type thing, an intense-type pain in the inside, upper part of my left leg.

I still didn't think about any kind of a bone problem. This went on for a year but it had been bothering me for two years. You know, you put things off. Every time I went in, it would be a great expense and they still didn't find anything. So Thanksgiving Day, I clipped my little toe nail on my left foot and it got infected. That night, it felt like somebody had lit a hot coal inside of my ankle. It was a pain like I had never experienced. It wasn't your standard type, ache-type pain. It felt like it was hot inside, that type of pain.

I thought I'd walked crooked on it but surely nothing would hurt . . . I'd never even felt that type of pain before.

I finally went back to that same doctor and said, "Look, I don't know what I've done to myself or what's wrong, but something is wrong with my left foot. I can't walk, I can't work, I can't get around and I'm doing injury to my foot by walking on it this way." With my sock on my foot and my shoe on my foot, he immediately diagnoses it as arthritis in my ankle. His logic was, "You're overweight. There's too much weight on your foot." Well, I've always been overweight. What would be overweight for somebody else would be skin and bones for me. I always weigh about 200 pounds.

He said, "You're going to have to take that weight off. How do you want to take it off?" I said I'd go without eating but he said I'd have to take it off quick so he gets me a big prescription of "bennies" to make me lose weight. What are they, amphetamines? Uppers?

Well, I took 'em for a couple of days and said, "I'm not takin' 'em any more." I just don't take drugs, not even aspirin. They were doing me more damage than I was hurt. But the pain got so intense by this time that I really couldn't walk without the use of a cane. It was hard to barber. I sat on the back bar. I stood with my right foot on a rubber mat and then I put my hip on the back bar where you put your tools and then turned the chair to accommodate that position. I was actually off my leg that way, and whenever I'd sit down I would elevate my foot.

The doctor gave me this anti-inflammatory drug; I can't think of the name of it, starts with a "B"; it's extremely hard on your system to take it. I knew that it was hard on my stomach but I'd just as soon have an upset stomach and be able to walk. So I took this stuff for seven days, and everything was fine, you know. The inflammation was out of the foot and I was able to walk.

After the seventh day, I went off the drug and in the eighth day I was on fire again. Well, a prominent bone doctor in town is a friend of mine. He came into the barber shop where I work and I went to him and said, "I'm not fishin' for free medical advice but I've been to a physician," and then I told him what the deal was. He said, "Well, you can't treat something through a sock. I'm not overriding anybody's diagnosis, but I'm advising you as a friend. You'd better get something done about it if it's the type of pain and inflammation you say it is." He suggested an orthopedic specialist that specialized in foot disorders and what have you.

So I called, trying to get into see him, but they told me it would be two months. I told the girl I just couldn't wait that long, somebody has to see what it is and see if I'm doing serious, lasting injury to my foot.

By this time, my mental state was just wrecked, not knowing what it was or if it was a bone infection or whatever. So I called a friend of mine who'd had a bone spur on his foot and he told me a podiatrist had attended to his bone spur. I checked around on this guy from people I knew who had foot problems and then I called and got an appointment for a week later.

Well, I'd never heard of a podiatrist before, I didn't even know what a podiatrist was. I just wanted somebody to look at my foot. Sometimes I had to use a cane because, especially after work, I just couldn't put that much weight on it.

The podiatrist looked at my foot and said, "Oh, it looks like you've got a problem there." He grabs ahold of my foot, pushes the bottom of it up and you could just hear it pop. You could hear it snap.

He said, "I'm going to x-ray it, but I know what's wrong with it. Your metatarsal arch has fallen. You have a joint which has fallen so far, you've walked on it so long, but you won't have a problem once I tape this up. This is not a serious problem but it needs to be corrected."

You could hear the bone crack but it wasn't painful. As a matter of fact, it was the first time I'd had relief in three months, at least. You know, after awhile your body learns to accommodate pain, extreme pain, and that's what I'd had for three months.

The whole thing was just ridiculous. When you stop to think about it, to have spent so much money in the G.P.'s office, you know, all of the drugs, and some of the drugs had been harmful. Plus, I'd been taking aspirin by the bottleful, thinking it was arthritis and I might get some relief.

The podiatrist pushed the bone back up in place, put my foot in the whirlpool for 20 minutes. I could barely stay awake, I had so much relief. He taped the foot and put a cotton pad under it to brace the arch back up in place. I got immediate relief, immediate relief.

And not only that, when he taped everything in place and pulled the foot in, I could bend my foot. Before when I walked, I lifted my whole foot. I never bent my foot. Immediately, my foot bent as I walked. Now, I walk differently. I used to walk on my right toe and I had to buy new shoes every 90 days because I wore the right shoe out in the toe.

He made your standard issue plastic arch supports that fit under the arch and pull the back of it in. I have to wear them all the time because it becomes real painful to walk without them.

As he was examining me, he asked, "Do you ever have pain up in your crotch?" I said, "Do you mean pain like prostate trouble, or somethin'?" And he said, "Yeah, I would imagine that you have experienced a lot of difficulty in your upper leg because of this. You've got all of the upper muscles of your legs really in a bind here. I don't see how you've been able to do long distance walking or prolonged standing." And I said, "You wouldn't believe what I've spent for drugs and examinations in the last two years over this pain in the upper part of my left leg."

Since I visited the podiatrist, it just isn't a problem. It's non-existent. No more pain.

I used to walk on one toe. I've got a closet full of shoes with the right toe worn out. I was a ballet dancer and didn't know it.

All of this time, I was having pain in my right foot as well as my left foot but I never noticed it because my left foot was just on fire. When I got the left foot straightened out, he said we'd have to do something about the right because it was almost as bad. It's an hereditary thing.

I saved enough money in shoes to pay the podiatrist.

The G.P. is still my good friend but I'm changing doctors. You know, after a while he hated to see me comin'. He wanted to give me the sugar pills they give the little old ladies because there was nothing wrong as far as he could find.

A month ago, I was nearly dead with the flu and I said to my wife, "Oh, God, call him, but if he prescribes arch supports, just don't even have him call it in."

33. Ruptured Disk

We drank coffee in their huge, eat-in kitchen while his wife finished the supper dishes. They live in a comfortable house on an acre plot. It is reached by traveling a graveled street which the city forgot to improve as it was building the subdivision which now surrounds their home. There is an old swimming pool in the backyard; brilliant annuals in random plantings surround it.

He is an administrator who works for a city-county educational institution. He is in his 40's, has dark hair, smokes cigars. His current physical problem is a second episode of a similar difficulty experienced eight years before.

- **Back Injury**
- **Ruptured Disk**
- **Laminectomy**
- **Surgical Correction**

I think my case is interesting because it is something you can put up against how you were treated eight years ago as opposed to today.

I had a bad disk, a ruptured disk, eight years ago. It took several months before it was diagnosed. I had gone to a chiropractor for approximately three months and the chiropractor finally decided it was more than he could handle so he recommended this orthopedic surgeon who diagnosed it very quickly as a ruptured disk.

I usually don't got to chiropractors but somebody recommended this particular one and suggested that he might be able to help me. He gave me what he called "manipulation." And he was a good man. I really do still have faith in him. He would work on my back and it would seem like it was all right and he'd say, "I think that did it." But then I'd get up, walk out, get into the car and find out that it didn't work, that I still had this terrible pain down my left leg. It went from my hip clear down to my ankle. The pain was primarily in my hip. The chiropractor kept saying that he felt it was a dislocated. How'd he put it? I can't remember what he said it was. But he worked very hard and I went through this for about 15 treatments and realized that it wasn't working. And he did, too, about the same time. He said, "I don't think I can help you," and turned me over to this orthopedic surgeon.

The surgeon put me in the hospital, in traction, for a week. He had my legs up with weights on them and so on. I realized then that this wasn't going to do it, either.

So he gave me a mylogram which means that you drain the fluid from the spine and put in some dye and you check it through some kind of x-ray or fluoroscope or whatever. He determined that I had a ruptured disk in the left, bottom side. He performed what they call a laminectomy about two days later.

It turned out that the operation was performed on a Saturday and the doctor evidently left town right afterwards; at least he was out of range of the nurse. He had prescribed certain anti-muscle-spasm drugs for me at the time and three hours after the operation, about noon or shortly thereafter, I started having terrible muscle spasms. I was given the drug he had prescribed and the head nurse said to me, "The doctor has prescribed this much and that's all you can have."

These huge muscle spasms were like a massive electric charge, starting from the base of the neck, going all of the way down my spine and then shooting my legs out like an arrow, both of them. The muscle spasms increased and it ended up that for 24 hours, from noon on one day until noon the next day, I had them. They would shoot my legs out straight like an arrow. It was like being on a roller coaster and not being able to get off.

The nurse kept saying, "I can't do anything about it." My wife stayed with me that night and she would hold my hand when I would have these terrible muscle spasms. Near the end, they would occur about every 10 seconds. They were like labor pains. I think back on it today and I wonder how I survived it. It was the worst. It wasn't pain, it was something you can't describe, like an electric shock every 10 seconds, a terrible electric shock.

I kept telling the nurse, between those muscle spasms, to get ahold of the doctor. I couldn't understand why he had prescribed such a small dose of drugs. Anyway, he finally showed up on Sunday about noon. I told him what I was going through and that the drug he had prescribed was not right. Maybe it was my weight. I drank a lot, I admitted that. I said to him, "Maybe you don't know I drink martinis, I drink whatever, and maybe that has something to do with it. All I know is, you're not prescribing the proper amount of drug to stop these muscle spasms." I don't know whether he doubled the dose or whatever, but within about a half hour I stopped having the muscle spasms. I had survived it.

I did everything the doctor prescribed after that and I healed very fast. Bones I've broken heal rapidly, wounds heal up fast. I'm just lucky that way. I was in the hospital about a week and then spent three weeks at home recuperating. I did the exercises prescribed, very minor exercises for your back, where you lie on your back and bring your legs up to your chest and try to bring your bottom up without using your legs. I did this for years and it seemed to help.

That was eight years ago and the years went by. This year, I went outside with my son, it was in February, and we fell on the ice. My son is five years old and he weighs about 40 pounds. My big concern was to try to prevent his being hurt. My son has cerebral palsy and he can't walk. He's in a cerebral palsy center during the week. We have him home on Friday night and Saturday night and take him back on Sunday. When he's home, I take him out after dinner to look at the moon and the stars and so on. That weekend on Saturday night, I took him outside and the only patch of ice left, I fell on it. I flung myself backwards and twisted so that he fell on me. He didn't get hurt but I knew as soon as I fell that I was really in bad trouble. Obviously, I had hurt a disk again because it was the same feeling I'd had eight years ago.

Sunday, I went to the emergency ward at a hospital here in the city. I called my doctor, a general practitioner, and told him I thought I was really in bad shape. I was hurting bad so he said to go to the hospital and have them check me out. He didn't volunteer to meet me over there.

A resident doctor examined me and immediately gave me x-rays for my hip and on down. At the same time I had fallen, I'd hurt my right elbow and he was more concerned about my right elbow than anything else. They put an Ace bandage on it. He said, "If you had come in yesterday, I would have given you stitches in your elbow." Well, I was not concerned about my elbow, I was concerned about my legs and my spine because that's where I hurt.

He checked the x-rays and said he couldn't see any fractures. Well, you cannot see a ruptured disk on a regular x-ray and I tried to tell him that but he was not interested. He said simply that I had a muscle strain and that I should stay home for a couple of days and I'd be all right. I knew he was wrong but what do you say to a doctor? That's where it gets interesting. I said I thought it was a disk and he said, "No. No way." He was more interested in the elbow. That's where I really get mad at doctors, when they start telling you where you hurt. And when you tell them what you think, they look at you as if to say, "Who the hell is the M.D. here? I am the M.D." Like Richard Nixon, "I am your President." You know? So I didn't argue with him. I just left, but the pain didn't. It just kept getting worse.

So Monday, instead of calling my family doctor, I just went back to the orthopedic surgeon I'd had before.

I called the nurse and she was able to tell by my voice over the telephone that I was really in bad shape and she did not argue with me when I said, "I've got to see the doctor today." Now, you've probably called your doctor 20 times in your lifetime and his nurse has said he's tied up for two weeks, or three weeks or six weeks and can you make an appointment for such and such. But all I had to do was tell this nurse I was in bad shape and she said, "You can come on in here at 1:30." She worked me in and I'm grateful for that, I really am. That nurse really knew.

When I got there, I didn't wait more than two minutes to see the doctor. He had me walk on my toes and he stabbed me with his little pins in my feet. I didn't have to say to him, "I think I broke a disk." He knew it that quickly. He's a good doctor.

He said, "I'm going to enter you in the hospital tomorrow and on Wednesday you'll have a lung scan and an EKG."

"Why a lung scan?"

Well, I'm 47 and eight years ago they wouldn't have worried about that, but now I'm 47 and he decided that he'd have to operate. He knew it. It's just instinct. In fact, he'd already reserved the operating room for Thursday and said to me, "If it turns out that I'm wrong, we can just cancel the operating room time, but I think you've ruptured another disk." The lung scan and the EKG were to see if there was something wrong with my lungs or my heart and if I could tolerate the surgery. They didn't want me to pass out on the operating table or if I did, they wanted to know what to do. If your lungs are not good, if you have emphysema or something like that at age 47, they'd better have the oxygen ready. So I accepted that, even though I know that an EKG will just say that you haven't had a heart attack. You can take an EKG and pass it and walk out and drop dead of a heart attack two minutes later.

When I went into the hospital, the nurse on duty started telling me about the room: this button you press to get the nurse and this button you press to get the TV on, that sort of thing. It was a very perfunctory briefing. She was being observed by a young nurse, I don't know what you call 'em, an apprentice nurse or whatever. The duty nurse was being very tense and she was giving me the briefing very fast, like you get in basic training in the army. And I kept stopping her to ask which button did what. She said, "I hope you got that." And I said, "Well, I haven't exactly." Then she asked me about my diet and I said I was on a low cholesterol diet. She started writing that down and the apprentice nurse said, "That's C-H-O-L. . . ." And the duty nurse said, "I know how to spell it but I've never had anyone looking over my shoulder before." I saw this tension between them. Later on this nurse kept coming into my room — but let me go back a bit.

When I had my mylogram, which is kind of a traumatic experience — it's almost like an operation because you have to hold your head down straight and then you lie flat on your back for six hours after that so you don't get terrible headaches while your spinal fluid is rehabilitating itself, you know, getting back in there. While I was lying down there having that mylogram, I watched it on the monitor. Now, everything is a little bit more sophisticated and I was able to watch the needle go up my spine. Eight years ago, even if

there had been a monitor there, I wouldn't have been able to watch that needle drain the last bit of dye they had put up my spine. I was damned grateful for my maturity. The first time, I couldn't have watched this, but now I am able to do it. I don't have the tension I had then. I was able to look at this, as though it was happening to someone else, you see, and I felt very damned macho about it. Not everybody can be there and watch a needle go up their own spine on a TV screen. I was fairly well anesthetized but I could feel it, though. It was like little needles and it wasn't bad. Not enough to hurt me. I think I have a high tolerance for pain since I've put up with it quite a bit. I'm not saying that to brag; I'm saying it because that's the way it is. I don't scream unless it's really bad and the only time I can remember screaming is when I was going through those muscle spasms I was telling you about. I've had my finger cut and a guy stitched it without any anesthetic at all. It hurt like hell, but I was able to tolerate it. I realized from that that I have a fairly high tolerance for pain.

The doctor found out what he had suspected on Monday: the disk on my right bottom side was shattered. It was not only ruptured, meaning that it cut away from where it was attached, but it was shattered into bits and pieces. The doctor was writing all of this up and I was lying there waiting for them to haul me back to my room — this was before the operation — and the doctor said, "Do you have anything you want to say?" And I said yes and told him about my previous experience eight years ago. I said, "You were gone. It happened on a weekend and I'm damned glad this operation is going to take place during a week day. I do not want those muscle spasms. I want you to prescribe anti-muscle-spasm drugs which will prevent this happening again." He's the kind of a person who will not give you any indication, with his eyes or his hand or his mouth, that he has understood. He hears you, but he won't say, "Was that the way it was? Well, I'll do such and such." He just simply does it. He won't talk to you. So I said to him, "Are you hearing me?" And he said, "Yes, I'm hearing you."

I also said, "And I don't want my bowels paralyzed the way they were before to the point that when I was finally able to go to the bathroom, I was unable to go." So I made it very clear and I feel that this is what people have to do to their doctors and their nurses. They shouldn't talk in the terms the doctors and nurses are used to using. Forget about the jargon. Simply say, "I don't want my legs to snap out the way they did before. I don't want my shit to come out the way it had to come out before. I don't want to have to reach up my ass and pull out the shit the way I did before."

The operation this time went well except that after the surgery, when I asked for the shot, the anti-muscle-spasm drug, this time before I had any spasms, the nurse said it wasn't on the orders and she couldn't give it to me. Well, I told her to get ahold of the doctor and get it ordered so I could have it. This seemed to upset her but I sure didn't want to be without that medication. Apparently, she got in touch with the doctor because not too long afterward she came in and gave me the shot. But my daughter, who was there with my wife, went past the nurse station and said this same duty nurse who had admitted me and the one who I asked to get me the shot was crying

my daughter overheard her saying, "Nobody tells me anything around here." This was on the evening shift so maybe somebody on the day shift failed to instruct her about the shot I was supposed to have.

Anyhow, I got along well and was out in about a week. The doctor told me what not to do while recuperating at home. He said I shouldn't bend and shouldn't lift anything and so on. When I asked him about having sex, he said, "Don't do anything until you come back and see me in two weeks." So I said to him, "Is that part of the instructions or is that a proposition?"

I've been home three weeks now and I'll be going back to see the doctor tomorrow. I still have some pain but it isn't bad like it was. It is more than I had the last time, though, so I don't know. I'll just have to wait and see whether this pain down my leg goes away.

The bill hasn't come in from the hospital yet so I don't know what it will all cost. Of course, I have insurance at work. When I left the hospital, they had me stop at the business office. The cashier asked me to pay $50 to cover part of the bill which the insurance won't pay but I told her I couldn't pay that much and wrote a check for $25. And she was very nice about it. But I was surprised I had to go by the office at all.

At work I have to handle the insurance for the employees and have had occasion to talk with a number of hospitalization insurance companies. And I'm convinced that in the next two or three years we're going to have to have some kind of national health insurance. The costs are going up so fast that nobody can afford to buy it anymore. Companies can't afford to buy insurance for their employees. The doctors' fees and the hospitals' charges are going up so fast that the insurance companies, when they go up on their rates, it isn't just 10 percent or 15 percent, it's 30 or 40 percent. And people can't afford it. Companies can't afford it for their employees. Pretty soon, the only way anybody will be able to afford to get their hospital and doctor bills paid for is through a government program, some kind of national health insurance. In my opinion, that's where we're headed and there's just no other way.

> *No costs have increased more rapidly in the last decade than the cost of medical care. And no group of Americans has felt the impact of these skyrocketing costs more than our elder citizens.*
>
> John F. Kennedy (1917–1963)
> Address on the 25th Anniversary of the Social Security Act, August 14, 1960

34. Arthritic Hip

Career military people tend to return to government once they have retired from active duty. This former Air Force colonel is in a federally-financed regional health program loosely tied to the state medical school. He is tall, spare, white-haired, in his middle 50's. Only by self-education was he able to select the kind of surgical procedure that he needed to get a successful solution to his health problem. The timing of it was almost pure happenstance.

- **Weak and Painful Hip**
- **Arthritic Hip**
- **Charnley Procedure**
- **Artificial Hip Operation**
- **Artificial Hip (Prosthesis)**

Back seven years or so ago, I noticed that when I'd try to climb a stepladder and put the weight on my right hip it would become weaker, particularly when I took a big step. It bothered me a little bit during the next two years.

I retired from the military after that and continued to have increased discomfort in my hip. Then I had a fall while I was playing tag with my daughter. One of the dogs cut in front of me and I went sprawling down the street. From then on, it began to get worse. This was three years ago.

If I played handball or anything, I would limp for two or three days. The irritation would give me considerable pain. When I was seated or inactive, there was a constant dull pain but it lessened when I would lie flat, but during the day I would notice the pain. I noticed the pain to such an extent that I started treatments with a doctor, an internist.

He treated me for about a year and it wasn't getting any better. I was on 12 aspirin a day plus four andocin, which is a drug they give for arthritis, and I still couldn't do the things I wanted to do. I had to stop playing handball. I was swimming to keep my muscle tone up. I could do things like swimming where I wasn't putting any pressure on my hip, things that weren't weight-bearing.. But if I'd go out and play golf or play handball, I regretted it for the next couple of days. Before I started treatments with the doctor, why I had reached the point that the pain was of such extent that it would take me maybe 10 minutes to stand up at my desk at the office.

I started the treatment at the outpatient department of the University Hospital. The first diagnosis was that it might be gout and they started giving me various treatments for gout but subsequently I was turned over to this internist whose specialty was arthritis and who treated me medically for arthritis.

He treated me with the aspirin and andocin, changing from gouty medicine to arthritic treatment. One thing that happens when you have osteo-arthritis is that your uric acid content goes up high because of the inflammation and soreness. The 12 aspirin will bring down your uric acid count to normal levels, whereas 2 or 3 aspirin will bring it up.

This treatment went along fairly well but I continued to get wear and tear on the hip joint. My right leg became about a half inch shorter than my left leg and it was becoming somewhat atrophied and smaller in circumference. And the constant pain was continuing.

I read in the paper about a hip operation that a local doctor was doing and I also saw a friend who had had this operation successfully, so I decided to see this doctor, an orthopedist. He took x-rays and recommended that I have this operation for the Charnley total hip replacement. That replaces the ball and the socket.

After I'd had his diagnosis, my job situation changed. I knew they were going to reduce the staff where I worked and I had some sick leave coming. The doctor here couldn't take me until late in the summer so I went out of state where this friend of mine had had his operation. His doctor had actually been to England and received his training under Dr. Charnley, who invented the process. So it was a question of timing. I didn't want to be looking for a job while I was recovering from an operation so that's why I went out of state.

"What did the doctor say would happen if you did not have this operation?"

It would continue to get worse and would eventually reach a point where they would not be able to correct it completely. I don't know that it would ever have completely grounded me, but it certainly prevented me from leading a full and active life. I had to continue to give it less and less strain. Even taking a walk was uncomfortable. I couldn't walk without limping.

I reported down to this hospital in the adjoining state and the doctor reviewed my case and the x-rays. He also recommended that I have the operation. This was on the nineteeth, he did all of the work-up on the twentieth and I had the operation on the twenty-first of March.

I'd made all of the arrangements in anticipation that I would have surgery. I was in the hospital two weeks and I left there walking with a cane.

When they prepared me for surgery, they gave me a shot of something in my room. I recognized the lad who came for me and I said to him, "I don't need any help. I'll get on the table myself." And that's the last thing I remember.

When I became conscious after the surgery, I was in my room but I had been in the recovery room for an hour and a half or two hours. The operation took a little over three hours. They had three doctors working on it. That's all they did, that type of operation.

The prosthesis is made of stainless steel, for the ball, which is something like a railroad spike. They cut off the head of the femur and drill a hole in there and cement it with dental cement. They use a dental cement to cement in a tempered, plastic socket after they have reamed it out. A liner. It is supposed to be good for ten years of extensive wear and then if it had to be replaced, the only thing they would replace would be the liner.

This operation, which was originated by Dr. Charnley in England, is performed successfully on miners and dock workers who go back to heavy-duty work. I've been very pleased with it.

One of the things they have to be very cautious about is infection, so after the operation I was given great amounts of antibiotics. It took three blood transfusions for the operation and I was on intravenous glucose for two days afterwards, or maybe it was just a day because I began to eat right shortly. And I had no dietary restrictions.

After surgery, my elimination system went to sleep and I fought that for some time before I realized I could ask for an enema and not go through that phase. Some people that have had trouble, not from the operation itself but from the postoperative condition, well, there were a couple of women there who developed a heart condition because of the strain which the postoperative situation placed on them. They had them in intensive care.

I had the operation on Thursday and by Sunday they had me standing up at the bed. On Monday I was taken down by wheel chair to do physical therapy which involved parallel bars and exercises on a flat board, lying on your stomach and raising your legs, holding them stiffly without raising your hip.

What happens in the operation is it takes about a nine-inch incision into the hip, the gluteas maximus, on the side of the hip. They pull the femur out, which is quite a stretching operation and quite a shock. By the time they put my hip back together, I had the strangest feeling when I stood up, I felt like I was lopsided due to the fact that I had both legs the same length. I was used to having one leg shorter than the other but now I felt like I was standing lopsided when I was really standing straight.

The extent to which they have to make the incision and pull the leg apart causes quite a trauma to the muscles, the leg muscles there. They lose their firmness, they lose their muscle tone. The main object of the physical therapy is to rebuild the muscle tone in order to hold the prosthesis in place.

The main thing they caution you about during the recovery period is being careful when you get out of a low chair or settee, not to put any weight on the leg on which the operation was performed. You have to watch it for six to eight weeks.

So what they do in physical therapy is to strengthen your muscles and at the same time teach you how to walk with a cane. You start off with a walking bar and practice with that three or four days, short periods of time. Then they teach you how to use a cane, how to climb stairs, how to go down stairs. By the time you have passed all of your tests using a cane properly and can walk a reasonable distance with a cane, then you're released.

After I left the hospital, I used a cane about six weeks. When I returned for my postoperative examination, six weeks after I went home, the doctor told me to throw away the cane which I did, and start walking completely without it.

I'm back playing handball two or three nights a week. When I have time, I play golf, swim, do anything I desire to do, no pain, no medication. The only thing I notice is that if I am in a strained position, on all fours, I'll feel a muscle pop in my hip. I've mentioned this to my doctor and it's nothing. I had my recent x-rays sent to my doctor out of state and he assured me that everything is in fine shape.

"Do you have any problem in any of your other joints?"

I get a little tennis elbow occasionally, playing handball, and I did have a little bursitis in my left shoulder as a result of the pressure of using the cane, but that's all gone away.

I highly recommend the operation.

In the hospital, I had a very fortunate situation. I had a small private room with a couch in it and my wife stayed with me for the whole two weeks. If there wasn't any response when I needed something, why, she'd go get it. That occurs sometimes, especially in the evening. It's a teaching hospital and they had . . . some of the assistants might have left a little to be desired, but, by and large, I don't have any complaints.

It's quite a relief after a couple of years of constant and increasing pain. We sold our house because it was just too much for me to mow the lawn. I could bicycle; it was easier to do that than walk. It didn't put the strain on the hip joint. It was very fortunate that I did continue to exercise and maintain a muscle tone. I'd recommend anyone going into this operation to prepare himself physically and definitely concentrate on rebuilding muscle tone post-operatively because this is what makes the operation a success. They give you a set of exercises that you perform during the post-op period at home, the exercises that are demonstrated during the physical therapy period of your training in the hospital. Only I failed to mention that they are very emphatic that you don't cross your legs after the operation. For the time you are in the hospital and during the postoperative recuperation at home, you constantly sleep with a couple of large pillows between your legs. You can sleep on your back or your side but you have to move those pillows with you.

"Is that hard to get used to?"

No, no. I didn't have any trouble. He never told me what would happen if I crossed my legs but I assumed that the hip joint might come out of the socket.

When I was in severe pain, I almost made the mistake of having the operation done by a doctor who evidently was not aware of the Charnley process and who wanted to pin my hip, which meant I would have been in a cast for six months and I'd never have been able to do the things I'm doing now. Pinning is sort of old-fashioned for this type of problem and I was really discouraged that I wouldn't have any use of my leg for six months. What they do is put a pin in and reorient the pressure point so the pin would hold the hip in place and you'd be putting pressure on another part of the socket that wasn't as worn as the normal point of impact. I'd have been in a walking cast, unable to use my leg in driving.

How close did you come to that kind of operation and why didn't you go ahead with it?"

I came close enough to get the diagnosis. This wás about a year before I had the Charnley operation. As I said before, I saw this article in the paper about it and also saw this friend of mine who'd had it successfully and he was so enthusiastic about it and so active, without any restrictions, I felt I'd like to see whether or not the operation would be suitable for me.

"The fact that you had a friend like that was pure luck, wasn't it?"

Yes. After I'd read the article, I was half inclined to investigate the process. Then I learned about this friend who had been in an automobile accident and had gone through the process of having his hip pinned, which had caused him no end of discomfort. This was before he had the Charnley procedure. Due to his injury, he did have one leg shorter than the other, a condition which could not be overcome by the Charnley operation. I believe this could have happened to me if I had waited longer and the leg had gotten shorter and more atrophy had taken place. Then I would not have recovered fully, as I did. My advice is, don't wait too long to have it done but don't rush into it too soon.

35. Bunion, Hammertoe

He is a trucker now but used to be in aircraft and automobile engine mainte-nance. This background prompts his comparison of health professionals and engine mechanics, observing the obligation of each to produce satisfactory results.

He is about 40, ruddy-complexioned, energetic, curly-haired. He is smart in the ways of the practical world and has a deep sense of responsibility.

- **Bunion**
- **Hammertoe**
- **Bunionectomy**

Doctors are body mechanics of the human body. If you take your automobile to a service dealer and have a problem repaired and immediately after pulling out of the garage you find out that problem is not repaired, you go back and that dealer will stand behind his repair guarantee. I think that doctors should stand behind their guarantee. Of course, it don't work that way. Doctors don't guarantee nothing.

When I was overhauling aircraft engines, you don't have room for mistakes just like doctors don't have room for any mistakes. I'm sure they are concerned when they finish an operation whether they've done it just right. But that's an afterthought which doesn't do a damn bit of good. I used to think that about engines I'd overhauled, whether I'd done it perfect. But that engine was already gone, flying people around the countryside. At that point, it didn't do a damn bit of good to think about it. One of the things that upsets me is that doctors don't stand behind their work but we have to.

My foot problem started when I was about 15 years old. I accidentally shot myself in the left foot with a .22 and the bullet barely creased the toe next to the big toe. Eventually, that toe turned into a hammertoe. About two years or so later I had to have that toe operated on and straightened out to prevent it from rubbing the top of my shoe. They took the middle joint, scraped each end of it, and made it grow together as a single bone. The last joint of that toe still turns downward. It's flexible enough to move if you use an outside force but it has no muscle power to move itself. They told me that was better than having the whole toe made as a solid bone. It has functioned well, but the last joint, which turns down, gives me toenail problems, doesn't grow properly.

The doctor couldn't say that the gunshot wound and hammertoe was a contributing factor to the bunion. Between the bunion and the wounded toe there was also a bone spur on the joint. The bunion formed on the outside of my big toe, away from the hammertoe.

It is not common for men to have bunions. That's more of a lady's disease, according to the doctor. He said that he performs ten bunion operations on women for every one he performs on a man.

A bunion takes a while to create itself. The bunion was there a long time before I had it operated on, due to my lack of knowledge of what a bunion is. A bunion is not something that grows on the side of your foot that you cut off. The doctor explained it to me and that's something good I can say about him. He was very patient in explaining the problem in a manner that I could understand what was wrong. After x-rays, the doctor showed me that a bunion is an improper bone growth. It may or may not have been caused by the bone spur. Normally, though, bunions just happen by themselves.

He operated, performing what is classified as a modified McBride bunionectomy. It was a total success as far as the bunion was concerned. The bunion is a misalignment of the bones of your foot. They go into your foot, open it up, and realign the leaders and the bones, sewing the leaders to hold the bones in place.

The bone spurs were on the toe with the previous surgery. He took them off to keep them from creating an irritation. This was not a successful operation. What it did was it left the joints rough. So I wound up with rough joints and no bone spurs, which was of no great help. I still have a constant irritation but not as much as what the bone spurs were.

I was in the hospital five days after the operation and after that, I was in a cast six weeks. Even after the cast comes off, you just don't walk on a foot that's had one of those operations.

It was a funny cast. It came up to the knee for the first six weeks. Then the doctor removed that cast and put another little deal that looked like a plastic shoe on me. He put a tennis shoe with the toe cut out and a built-up heel over that. The reason for this was to get the foot back into operation as soon as possible.

Headaches are bad but I don't believe you can have any worse hurt than in your feet. It's an old wive's tale that if your feet hurt, you hurt all over. This is true. All of your weight, all of your blood, all of your natural body fluids will contribute to your feet hurtin'. There ain't nothing that hurts worse than your feet.

I was off work for three months. That is an absolute necessity. We had a very good workmen's compensation set up. You had to be off three months before it paid a penny. I didn't get a penny. In three months, almost to the day, they let me come back to work.

There is no doubt in my mind that within two years, I'll have to have the right foot operated on for bunion. I see it coming. I'm going to call the doctor and ask him if I can have premature surgery, but I'll probably do it just like I did the other one, put it off until I can't stand it no more.

While I was in the hospital they gave me medication for the pain but I'm not much for takin' medication. Addiction. I'm afraid of it. I'll put it to you this way. I spent four years in Vietnam in combat. I saw addiction to drugs of all kinds. Now I'm addicted to alcohol. I like that. But I don't like painkillers for another reason. If your body's hurtin' you, you've got somethin' wrong with you. Then it's best to go have somethin' done about it. Of course, the pain after an operation, that's going to hurt you. That's true. You've got to suffer some pain, you've got to expect that.

I have no complaints about the way I have ever been treated in any hospital. I know that there are times that I could have been treated better but them people have got problems just like the rest of us. Ninety percent of the time I've been treated excellent and when I wasn't I figured there was somebody else who needed a little more treatment than I did.

What would help would be a better, straighter way to be dissatisfied with your health service. Suppose I go out here and pay five or six hundred dollars for an operation that is not successful; then I should have a way to get the results that I want short of a malpractice suit. A malpractice suit hurts all of us, the doctor and me. Next time I go to a doctor I'm going to have to pay more so he can pay for that malpractice suit some patient brought against him.

I'm not the least bit bashful about tellin' a doctor I don't think he's a bit better than I am. He goes to the school, he studies, he learns and I expect as good a performance out of him as he expects out of me. If a doctor brings me his car and I fix it and two days later he brings it back because it don't work, I'm not going to say, "Well, contact my lawyer if you don't like the way I did it." I'm going to say, "Bring your car in here and let's see what's wrong with it."

Used to, in the old days, you'd sit out there in the doctor's waitin' room for about an hour after your appointment and you'd get called in and see the doctor and then you'd go on about your way. Now, you go to the doctor's office and you sit for about an hour past your appointment and then you get up and go sit in the examinin' room or the shot room for another 15 or 20 minutes before the doctor comes to see you. This irritates me. In the old days, I believe that people entered the doctor profession out of compassion and caring for other people. But not one person in 10 believes that they do today. They enter the profession for the money.

Recently, I went to a doctor who requires a urinalysis and a blood analysis if you haven't seen him in the last two weeks. You get those lab tests before you even see the doctor. That's $18 right there.

This happened when I attempted to change doctors and I got worse than I had before. You know that old saying, "Take care of the boss you've got, the next one might be worse." So I went back to the same one I had. Where do you go to look for a good doctor? You can't afford to change doctors because everyone of them wants to take a blood test, chest x-rays, urinanalysis, they want to do a complete physical on you. They charged me $50 and I wasn't any better in two weeks so I went back and it was $32. It was $82 and I was still sick.

The last couple of times I went to the doctor, I didn't get to say anything! I told the nurse out front what my problem was and the report's settin' on the door outside the examining room and before the doctor walks in, he's done read it. He comes in, says, "Let's listen to your chest. Okay. Breathe deep. Okay. Let's check you right here. Okay." He goes out the door, tells his nurse, "Give him a shot. Three of these here pills. Two for next week." And so on and so on and he's gone. I didn't have the opportunity to say anything. The doctors don't have time to talk to you. Trouble is, they've got five more patients out there than what they've got scheduled. They've got to rush you up so they can work them there in.

XII.
Blood Flow

The blood is the life.

The Bible
Deuteronomy 12:23

36. Arteriosclerosis

He is a wiry, energetic, talkative entrepreneur in the business of buying and reselling used equipment for industry and business. This crew-cut, 62-year-old salesman is a decisive, quick-minded dealer who warehouses his goods in a suburban industrial park in a Sun Belt city. He is a widower. He has such an overwhelming zest for living, despite serious medical problems, that you get the feeling he can survive anything. He accepts his finiteness philosophically.

- **Arteriosclerosis**
- **Cardiac Bypass Surgery**

About ten years ago, I had an occasion to be more or less paralyzed from my legs down due to numbness, lack of circulation, I don't know what. All of a sudden. It being a Saturday afternoon and not being able to get in touch with any medical people, I called a naturopathic or chiro, a friend of mine. The chiro asked me to come out and he'd do what he could to help me.

First, before he touched me, he took some tests and discovered, electronically, that I did have no circulation in my lower extremities. There was nothing he could do for me but he had a friend who was an osteopath he thought would be able to help me. The osteopath checked me out and verified what the chiro found: that I had no circulation in my legs and that was the reason my back was hurting and my legs were numb. So he had me admitted into the osteopathic hospital. I was 52 at that time.

The osteopath and three other doctors in the hospital were confused at what was causing the stop in the flow of the blood to my legs. So we finally agreed, the doctors and myself, that they would have to do an exploratory surgery in my lower abdomen. I agreed to this and we went through with it. It was very successful because I found out, four years later, they had reamed my lower arteries in my legs to get the blood to flow in my legs. They had reamed them out.

"You didn't find this out for four years?"

Not until after I hit the American Medical Association people *(names a group of cardiovascular specialists).*

"Didn't you find this a little strange?"

I felt so good after the reaming of my legs and was able to continue the operation of my business, go horseback riding, whatever I wanted to do, that it didn't concern me. There were 24 inches of stitches on my legs and lower abdomen, 12 inches of scars on both legs. But they failed to tell me, never did tell me what they did. I felt so much better, I didn't argue with them.

Four or five years later I started having severe pains in my back and I went to Dr. Johnson, a medical man, an orthopedist at the bone and joint hospital. He x-rayed me and discovered I had three missing disks and two misplaced vertebraes from an old injury. He said, "You do have a back problem but I think you can learn to live with it if you get this other problem taken care of. You have a complete closure of the main artery from your aorta to your legs. There is no blood flowing. It's just like a faucet, damn near closed off." I said, "And you can't help me?" He said, "No way." "What do you recommend?" "Vascular arterior by Dr. Ellison or one of his cohorts, who are the best in the country. I'll send you to them if you are willing to go and let them check it out and verify what I've said." I says, "Fine. Give me his number. I'll talk to him now. Make an appointment. I'm ready." I was hurtin', severely hurtin'.

Dr. Ellison's group verified what Dr. Johnson told me. They took their x-rays and explained it all to me in a sensible, mechanical manner, which I understood. "What's it going to take to get this thing on the road?" I asked and the doctor said, "Well, we're booked pretty heavy with bypasses, open heart surgery. It's liable to be two or three weeks." On Thursday morning I got a call from Dr. Ellison who said, "John, are you still hurtin'?" and I said, "I am, Doctor. But thanks to the bourbon and the aspirin, I'm making it." That's just what I told him. He says, "Okay. See what your wife says. We've had a cancellation and I'm scheduled for surgery with an open operating room at eight o'clock tomorrow morning." I said, "I'll be there. I don't need to ask my wife. I'll be there." And I was there.

He ripped me open and gave me the "Y" arterial bypass, the upside down "Y" as he referred to it. That was eight years ago and I've been in pretty good shape ever since. Except, 30 days after surgery, my wife cracked up and had a nervous breakdown in an airplane over Wichita. And, God willing — and nobody but God alone gave me the power to do what I did at that airport — she broke and ran from me for a quarter of a mile and I chased her and caught her. Thirty days after surgery! I caught her and finally got some help from a security guard at the Wichita airport. She cracked and became berserk and we got her into a hospital there and finally brought her back here in an ambulance. And I went on back to work.

"How did the bypass surgery make you feel?"

It made me feel very good, particularly after the first six months when I became adjusted to it. I was out bowling 30 days after open heart surgery. Physically I felt good.

I sold my business and got out of the situation I was in. I sold my company to my employees, gave 'em ten years to pay me for it. I felt like I might live another year or two. I got rid of the pressure.

I had a bad experience while I was in the hospital and Dr. Ellison knows this. The medication they gave me in the recovery room, I reacted to it. I should know what it is so no one will ever give it to me again. I went up to "high C." The doctor said I wasn't allergic to it but I reacted in complete reverse. I don't ever want that medication again.

The drug was to knock me out after surgery, in the recovery room, and instead, I became a raving maniac. They ended up putting me in a straight jacket and tying me down. I took off for one really wild trip that lasted for 24 hours.

"What kind of sensations did you have?"

Would you believe that the Communists were trying to get to me? That at one time I was scheduled for slaughter at the local packing company? I remember all of this very vividly. It was so clear. My father-in-law came in from Kansas City and I knew he was a deputy sheriff. I said, "Boy, I'm glad to see you! I hope you've got your gun on you because I'm going to shoot my way out of this goddamn place." That's the kind of a wild person I was. The nurses, they got kicked, they got slugged and when I went out of the hospital, they said they couldn't believe I was such a nice person after what they'd been through with me. But I mean I kicked 'em; I mean I just slugged the hell out of the doctors, interns, anybody.

I have been in several different hospitals in the country where, if they give me the wrong medication I seem to get built up to "high C." For seven days and seven nights in one hospital on the West Coast I was in a terrible nightmare; no eating, no drinking, no water, no nothin'. I came out of it on the seventh day and asked the head nurse what was good for an overdose of pheno-barbital and ammoniated mercury. She said, "For any overdose, it's water." I said, "Bring me a gallon." She brought me a gallon and I said, "Now, bring me a urinal." So on that seventh day, unshaven, unkempt, I sat on the side of that bed and drank gallon after gallon of water and kept pissin' that water right on through. In three days, I was out of that hospital. But they gave me the wrong medication and I know that. I've been in the drug business; I know something about some of this stuff. Whatever it was, it sent me off to "high C." That's what the boys in the army tell me. When you get built up to high C, you can imagine anything. That trip I took in the hospital was the worst I ever had. I was fighting the battle of Waterloo all by myself, I tell you.

After I got out of that trip, it was all right. But while I was on that trip, the doctor said it was a wonder I didn't bust loose everything he had done.

On the eleventh day I was fightin' to get out of the hospital but my doctor's mother died over that weekend so he wasn't there to let me out so I stayed in 15 days altogether.

You have to live day by day and not worry about it. If it's God's will that you go tomorrow, you go tomorrow. I am not a religious person, but I do fear God.

Dr. Ellison caught me doing knee bends on the fourth day in the hospital room. His words were this, "What in the hell do you think you're doing?" I said, "I'm checking your plumbing, Doctor. It if don't stand up, I want to know it before I leave the hospital." He laughed and said, "Okeydokey," but he stopped me from doing those knee bends any more, I can tell you. I had 72 stitches in my belly and was doin' knee bends on his reputation and he didn't like it.

"Have you had any recurrence of symptoms?"

I get chest pains if I'm too tense and get goin' too fast. Right now, I'm undergoing severe back pains, muscle spasms. As soon as I get my business here in order and pay off a $10,000 note at the bank and get kinda squared away, I'm going right back in the hospital for a checkup because I think I've got the same thing reoccurring. My back is killing me. I don't know whether it's the vertebraes, my legs are all right, or the missing disks or more hardening of the arteries. I don't know. That's why I'm going for expert advice, x-rays and checking. I'm going to two or three different doctors to get an opinion. It's been a laughing joke with my family. Knowing me, they say, "What are you going to do, Daddy, go out for three bids to see who'll do it the cheapest?"

I'm not afraid to get several opinions. I can talk to a doctor on his own level. In other words, it's my body he's going to be whackin' on, so I want to know what's going on. The osteopaths, the chiros and the medical people of this city will tell you that I'm not bashful one damn bit.

I had plenty of insurance on this last deal. When my wife died of leukemia in the '50's, I didn't have any insurance and it bankrupted me. I lost my wife, my home, my car and everything. That's why I'm an insurance nut now. This bypass surgery cost close to $3000 and the insurance paid all of it but $15.

I've done okay, but no thanks to government, social security, medicare, medicaid, or anything. It's because of my own practical experience that I've been able to survive. I've had to help so many people in my business, help them get their hospitalization, keep them covered for the maximum. People are so gullible. They need somebody to watch over them. I wanted my employees to be sure and have adequate life insurance and hospitalization. The right kind of coverage. They'd believe anything any of these salesmen would tell them about insurance, hospitalization in particular. In other words, they'd say they had hospitalization, Blue Cross. Well, Blue Cross won't cover half of the expenses today. One time, our insurance company paid $35 a day for hospitalization. Today it's a hundred to a hundred and a quarter. You've got to keep updated, keep bringing the premiums and the policies up the way they're raising prices. The reason for this is, the doctor finds himself with his own insurance problems and has to keep raising his prices. Consequently, the doctor is just like the bankers, getting richer and richer by the day. There is no question about that.

This is why I want dollar for dollar value. This is why I want, you might say, three bids if I go back to surgery again. And I want the doctors to tell me for sure what they think and know is wrong. I'm trying to evaluate their knowledge and their prices. But the doctors in this state are ripping off the poor stupid jerks who are working day by day making a living for them. One of my doctors said to me, "Why don't you do like I do, take a week off every month and go to Acapulco, go to Hawaii, take a vacation?" I said to him, "Doctor, I don't have that many suckers paying my way." That's just what I told him.

He was ripping me off for 60 bucks every 90 days and insisting I come back after surgery. Do you know what? After a year, I called up and cancelled my last appointment. I told her to tell him I didn't have the time to devote to help him make his next trip to Hawaii. It's a rip-off.

To them, a person, a human being that comes in their office is nothing in the world but another cadaver. There is not an honest-to-God true doctor that I've met.

"How do you reconcile that statement with your enthusiasm for the good results you've gotten from Dr. Ellison's work?"

I asked him how good he was. He said, "I'm the best in the business," and I said, "You'd better be." He said, "Why?" and I said, "If you're not, I'll come back and haunt the hell out of you."

Today, that same bypass job I paid $3000 for is $10,000. It's ridiculous. Their costs haven't gone up that much. There's no way.

I've seen 'em make so many mistakes. I know they don't intend to but they all try to take care of just one more customer, try to get another $10 a day!

> *A physician ought to be extremely watchful against covetousness; for it is a vice imputed, justly or unjustly, to his Profession.*
>
> Thomas Gisborne (1758–1846)
> *The Duties of Physicians*

37. Stroke

This quiet, white-haired lady is well into her 70's. She is genteel yet forceful, knows her own mind. She and her husband live in a garden apartment in a Midwestern city but are moving to California to be close to their children and grandchildren. She is clear-witted and it is obvious that she loves life but she is not afraid to let go of it. She demands appropriate attention from the medical profession but she takes her infirmities with good humor and a shrug. Her daily routine involves much pill-taking but she doesn't have total confidence in the efficacy of the drugs which have been prescribed for her.

- **Stroke**
- **Cerebral Vascular Accident (CVA)**

I had a stroke and they took me in an ambulance to the hospital. John *(her husband)* was already in the hospital; he was taken in on Sunday and I was taken in on Thursday.

They let me lay in that downstairs emergency room; they couldn't get the doctor. My doctor was out of town and the doctor they were calling didn't come.

It was a light stroke. I woke up early that morning, at six o'clock, and planned to go see John in the hospital that day. I did a load of laundry at six o'clock in the morning and brought it home. Then I fixed my breakfast, half of it, my fruit, my pills; I take more pills than anybody I know. I have poor blood pressure and poor circulation, high blood pressure. I didn't have a headache, there was nothing wrong with me. I drank my juice and went into the kitchen to fix my cereal and put my toast in the toaster. Before I could turn the toaster on, I thought somebody clubbed me on the back of the head with a baseball bat.

I grabbed ahold of the sink and held onto it but I don't remember doing it. It must have knocked me out. When I came to, my hands were so clinched on that sink, I had a hard time getting them off. I was dizzy but managed to get to a chair which was only a few steps away. I sat there for a while and then I wasn't as dizzy as I was to begin with. I went to the bedroom and lay down on the bed and I must have passed out again. I didn't come to until eight o'clock.

I was expecting a friend at eight o'clock. She was coming to pick up some letters to take them to my husband in the hospital, so I sat down and waited for her. When she came in and looked at me she said, "What's the matter with you? You look funny." I began to tell her what was wrong and she said later she could understand half of what I said but half she couldn't. She telephoned her friend who's a nurse and told her what was happening and the nurse said, "It sounds as though she's had a stroke. I'll be right over."

Our family doctor was out of town so his answering service told my friend to call Dr. Brown who was taking his place. Well, Dr. Brown is a brain surgeon or brain doctor so that was who they took me to the hospital to see and let me lay down there until they finally found him around eleven o'clock. I got to the hospital before nine. A nurse came and stood beside me and wouldn't let anybody see me. I got my purse; they gave it to me so I could pay the ambulance $40 but they wouldn't let my friend in to see me. She was going to stay until they got me into a room. I kept drifting in and out and I'm not sure when I got to my room.

I told the nurse, "I don't want this room. I want a room upstairs where my husband is." They didn't let me see a doctor or anybody or if one did see me, I was passed out.

My doctor said I was paralyzed for three days on my left side but he lied. I couldn't have been paralyzed because I got up and went to the bathroom. If I'd been paralyzed, I couldn't walk.

I was out when they took me down for the brain scans. They washed my hair. I had just washed my hair the day before so I said, "What are you washing my hair for?" And they said it had to be washed and wet for the brain scan. Then they put some kind of glop on it, looks like brown putty. And they never washed it off. I was there nine days and that stuff was glued into my head all that time.

During the nine days, I'd be out and in. I don't ever remember seeing Dr. Brown and I got a terrific bill from him.

"What kind of medication and treatment did they give you?"

Nothing. Nothing! They put me on a diabetic diet and left it by my bed. I didn't eat half of it, couldn't. And nobody fed me. I asked one of the girls to feed me. They didn't even give me a bath. On mornings I couldn't bathe myself, I got no bath.

A nurse came in and said, "You aren't eating." And I said, "I can't eat it. I wouldn't feed a dog that stuff that's brought to me." I tasted it and, oooh, it was terrible. I lost 20 pounds. I was glad of that. That was the best part of it.

I can't tell you how long I drifted in and out of consciousness. It must have been several days. But when I had to go to the bathroom, I'd always come out of it and go to the bathroom. No trouble with my left side at all. And as far as my speech was concerned, I don't know about that because I didn't have anybody to talk to. Nurses would come in every once in a while, but they never said anything. I got a lot of long distance telephone calls I couldn't talk to. John would talk to them, my two sons and my ex-husband called me up. By the time I went home, my speech had cleared up.

After I got home, I had a nurse for seven weeks. I don't know what for — the doctor wanted me to have a nurse — unless he thought I was going to have another stroke. I paid her for the full week, but I'd only keep her three or four hours a day and then send her home, so I could take a nap. She did nothing for me. She finally got disgusted, just sitting and reading. She offered to do the laundry and then she offered to clean the apartment. She was here seven weeks and she did nothing for me.

"Why did the doctor think you needed a nurse?"

I don't know. He said if you want to go home, you can go today if you get a nurse. I wanted to go home whether I had a nurse or not. I never did know why I had to have one.

My head hurts me every once in a while. I live on pain pills. I don't have a headache. I have a hurt in my head on the left side. It's a pain on my left side and I take a pain pill and it goes and sometimes I don't have another one for a day and a half or two days. The doctors said the x-rays didn't show where it was or what it was and the brain scan showed something on both sides but I don't have any pain on the right side.

Husband: Let me explain that. When I was in her room, the doctor and his assistant were discussing her reaction to the brain scan and he said the first brain scan showed the left side was affected, the second one showed the right side was affected and they are uncertain which part of her brain was damaged. He suggested that the next thing would be to get her a very severe test with blood coloration or something. They shoot colored blood through the brain to see what happens to it. He said it was very severe and I thought she'd had enough of that brain business, so I said, "Let's not do that. I'll take her home and let's see how she reacts to being home," which the doctor agreed was all right to do.

Patient: As they were getting me ready to take me back to my room, I heard one of the technicians say that the brain scan machine wasn't working good. Take it from there, brother. I'm through with hospitals. I'm done with doctors, hospitals and pills. I take 18 pills a day. My pill bill for 3 months is $268. I send it to Blue Cross and Blue Shield.

When I asked the doctor if I had to take those hydrogen pills under my tongue, "Can't I just take them?" he looked at me and said, "Well, you don't want to die, do you?"

Everybody's got to die. I don't see why they make such a fuss over it.

> *Despise not death, but welcome it, for*
> *Nature wills it like all else.*
>
> Marcus Aurelius (121-180)
> *Meditations,* IX.3
> (tr. by C.R. Haines)

38. Fainting Spell

Some people would call him a health nut. He is tall and balding, a health enthusiast who has chosen long-distance running as a hobby as well as a way to keep in shape. Perhaps his thin, even gaunt physique is the result of his running; perhaps he is naturally weedy and linear.

He is around 50 and his children are either out of college or will soon graduate. His job with a large oil company keeps his family in upper-middle-class comfort. His sense of humor is a delight and readily emerges in the retelling of this episode which has become a classic tale in the family and among their acquaintances.

• Fainting Spell

One of my buddies had a heart attack right as we were going into the game of the century between OU *(the University of Oklahoma)* and Nebraska a few years back. You may remember that game. He had it as we walked through the gate at the game. He sat down and had his heart attack right there. It just ruined my whole day.

I got him to that heart deal at the northwest part of the stadium. I carried him in because he was turnin' green on me. I said, "What's the matter with this guy?" They laid him down, gave him some treatments and said, "He's having a heart attack." How tacky of him. They threw him into an ambulance and took him to the hospital.

Later, he had this bypass surgery and now he's doing fine. We ran over to the hospital right after he'd had his open heart surgery to see him for a few minutes.

Wife: We could only see Bill for a ten-minute period so when we got to the hospital, Bill's wife motioned for us to come on in. June was talking, that's his wife, and I realized that we shouldn't stay long. Also I could see that Frank was getting a little pale, so I said, "Let's go on out; we've been here for our time."

Husband: Bill had tubes coming out of him at all angles. He had his pajamas open and the scar on his chest where he'd been sewed up was about eight feet long, looked like. My old buddy. And beside him was this huge bucket of blood. Oh, a bathtub of blood. Pumping blood in and out.

And that did it. I made a mental note, "Now, I'm not going to let this bother me, the odor in here and all of this blood." But I began to get faint anyway.

Wife: I had gone on out and sat across the hall and I looked up and saw Frank at the door. He had something in his hand which he was concentrating on real hard. I said, "Are you all right?" And about that time, he went down and hit his head on the corner of the door.

I went over and started to get ahold of him. There weren't any nurses or anybody in the hallway. I started lifting his head and got blood on my hand. Just then, a nurse came around the corner, looked at us and said,"Oh my goodness, what's wrong?"

Husband: She thought I was having a heart attack because I was on a heart ward, see. Pandemonium broke loose. People were running everywhere.

Wife: She said, "I'll get a wheelchair." and disappeared running. I said, "Oh, it's all right. He faints easy." Well, she came back with the wheelchair and they got him in it. He was awake, and just as she started down this great long hall with him, he kind of fainted again and threw himself back in the wheelchair.

Husband: When I felt the back of my head and realized I was bleeding, I fainted again.

Wife: The nurse yelled at another nurse down at the end of the hall.

Husband, (quoting nurse): "We've got a bad one here."

Wife: The nurse thought Frank had had a heart attack, I guess. Well, our friend June, who was very tense, worrying about her husband, was still in the room. The nurse came running, a little man in a white coat came running and they started hooking him up to take his blood pressure. I turned to June, who was just coming out into the hall, and when she saw all of the commotion, she said, "Who is that? Is that that big fat man I saw come in here? Who is that down there?" And I said, "It's all right, June." But she repeated her question, "Who is that?" And finally I said, "It's Frank."

Of course, she had been very tense all day and when she heard it was Frank, she said, "Frank."

Husband: I just did it to relieve the tension, you know.

Wife: And then June started laughing and I began laughing, too.

Husband: And I said, "Damn you, girl, what are you laughing at?" And June said, "The perfect specimen. Look at him." She was laughing hysterically.

Wife: I wasn't too concerned because Frank had just had a physical; he had been running every day and he kept telling us constantly how healthy he was. They wouldn't let him up even though we told them he was all right.

Husband: Well, I am healthy. In fact, the last time I went to my doctor to take a physical, he didn't believe my pulse rate.

"What is your resting heart rate?"

Thirty-eight. And, of course, these doctors haven't been around long-distance runners much. When I got on the treadmill for about 15 minutes, I didn't work my pulse rate up much. I didn't hardly break a sweat or anything and the doctor came in and said, "Well, this thing's not working. It's not reading right," and began pushing all of the buttons on the EKG machine. I said, "Everything's working, Doc. Get me off this stupid thing." They had electrodes on me and all that jazz.

He came back about 15 minutes later and brought a couple of interns with him and pumped up the treadmill as fast as it would go. Again, he said, "This thing is not working." And I said, "Hell, it's working. Don't you ever take care of people who are in good shape?" Bunch of quacks. I was giving him a hard time. He brought in a couple of nurses and they were all looking at the printout. My pulse rate wouldn't go up very high, see? I was just going slow on the treadmill. Finally, he concluded that the machine really was working.

He sat down afterward and said, "Well, I thought, Mr. Jackson, that you had set some kind of a record, but I looked up my records and you are second. A couple of years ago we had a little old schoolteacher in here and she's got a better heart than you have. And she smokes a pack a day." So I said, "The hell she has. I'd like to see that little old gal."

We've got a guy in our running club whose heart rate is 28. He's a nationally-rated marathon runner who, in fact, tried out for the Olympics. Most of the marathon runners' pulse rates are in the 30's. Their hearts are beating so slow you think there is something wrong.

I guess if my own doctor doesn't believe me, I couldn't expect the doctors and the other people at the hospital to. And they didn't.

First, they put me on that stupid wheelchair and then, when I fainted again, I just kind of drained right out onto the floor. I was weak. I was sick. That atmosphere. There I was, back on the floor again, limbo. Then they picked me up again and put me on a long stretcher and strapped me in. They must have thought I was going to fall off. There were a lot of people around. It was very embarrassing.

Wife: Yeah, Frank attracted quite a crowd for no one being there when it happened. They wheeled him on down to the emergency room so they could sew up his head.

Husband: And I kept saying, "I'm in perfect shape. Get me out of here, damn it." And June was walking along just laughing hysterically. I was really amusing her. Maybe I should have sued them. They ought to have had rubber bumpers on the corners of those walls.

Wife: No, it was a door.

Husband: It was the corner of the wall, the tile wall.

Wife: No, it was a door. I was there; you weren't conscious.

Husband: Anyhow, I thought Bill was going to get up out of bed to see what all of the commotion was about. I was stealing his thunder, you know. He was the patient.

Wife: When we got down to the emergency ward, I had to go over and answer certain questions, name, address and all. June came down with me and we kept laughing about Frank's fainting spell. The little girl at the desk said, "It's not often we get people who are laughing when they come to the emergency room.

Husband: Everyone was having a ball but me.

Wife: They had taken Frank's heart beat all along and they sewed up his head and I kept thinking that they'd bring him out and tell us we could take him home. We hadn't planned to stay long. Every so often a doctor would come out and I could see him run through this heart beat thing. Of course, they didn't know he normally had a very low pulse rate so they kept him in there.

Finally, they got ahold of Frank's doctor because they didn't believe his pulse rate. They had to check it out with his doctor.

Husband: The doc in the emergency room didn't believe me. But I said, "I'm all right, see. You guys need to quit this clowning around and let me out of here." But I really wasn't feeling too good; I was kinda sick at my stomach.

Wife: Finally, after the doctor kept him another 30 or 40 minutes, he said we could go home. By this time it was eleven o'clock and he'd fainted about 8:30. But they took good care of him.

Husband: I've been embarrassed many times by June and my wife telling this story. This story used to take about eight minutes for them to tell but each time it gets longer. Now it's up to about 20 minutes. Same story, same incidents. The best thing about it was that it relieved June of her tensions. She was about to have a stroke worrying about her husband. I thought we were going to lose her. Now, June tells that story and just screams. But I don't think it's very funny.

> *A good laugh and a long sleep are the best cures in the doctor's book.*
>
> Irish Proverb

39. High Blood Pressure

This young architect heads a newly-organized firm with offices in the Southwest and in San Francisco. He is curly-haired and has a tendency to gain weight now that he has stopped smoking cigarettes. There is always a flicker of a smile playing about his mouth, ready to break into a grin. It gives him a boyish appearance.

Because he is specializing in the design of health care institutions, his projects and consulting assignments take him on flights to cities all over the U.S.

In 10 years, he plans to buy a boat, take two years off and, with his wife and two children, circumnavigate the world.

- **Weakness**
- **Chest Pains**
- **High Blood Pressure**

My blood pressure problem is not new. It first occurred about a year and a half or two years ago during the period of time we were trying to finalize the construction of Memorial Hospital. I was working somewhere around 80 hours a week, being at the building site itself sometimes almost 24 hours straight, whatever. I began to feel very weak and often had pains in my chest and generally didn't feel well.

Went to my doctor who's a general practitioner. He checked me out, told me I had high blood pressure, that my blood pressure was 150 over 110, as I recall. The 150 didn't bother him but the 110 scared him to death. He told me to start taking the white pills. He didn't tell me what they were, just that they were good for me. He told me they would lower my blood pressure if I took them like a good boy and I might live.

I did so. Ninety days later, I returned to the scene of my examination and was told that I now had blood pressure of 130 over 87, or something, that I was doing marvelously well and that I could take these another 90 days. If I wasn't feeling well, I could come back, but if not, not to worry about it. He said that I had pretty well cured myself at that point.

So I took another 90 days worth of tablets and forgot it. Stopped taking the tablets.

Approximately three months ago, I was not really necessarily feeling bad; I just wasn't feeling real good. I had been working for myself about four months, living on airplanes, at a very rapid pace, working many long hours, eating terribly, sleeping worse. My wife determined it was time for me to have a checkup and made certain conditions upon our relationship which caused me to want the checkup. And I had a checkup.

Upon having a checkup, I found out I was back to having high blood pressure again. This time it was 150 over 104. And he gave me the pills again. He did a rather thorough check of my body which did not impress me because he did not use all of the machines and tools I knew were utilized in Memorial Hospital for a complete physical. But he told me, based on his examination, that my heart was in good shape and all I had was high blood pressure.

Since I now knew that I had high blood pressure, I began to notice other symptoms. Like pains in my chest and other things and at that point I became concerned that maybe I had a bad heart or some other problems that my poor old general practitioner couldn't find out about, because all he did was thump me and listen to me just like G.P.'s have been doing for a few hundred years.

So I decided to journey to a prominent group-practice clinic in town and consult whom I believe to be the state's leading cardiologist. He checked me out, had me run on a treadmill and did all kinds of things; gave me what I consider to be a very thorough examination, especially upon receiving his statement.

"What did it cost you?"

One hundred and sixty dollars. He informed me that I had a very good heart, that I was healthy, and the general practitioner who had charged me $12 was correct in everything he had told me. He said I had high blood pressure but other than that I had no problems. However, he did inform me that high blood pressure was a serious thing if it was not hereditary. If it was hereditary, all I had to do was take those white pills for the rest of my life. He informed me to check with my family, because I did not believe it was hereditary. He told me to inform my mother and father how serious it was, that I know. If it was hereditary, they probably couldn't cure it and I'd be taking pills the rest of my life. If it was not hereditary, I probably had something else wrong with me and I'd have to go into the hospital for three or four days of extensive tests.

I contacted my parents that night by telephone and they reluctantly told me that, yes, my father has had high blood pressure problems and so has my mother, for many years. I also found that they think that their parents, my grandfather on my father's side and my grandfather on my mother's side, both had high blood pressure problems, too.

Faced with that information, I have not proceeded with the three days of tests. Now we know that I have hereditary high blood pressure and I will continue to take my white pills until they run out. Then, I'll go back to the cardiologist and have him check me again. I'll run out of them in another 60 days because I still have some I didn't take the last time.

One interesting thing, though, was that when he informed me that there really wasn't a damn thing the matter with my heart and that I was really healthy with the exception of this high blood pressure, I immediately felt a helluva lot better than I had for days.

"Have you had any chest pains or other symptoms since?"

Yes. Last week, when I ate at a Bohemian restaurant in Chicago, I had some pains which I determined right away were heartburn. But they were similar to the ones I had had before. When I got back to the hotel, I pulled out the antacid tablets which the cardiologist had given me for that type situation.

I'm also losing some weight which the cardiologist told me I had to do. He informed me that people with high blood pressure are more susceptible to heart attacks and so are people who are overweight. He did not threaten me or scare me. He treated me as though I was a grownup. He told me that through a long and full life I'd be taking those pills, until my long and full life came to an abrupt end. I take them every day, one each morning. A pill a day keeps the cardiologist away.

Unlike other times when I've been examined, at every step of the way through the examination, the cardiologist explained the reasons for everything he was doing, what he was trying to find out. And when he got all of that information, he explained to me what it meant, how he was evaluating it and why I had run on the treadmill, what that did and how that information assisted him in making a second check on the decision. He explained all of the tests I would have to go through if I didn't have hereditary high blood pressure, what types of things they were designed to find out. He said my high blood pressure could be caused by bad kidneys or all kinds of things. He was very thorough in his explanation, what might be the matter and why he was doing what he was doing.

I assume that he was being this thorough because we had a working relationship in designing the hospital and he had some respect for my intellect, contrary to the normal give-and-take between a doctor and a patient where the doctor doesn't always feel that the patient has a lick of sense when it pertains to anything important.

The general practitioner, on the other hand, just told me what it was and didn't bother to talk about anything else. He didn't have time because he was only charging me 12 bucks. He had to get me in and out of there.

The cardiologist gave me no diet instructions except to tell me that I was too heavy. More important, he said, I was in terrible physical shape for somebody my age, 32. He said I looked terrible. He said if I didn't do something about it now, when it wasn't causing me problems, that in 10 years I'd really have problems. I'm nine or 10 pounds lighter than I was and I need to be 10 pounds lighter than I am.

"Now that you have gone through this thorough examination, do you get favorable vibes from your wife?"

Yes. She's not afraid to overly excite me.

"What did you think about your bill of $160?"

I was amazed but not quite amused. However, I felt I got my money's worth and I don't recall that the doctor ever questioned my architectural design fees.

> *It is a distinct art to talk medicine in the language of the non-medical man.*

> Edward H. Goodman (1879–)

XIII.
Pump Problems

*The heart . . . moves of itself and does not
stop unless forever.*

Leonardo da Vinci (1452–1519)
Dell Anatomi, Fogli B
(tr. by Edward MacCurdy in *The Notebooks
of Leonardo da Vinci*) Vol. I, Ch. III

40. Heart Attack

The demands of his business, supplying specially designed equipment for laboratories and similar operations, involve critical attention to the details of use and fit and a hundred other specifications. This advanced degree of meticulousness is necessary for the survival of his business and his personal survival as pilot of his own airplane. His appearance, his language and his demeanor all reflect this lifetime habit of thoroughness. He is a Midwesterner in his middle 50's.

- **Heart Attack**
- **Myocardial Infarction**
- **Bypass Surgery**

I was in the hospital on three different occasions, but I think the one that would be significant would be the last time which was for surgery. First, I went in because of the attack. I was in for 10 days. Then I went back in for two days so that they could perform coronary angiography. Then it was determined where the trouble was and how they would go about dealing with it. And then the third time, which was the heavy incident, this was the surgery.

I was playing squash and I got a pain in the wishbone and not an excruciating pain. It was not excruciating but it was persistent. Wouldn't go away. And with my usual brilliance, I continued to play. Played the full 45 minutes. And then, to compound the felony, I had a massage. I later learned that was probably the worst thing I could have done. In the massage process, there's a tremendous amount of hydraulic pressure that is generated by the masseur. I didn't need that.

I finished the massage, showered, got dressed and I wasn't thinking clearly. I still had this discomfort; it was quite a bit of discomfort so I called my wife and asked her to make an appointment with our physician, that day, if possible. I played squash at noon.

Apparently there was that about my manner of speech that triggered her suspicion because she wanted to know what the hell was going on. She said, "What'll I tell him is wrong with you?" "Well, I've got some chest pains."

I'd never had this kind of pain before and nothing to lead me to believe I had any heart problems. In fact, my cholesterol was extremely low, so low that

I was rejected for the lipid research program at the medical research foundation. Yeah, they turned me down. They sent me a form which said, "Your cholesterol and triglycerides are too far down the line, we can't use you."

Anyway, my wife persuaded me that I should go to the emergency room of the hospital. So I did. I drove there. By the time I reached there, the pain had subsided and I felt embarrassed. I wasn't really going to go in, but then I felt that that would be pretty foolish. So I got out of the car and by the time I'd made the front entrance, I was right back in trouble. So I went into the emergency area and all I had to say was "chest pains" and I was getting all of the attention in the world.

The first thing I knew, a physician there said, "You have had a heart attack and we're going to keep you here." Which they did, for ten days.

I was only in the CCU *(coronary care unit)* four days and then I was put in a room on a wing which is pretty much reserved for heart patients. For about three days there I wore a portable transmitter, which was monitored up on the seventh floor at a central monitoring area. It's a transmitter that transmits my beat to . . . it's telemetry they have on the seventh floor that picks up the signal, the transmission. If there are any aberrations, they pick it up and the nurse comes in.

My family physician assigned a cardiologist to me and he told me what had happened. There was a mild cardio-infarction, very mild. He said, "I believe you have coronary artery disease and I think you're a fine candidate for bypass surgery and he explained this to me.

"When did the pain stop?"

Oh, the pain stopped before I ever left the emergency room. I never felt it again. They gave me plenty of drugs, the pain stopped and I just sort of took a vacation in the hospital. The doctors knew there had been damage and they felt that scar tissue needed to form before I could be released. In the meantime, they did other tests to try to support their conclusion that I was a candidate for bypass surgery. The cardiologist is 40, no more, and he thinks aggressively and I formed instant rapport with him, after he had explained to me the full dimensions, where I was, or where he thought I was and what he thought could be done.

About a week after I was discharged, I went back in so they could perform the angiograph and it confirmed exactly what he suspected. In fact, I watched on the videotape. I watched the process and as a layman, I could determine that there was one artery that had two critical blockages. And there was one artery that was just out of business. The dye would come down just a little ways and then, nothin'. It was completely blocked off.

So this confirmed precisely what he suspected and he laid out the options for me again. I forget whether he called this condition, athero-sclerosis or what's the other name?

"Arteriosclerosis? That's the same thing, isn't it?"

No, no. There's a subtle difference. This is something I learned in my stay there. But this seemed not to be important to him.

We agreed that this was the way to go so then there was the question, who is going to be the surgeon. It turns out that there's at least five guys in this town that do this surgery. In fact, these five have formed a corporation and this is what they do.

I did some research on my own with a friend of mine who is at the medical center and he said, "Well, if you could get a guy by the name of Harrison to do it, I think you should get it done right there because he's the best there is." Well, when I mentioned the name Harrison to the cardiologist, why his eyes lit up like a Christmas tree. You know, that was his boy. But he didn't want to give me any guidance or direction. He would not disparage any of the heart surgeons except one. This one, he said, is a skilled mechanic but he's a prima donna and I don't think you and he would . . . I don't think you'd be comfortable with him. And as it turned out, he was right. I met this fellow later.

But anyway, we settled on this surgeon and he came to visit me and I was immediately comfortable, totally comfortable. He spelled it out in fairly harsh terms: this is what we do, this is what can happen and these are the odds against it happening. When he got through talking, I said, "Let's set it up."

"What are the odds?"

He said about 30 percent of the bypasses plug up. He also explained why this is so. He said that the key to the bypass thing is the flow rate they are able to achieve in the bypass. When they turn the juice back on, the cubic centimeters per minute is the key. They must have 30. Forty is good. Incidentally, as it turned out, I achieved 70 in one and 100 in the other. But not all hospitals have the instrumentation to measure this precisely. And I didn't know that. But many hospitals will go ahead without this apparatus because of, I don't know, some kind of chauvinism or keep up with the Joneses or something.

"Will you explain in your own language what bypass surgery is?"

Yes. In my language, they simply take good veins out of another part of your anatomy, in my case out of the left thigh, and they use those veins to bypass the blocked areas of the coronary arteries so that those areas are no longer in business. It's a plumbing job, strictly.

"What happens down where they took the veins out?"

Well, there's so much veinage down there, I find out, plus the fact that the human cardiovascular system has an inexorable thrust to expand, to develop collateral systems. This is what I did playing squash and this is why I stayed out of trouble as long as I did. The vascular system has this urge to extend itself and to find new channels when a blockage does occur, so that the loss of, well, I don't know what the hell it might have been, maybe a total of eight inches of vein in my upper thigh was of no great significance.

"Why doesn't the coronary artery do that?"

Well, it does, to some extent. I did develop fairly extensive collateral apparatus, but not enough, not enough. There's no way that you can substitute for those big coronary arteries, finally. If they quit working altogether, you're out of business.

The doctor explained to me what he was going to do and how he was going to do it and what some of the hazards were. I weighed the whole thing, made an assessment and decided how I wanted to spend the rest of my life. I said, "Let's go."

He said, "All right. I want to do it at a time of my choosing, when I can get all of my people in that room and when they have had a good night's rest and you'll be the first piece of business that day."

There was no way I could argue with that, so I was scheduled for May 29. I went in the hospital on May 28. My experience with the personnel and the system of that hospital were just . . . of course, I think it is accurate to say that when you go into any hospital for heavy surgery, you're seeing the best they have to offer in all areas: personnel, facilities, machinery, the whole thing. It was excellent.

The procedure took three and a half hours. And I got into a little bit of trouble. I was in the recovery room about 12 hours. Turns out I'm a bleeder and I didn't know it. The surgeon couldn't find the key to managing the plasma.

About midnight, all of my family was gathered in a room there and the surgeon was talking to them. My sister had come in from California and she mentioned sort of off-handedly that she and I both have this characteristic. We bleed profusely and easily. This was significant to him and he ordered an immediate rearrangement of the plasma management. He got into platelets, I think, a different kind of platelet. To make a long story short, that turned the trick.

But I was there a long time and I was in some trouble and some thought was being given to taking me back into surgery. The experience in recovery was a very profound one, and at the risk of sounding a little starry-eyed, I just have to tell you about it.

By the time I got around to knowing what was going on even a little bit, it was probably about eight o'clock in the evening. By then the recovery room was cleared out; I was the only patient in there. The fellow who was taking care of me was a young, bearded type. I could detect that he was unhappy and all of this came through to me in a subliminal way because they'd pumped me full of morphine. Nevertheless, I sensed this, I could perceive this. He'd make observations — I couldn't tell what kind of apparatus was there on the floor — take readings and write them down. He was kind of muttering to himself.

Then about ten o'clock, there were two other fellows about the same age — they were not physicians, they were technicians — and one of them said, "Well, it's about time for me to go off shift but I don't have anywhere to go. Maybe you'd like for me to stick around?" The bearded fellow was immensely relieved and said, "Yeah, I'd appreciate that." Shortly after that, the other fellow was also due to go off shift and he, too, volunteered to stay on. And all this time, I was using up a lot of blood.

"Did this alarm you?"

No alarm, but I was aware that it wasn't going right. Then, shortly, a woman came in and she came right up to me and took my hand and told me her name. Well, she was the supervisor of the recovery room and she works when she wants to work. As it later turns out, she is an immense person, has a wide-ranging reputation as being very competent in the recovery room. But, anyway, she hooked up another drain, up to that point I'd been swallowing blood, and she put in another drain.

Just before midnight, I perceived that this just wasn't going all that well, so I asked this woman, "Nancy, is this going to work out?" I wasn't afraid but I was alert to my condition. And she took me by the hand and said, "We're going to work it out." She was such a tremendous, vibrant person that I knew that that was going to happen. I know how corny this must sound but it was a moving experience and I'll never forget it.

The surgeon got this information from my sister about my slow clotting time and he ordered an immediate rearrangement of the plasma. This was done and they were all gathered around my bed. We were like a team and this was a campaign. I was a member of the team. I was the cause of all the trouble but I was also a member of the team. We were holding hands.

It was probably about 12:30 when one of the bearded guys looked down at this tube and said, "I just saw my first clot!" Then Nancy paid attention and said, "Yes, and I just saw another one and another one." We all knew that I was over the hump then.

They kept me in recovery for another three hours, to make sure, and then wheeled me up to ICU *(intensive care unit)*. From then on it was just routine. I was in ICU, I guess, three days and then back to my wing with the portable transmitter. I was discharged in a week. I didn't expect to get out that soon and, of course, I was delighted, but the surgeon said, "There's nothing more we can do for you here."

Discomfort? No. I hit the Tylenol and codeine pretty regularly but I can't remember any pain. I can remember discomfort and that would be as far as I'd want to go.

Now, the surgeon doesn't want me to do anything, even swim, for another month because they saw through the sternum and he's apprehensive about misalignment. The surgery was four weeks ago. You see, they saw the ribs off the sternum and put spreaders in there and it stays that way for three or four hours, which is traumatic. Then they sew you back together again. What it seems to have done to me is to inflame the pleura. I'm a layman, you know, making my own diagnosis, but that's the way it seems to me. I don't feel any bone pain or rib pain but it would be difficult for me to take a deep breath.

Everything from the recovery room on is anticlimactic. I came along very fast and Harrison kicked me out of there a week after surgery. I got out on a Friday, and the following Monday, I was driving my car. The way I get the picture, if they get a good flow rate through the bypass before they close you up, and presupposing that you are healthy before you have the surgery, you're home free. If you don't bust anything the first week and they get the flow rate they seek, which in my case was twice as much as I had to have, you're home free.

I have no restrictions. The day I got out of the hospital, the cardiologist looked me in the eye and said, "We're turning you back in better shape than you've been in years."

"Do you feel in better shape?"

I can't answer that yet because there is still some trauma. There's what I presume to be the pleura inflammation, which is subsiding, but if the little flashes that I get are any indication, he's absolutely right. I'll really kill 'em on the squash court! With a new plumbing system, I'll be hard to deal with.

I was so profoundly impressed by the package of health care they dished up there and by the cardiologist and the surgeon. We had rapport. There was no antagonism. I was a good patient because, you know, it's smart to be a good patient. Things go better that way.

At four o'clock the morning after the surgery, they started me on inhalation therapy. The young fellow who came around to administer it explained to me exactly why it was important and beneficial. He was knowledgeable, his training had been so complete that I could get with him immediately on the importance of it. He explained it graphically to me. I thought that was terrific. As uncomfortable as inhalation therapy is to a bypass patient, I plunged right into it with a will.

All of the personnel were well-trained. They knew what they were talking about. They laid all kinds of potassium on me while I was in there, in orange juice, straight. Well, I asked some kind of an aide, "Why potassium? What is important about that?" It turns out that potassium is an electrolyte and since the whole heart action is one of electricity, you need that. And there's one other element which she named and she explained exactly how that works electrically. And she was just a snot-nosed little broad. I thought that was terrific.

She was an aide, like, but she worked always in ICU, her specialty. She was not a registered nurse but she knew why I was taking potassium. And you know, that's an interesting thing that I encountered there and I think probably it's a condition in a great many hospitals. I noticed a lot of young men, a lot of them with beards and as I later found out, a lot of them had some college and some were college graduates. They were there in the capacity of technicians, they were not physicians or medical students even, and I wondered about them. Of course, in ICU, nights and days don't make any difference.You sleep when you're tired and there aren't any windows in there, anyway. During the long nights, I had a chance to visit with them and get acquainted. Now I know this sounds corny, but most of these guys I talked to were under 30, somewhat anti-establishment but they knew they had to do something to make a living within the establishment framework and they could do it there and find a kind of fulfillment. They had a degree of dedication which I found beautiful and amazing. They were highly trained, they knew what they were doing and why there were doing it. Highly motivated. A refreshing thing to observe.

I don't have any hospital insurance and the bill was mind-boggling but nobody'll ever hear me whimper about that. It was a bargain. As far as I'm concerned, it's the best bargain there is around. Of course, I haven't got the surgeon's bill yet, but nevertheless. Actually, the way it's set up, my little corporation pays all of the medical expenses.

"What do you think the whole bill will run?"

Well, I've got a nine-inch scar and I think it'll run about $1200 an inch! And it's the bargain of the century. I've got a whole new plumbing system and a new lease. Life. It never really belongs to you; some guys get to use more of it than others.

"How did they explain the fact that you have a low cholesterol rate and yet you build up boiler rust in your arterial pipes?"

The cardiologist copped out when I asked him that question directly. He took out his pencil and wrote down the name of a book that was written by a research physician on the West Coast named Friedman. He divided men into personality types, A and B. He has further correlated the incidence of heart disease with behavior.

"You're a Type A?"

Yeah. And he said, "We don't know, but that's the best thing we've got going right now." In my own mind, there is no question but what the cardiac disease relates to temperament but there's not yet enough data to support getting up on a stump and saying this is so.

In my case, I guess you'd say it is stress and tension, to the extent that those words are adequate. You know the syndrome, the type. I'm not kidding you. You know about the medical research foundation's lipid research program. I went in there because I thought I'd be making a contribution. They wanted men in certain age brackets, middle-aged, with a certain kind of history and I said, "I fit. And if I can be useful, what have I got to lose?" It might take me half a day every other week or something like that. I already knew my cholesterol was low but I didn't know anything about my triglycerides, which I found out was 84 which was extremely low and which alarmed me. So I got with my old buddy at the medical school, the one who later recommended the heart surgeon, and I said, "What the hell are triglycerides and what does 84 mean?" And he said it means if you have that kind of a count, you're in good shape. So naturally, at that stage of the game I wasn't worrying about any coronary insufficiencies. I thought I had it made for as far down the road as anybody could see.

I thought of my father, who died of a massive coronary thrombosis, and if he were undergoing that today, he could live, but 20 years ago, that was so radical, I doubt that there were three men in the country who would even take a whack at it. I don't think even DeBakey was on the threshold of that sort of thing back then.

The cardiologist told me an interesting thing when we started to talk about coronary angiography. He told me that there are more big corporations than you'd think that require an arteriogram on the people they are eyeing for promotion to the top bracket or next to the top bracket. It's a condition of the promotion. Now that's as plastic and cold-blooded as anything I can imagine and yet it makes total sense. At first blush, it takes you aback a little, but it's hard to quarrel with a policy like that.

"When do you get to pilot your plane again?"

If ever, not sooner than two years from the date of the surgery. This is FAA regulations. I've researched it a little bit, and nobody has been able to bust that so far. And even then, I may have to submit to more angiography to prove to them that the bypasses are effective, which would be okay. I wouldn't fight them. But it's ironical. If I flew tomorrow, I'd be in better shape arterially than I probably ever was when I flew before.

But summing it all up, I've always been a little bit distrustful of the word "luck." I know that if you work 12 hours a day, seven days a week, you tend to get lucky. But I think in this case, boy, I've been lucky in a lot of ways. One, the fact that I got into a vigorous exercise program and was given a warning. Incidentally, while they had everything exposed, they had an opportunity to examine the heart muscle and there is no evidence of external damage, so any damage which occurred is internal and therefore minimal. No scar tissue, which is gratifying and here, again, luck. Two, I was lucky I was in shape anatomically to be able to stand up to the surgery. In other words, I wasn't sick when I went in. I was healthy. I had that going for me. And three, I was lucky to be in this city where they have the kind of talent and facility I needed when my Type A behavior caught up with me.

41. Cardiac Arrest

This osteopathic physician is perhaps the luckiest man alive because, by pure happenstance, he was in the best possible place to receive prompt, professional attention when his heart suddenly stopped beating. He is one of the few people who have gone to the far edge of life and returned to this world.

He is a general practitioner, in his early 60's, soft spoken, dignified, capable. His office is across the street from the osteopathic hospital in a city of 600,000 in the Southwest. His wife, who is a registered nurse, works closely with him, making rounds of his hospital patients and assisting him in the office.

- **Heart Stoppage**
- **Cardiac Arrest**

It was a regular staff meeting. You know, all hospitals have a lot of problems with medical records. Ours had gotten into bad shape and the medical staff had asked me to take over medical records. In order to straighten things out, I was going to have to make a lot of doctors mad at me. They were taking the delinquent, incomplete records out to work on them and losing them and this and that. I had written a directive of three or four pages and was presenting it at that staff meeting.

Of course, it worries you. Doctors are kind of prima donnas, in a way, and I was worried and upset when I went in there because I knew I was going to have to tell them. That was really what I think triggered it.

"Had you had cardiovascular problems previously?"

Yeah, I had rheumatic fever when I was a kid, irregular heart rate, so I had lived with it for years. While the doctors were sitting there talking about the directive I had written, they started bitchin' and raising Cain; they weren't going to do this and they weren't going to do that. I noticed myself going into a ventricular fibrillation. I know the symptoms. My heart felt like it was beating up in my shoulder rather than where it is supposed to be. I was not really dizzy but I had a little chest pain. I started to get up to go out and take a nitroglycerin pill. One of the doctors next to me asked me if I was okay and I said I was. Then I fell about that far *(indicates that he had not completely risen from his chair).* The rest of it, they can tell you more about than I can. That's about the gist of the whole thing. I had classic cardiac arrest.

I'd carried nitroglycerin all of the time but I hardly ever had to take it. I had occasional angina, usually with emotional upsets. I found I could work pretty hard, still can, but you get me in an emotional situation and that will trigger them quicker than anything else. I stay out of those situations now.

When I regained consciousness, I was laying on the floor. They had put in a tracheal tube and had shocked me five times, I guess; I think the defibrillator was setting right in the room. That's where they stored it. The anesthesiologist and all of the specialists were there.

I don't know precisely how long I was unconscious. That is a part I haven't delved into. I didn't especially want to get into it. They say it was about 30 minutes.

I woke up before they realized it. Of course, I realized what had happened when I woke up but I couldn't talk because of the tracheal tube. They were trying to put a pacemaker into the femoral area (they had already tried putting one in from the shoulder). My bladder was completely full. I don't know how it got that way in such a short time but that is the way it felt. And they were leaning on it. My first interest was to try to get them off my bladder and the only way I could do it was through sign language because of the tracheal tube and they had the big breathing machine on me so I couldn't talk. When they saw me move, a big shout went up, "He's all right. He's alive." There must have been 20 or 30 doctors around me.

I never did get them to understand to get off my bladder but they did get the pacemaker threaded up through the femoral artery to where they thought they had it in the right spot in the heart. Then they picked me up, took me to x-ray and did an x-ray to see about the placement of the pacemaker. While I was there, they decided I was breathing on my own so they could take out the tracheal tube.

Then they rushed me into intensive care and hooked me up to the monitors. They were going to put a catheter in to relieve the urine but I didn't want that and told them not to so they let me get along without it. I was able to pass the urine all right but it was pretty hard to get going after it got that much involved.

The rest of it was really just care. They gave me Valium to settle me down and a solution of xylocaine to keep down the irritability of the heart. I didn't feel like I especially needed the Valium. They kept me down completely for three days before they allowed me to get up. They put me on Pronestyl which knocks out the extra beats, the irregularity. It's good medicine but if it's used over a period of years, it sometimes brings on a lupus-like syndrome which causes trouble.

When they first gave it to me, it was high dosage which agreed with me. I could tell that my heart rate was improved. For the first time in a long time, it was so I couldn't feel my own heart beat. Most of my life I have been able to feel my own heart beat, due to what, I don't know. I could practically count it most of the time. Most people can't do that. But because of that, I knew what my heart was doing more than most people ever do. I had the irregularity and extra systole. I've worked over the years with what's called a "by jimeny," where every other beat is an extra systole. It didn't cause pain; it was just a nuisance. I compensated all right with it over a long period of years. I think this was direct result of the rheumatic heart disease I had when I was a child. It was a severe case; my knees were swollen up and I couldn't walk for six or eight months. I was probably eight or ten years old. I'm 60 now. I was 58 when this episode happened.

Any severe emotional thing made my condition worse. Drinking too much would have an effect on it. If I had too many drinks, or more drinks than I ought to or just a few drinks some times, I'd notice that had an effect on it so I'd never drink too much. But primarily it was a tense emotional situation which would bring about these episodes.

When I was in the intensive care unit, they had me on the monitor, hooked up with the beeper. They cut the beeper off first, thinking that would help, but the monitor probably worried me more than it did me good. It gave them some information, but I've always felt like it is a good possibility that the monitors may do more harm than they do good. Where a patient is apprehensive. I don't really feel that I was apprehensive, but I was questioning the way they were doing it compared to the way I would do it. I didn't want the pacemaker taking over my heartbeat and running it when I felt it would do pretty good by itself if they'd just leave it alone. I thought they should have left the pacemaker set low enough so that if my heart rate dropped off, it would take over. I thought that it should have been handled that way. Instead, they were running the pacemaker at a set rate above what my heart rate would be. I was being paced instead of my heart doing its own job. I wasn't antsy about it except the fact that I've seen a pacemaker hit on a "T" wave and kill a patient. So I don't have all that much confidence that a pacemaker is the best, because I've seen it have trouble.

"How long was the pacemaker in your heart?"

Two weeks. I was in intensive care six days and then in a private room but still hooked up to a monitor for the remainder of the time I was in the hospital. They took the pacemaker out four or five days after they put it in but they had me on the monitor for two weeks. That's the way it was. They put a cardiac monitor on me with chest wall leads and kept track of that in the intensive care unit. The monitor was some distance away and when the leads would slip, which they always do, the nurses would come in, thinking something had happened to me. When the doctors took me off the monitor, they didn't tell the intensive care nurses they were going to do it and they came tearing in, thinking something had happened to me. When he took it off, it registered a straight line on the monitor and they thought something had happened, altogether I looked to them like I had died. And that was the doctor's fault. He should have notified the nurses what he was going to do. It wasn't important as far as my care was concerned, but it was pretty important from the nurses' standpoint.

It takes a long time to get back your strength. I took off a month and a half, didn't do any work. An intern came over and ran my office. After that time, I gradually got back into it, reregulating my life to see patients only in the mornings. Before, I had seen patients all day and then gone to the hospital for rounds. Now, I make rounds in the afternoon, but it has gradually gotten back to where I see almost as many patients in the morning, in three or four hours, as I used to see all day.

I wanted to continue with my job as head of the medical records committee and maybe as a result of what happened to me at the staff meeting, the doctors did do a lot better. One of the main culprits in the medical record situation was one of the doctors who had done me the most good. I had to kick him off the staff three or four times before he got straightened out. We are good friends but he was one of the worst offenders in the chart business. He manned the defibrillator when I had my episode, took care of the whole works really and was probably the most important one there. But I don't think that one person could have done everything, the way it happened. Somebody had to get the tracheal tube in pretty quick and someone had to do cardiac massage until they could get going. They broke about three ribs in the process but that is to be expected. And then they had to put in the pacemaker. And evidently, they had quite a bit of trouble because they had to shock me five times, which is a little unusual. So one person didn't do it. There was two internists there and the anesthesiologist who was good at getting the endotracheal tube in, breathing you and taking care of your biorespiratory problems. I was just really lucky it happened with the team I needed right on hand.

There have been some articles in medical journals lately about what happened to people who supposedly died, or whatever you want to call it, and were revived. You would expect a person to be real fearful but there is a peaceful feeling which you just don't have under ordinary circumstances. It was the most peaceful feeling at that time which you could have. I was not worried or apprehensive at all after I came to.

At some time during the period that I was unconscious, I knew I was laying there on the floor. I can remember it now, just as if I was conscious. I knew I was laying on the floor but to me, there was no one around me. There was no noise. I was laying there holding a box, which was maybe a foot wide, eighteen inches long and about a foot high. It was light, as though it had air in it, so I'm sure it was not because someone was pressing on my chest. It doesn't make sense but that is the part I remember. And the peacefulness of it all. That's the other thing.

I was holding this box and looking at it. I am color blind, but the way I would describe it, it was a dark tan and it had lines down the sides as if you would put a piece of tape over the center of it and run it all of the way down the sides from both ends. And it wasn't tape; it was as though it was all one piece. And it was shiny.

"Do you have any idea what was in the box?"

No. It was so light, like holding a balloon. It wasn't heavy at all. It was weird and it is the only thing that kind of worries me, afterward. It is hard to make sense of it, why it happened that way. You wonder what in the world it meant. If that box contained my good points, I sure didn't have many to carry with me. If it was my sins, I think I got it wrong. It was awfully light.

I don't believe the feeling of peace I experienced had anything to do with knowing that all those doctors were there taking care of me. I didn't think about what was happening or what was going to happen, one way or the other. It was just a serenity, a feeling of peace, and no worries, period. I wasn't worried about what they were doing except I wanted them to get off my bladder.

When you go through something like this, though, everybody is afraid you are going to die on them the next minute. It takes them a long time to get over that.

I've had less chest pain since the episode than before. I took the Pronestyl for about a year and because of the lupus-like syndrome, I was sure it was causing me problems so I dropped myself off of that and started on Inderal. They both do the same thing and Inderal agreed with me better. I still take it, in a little less dose than they advised me to, and I'm taking a lot less Valium than they had me on at first. I really cut it down because it was causing more trouble than it was worth and I didn't need it for the nervous upshot of it. I still take a small dose each day.

Thinking of the Valium, I wound up with a messed up sleep pattern. It is not because of emotion or anything but somehow, I can't sleep for a full night. For a long time, I'd wake up at three o'clock in the morning and I'd just as well get up because I couldn't sleep. I would be wide awake. It seemed like I didn't need the sleep. So I'd get up, read, write letters or listen to tapes or whatnot. And that has pretty well continued. Now I don't get sleepy before two a.m. and I get up by eight and I feel rested, just as though I'd slept as much as anyone else. A lot of times I'll get sleepy in the afternoon and take a couple of hours nap.

I also had vision problems. It wasn't double vision. It was flashing light images to the side or any place. And lines, as though I were looking through an ophthalmoscope grid.

I still have some heartbeat irregularity but it is pretty well controlled. I can't hear my heart beat as well as I used to because of the medicine. The medicine quiets down the beat to where I'm not conscious of it. If my heart gets to where I can hear it, I know I need a little medicine.

I have more trouble with memory now, not with medicine or dosages or diagnostic work or anything like that, but I'll forget a whole lot quicker than I used to. I don't think I've had any other mental deterioration except memory. It could be aging, but there was definite change quicker than you would expect as a result of aging.

I don't worry about things like I used to. When I know I have a real problem patient, I'll refer that patient to a specialist where before I would take care of him myself. The biggest part of your worry comes from the hospital work. I'd like to get out of taking care of hospital patients altogether and just do office practice. I went on the associate staff so I wouldn't have to go to meetings and be on committees. Up until that time, I was on all the committees, mortality, records, tissue, infection, the credentials committee; I was head of that one. I don't go to staff meetings any more because they turn out to be a big argument in a lot of cases. You know doctors.

There are other feelings of uncertainty. You sometimes feel that more things have changed with you than you realize yourself.

I sure would like to know what was in that box.

> *To preserve a man alive in the midst of so many chances and hostilities, is as great a miracle as to create him.*
>
> Jeremy Taylor
> *The Rule and Exercise of Holy Dying,*
> (1651), 1

42. Heart Attack

When a person suffers a heart attack, it is not unusual to hear his friends remark, "Well, I'm not surprised." Some people seem to be heart-attack prone, their compulsive behavior heralding what appears to be an inevitable event. But other people have heart attacks despite their laid-back lifestyle, their relative youth and other apparent contraindications. This man is one of those. He is a slim, soft-spoken, unexcitable, married man, only 42 years old — not the kind of person you would classify as the cardiovascular type. He is college educated, holds a well-paying, non-pressure government position. Of course, it is not possible to know what private stresses may have contributed to his medical problem.

- **Heart Attack**
- **Myocardial Infarction**
- **Bypass Surgery**

I was at my office at the time I first had a heart attack.

"How old were you?"

Forty-two. I was going through a complete physical checkup at the time. I really had not felt any pain or any one particular thing, it had just been a long time since I'd had a complete physical checkup, and for some reason, I felt the need to have a physical checkup of this nature. I had already gone through my electrocardiogram and some of the tests and was preparing for other tests later.

The first attack I had was very mild. I was talking on the phone at the time and I felt a pain hit my left arm, go up my arm and across my chest and down the right arm. It felt as if a bee had stung the marrow of the bone. It built up in intensity very similar to a bee sting and I was thinking to myself as I was talking on the phone, if this continues or gets any worse, I'm just going to have to hang up this phone and lie on the floor. But it went away. It eased back off and I felt normal again.

It felt as if the bone marrow itself was hurting. It went across the chest, possibly a little bit larger area at the center beneath the sternum and then down the right arm. The left and the right arm hurt equally. And the chest did also with the exception of the widening-out portion in the middle.

At any rate, I went on home and didn't think a lot about it, but as I was going home I sort of sensed or felt like maybe that was a light heart attack. But then I thought, well, it couldn't be because I just got through having an electrocardiogram and my heart sounded great. My EKG came out just fine.

It happened to be my son's birthday and we had given him a stereo for his car. After dinner, I mentioned to my wife, I said, "If I weren't going through a physical at the present time and if I hadn't had an electrocardiogram less than a week ago, I'd have thought I had light heart attack at the office today."

"How long did the pain last?"

Probably not over two minutes, because I was on the phone. It wasn't very long.

I think my wife said, "Oh" in passing or maybe it worried her a little bit, I don't really know. But I proceeded to help my son put the stereo in his car. I was in the back portion of the car, using a skil-saw, sawing a hole for the back speaker when I had the same thing happen again. Only this time, about eleven o'clock — the first one was shortly before five — it came on hard. It wasn't a build-up like before, like a bee sting. It still felt like a bee sting, all right, but there wasn't any build-up. It came on strong and hit clear across the chest, down both arms again, and a bit nauseating this time. So I let go of the saw and told my son I'd have to quit for the night. I'd had it.

Again, subconsciously, I knew what was happening. I knew I was having a heart attack. There wasn't any extremely fast pulse other than the adrenalin I was beginning to turn loose about that time, I'm sure, but I didn't have any other indications. I'd never had anyone tell me what to expect. I guess it depends on the type of heart attack you have as to what type of pain you may feel. Some people describe it like a heavy sack, a weight put on your chest. I didn't feel this. I felt only the sharpness of the pain up both arms and across the chest.

I went inside the house. My wife had gone upstairs to bed. I tried to communicate with her without climbing the stairs but I couldn't, so I climbed the steps and by the time I got to the top, I was on my knees.

I said, "Call the doctor. I'm having a heart attack." She ran into the bedroom to call the doctor and told me to get Don, our son, to drive me to the hospital and she would follow. That way the doctor would have a jump on us and we wouldn't have to wait 'til he got to the hospital. It was our family doctor, a general practitioner, but, unbeknownst to me, he wasn't in. I don't know how she got the doctor who took the call because he wasn't the one who usually takes our family doctor's calls when he's away. I think he was at the hospital then.

Then came a time of panic. Don was still working on the car. I felt like I was not going to make it to the car. I was sort of staggering and trying to get it across to my son that I was having a heart attack and I needed to get to the hospital. My younger son was there, too, and it seemed like it took forever to explain to people what was happening.

We have two dogs, a large collie and a small dog, a mixture. Both dogs followed me out to the car, jumped up into my lap and it was a real show trying to get them off of me and the door closed. The dogs apparently sensed that there was something going on wrong. The boys were trying to get the dogs off of me and they were still trying to get back in through the windows.

Then we made a scramble for the hospital, which took perhaps 10 minutes and all I could say was, "I'm hurting. I'm hurting." We came to a railroad crossing on the way and just as we got there, the crossbars were coming down. We could see that the train was quite some distance down the track so I told my son to go around the crossbars; there's a way to go around one and then around the other, to go right on through.

When we got to the hospital, with my wife having the presence of mind to call ahead, they were ready. They had a wheel chair out and were waiting for me. When they were wheeling me into the emergency room, the nausea which I'd felt earlier returned and even more so, and I was upchucking as we went along. It's silly but I was apologizing, "I'm sorry. I'm sorry." And they told me, "Don't worry about that."

They lifted me up onto an examining table and began to work on me immediately. I couldn't help but think at the time — strange and crazy things go through your mind at a time like that — as I looked up into the faces of some very young people, in their early 20's, I thought how efficient they are. There were four or five people working on me at once, putting I.V.'s in both arms, hooking me up to an electrocardiogram, giving me a shot of morphine.

The pain really didn't intensify. It reached a maximum when it first started and stayed there. I don't know that it ever got any worse or any better. The one shot of morphine didn't have much effect.

I couldn't tell whether the doctor was there or not. All I could see was faces. I was looking straight up and only those people looking down on me could I see. It seemed to me quite some time before I actually talked with the doctor. The attendants kept asking me how I was doing and I kept telling them I still hurt just as I did when I first came in the emergency room. They gave me another shot of morphine.

By that time, the doctor who apparently was there had read the electrocardiogram and came up to the side of the table. "Well, you've had one, all right," he told me. "By the description of your pain and from the electrocardiogram, it's more likely to be the lower, backside of your heart. If you had to have one, that's the best place to have it." That was some comfort, anyway. He said he thought I'd be just fine and sent me off to the cardiac intensive care unit.

The pain still had not let up, even with the second shot, but just about the time I got back to the CCU, the pain did begin to ease.

This was in a way a religious experience, too. I don't mean by that there was any feeling of, or seeing anything or hallucinating, or voices speaking. But you do have a feeling of closeness to your Maker because you are laying there, looking straight up. There's nothing you can do. It's too late for any great deeds that are going to help you at all. The only thing that goes through your mind is "Forgive me for whatever I've done before." You're sort of released, you let go and let your Maker have his way. There's nothing much to worry about. It's not a frightening experience; it wasn't for me, past that point. There's just no need for fright. It's useless. You just feel a waste to be frightened. Before then I was frightened that I wouldn't make it to the hospital. It was such a relief upon arriving before I was completely gone and was finally in the hands of others.

My stay in the hospital was a little over a month and six weeks at home after that. I was in the cardiac unit a little over a week. Then they put me into a room and I developed premature cardiac vacillations, or whatever it's called, and they put me back in the CCU for three days. I was so glad, in a way, that those happened one time while I was in a hospital because I'd had those all my life and didn't know what I was having. Premature cardiac vacillations means that the heart is beating or is "firing off" before it fills. In other words, it's pumping empty. It pumps two times in a row real quick then there's a delay there. Feels like it skips a beat but it really doesn't do that.

"Can you feel that?"

Oh, yes. It feels like, I'd always described it as being like a flopping fish in there. Up until this time, every time I had an attack like this, it would go away before I could get to the doctor. When I explained to them about it, none of them ever really gave me any satisfaction about what was going on. I had thought these were little heart attacks, but they weren't. But, believe me, they're frightening. They are more frightening than the heart attack. I still have them occasionally and they are still more frightening than a heart attack. It's an electrical problem of some sort, as I understand it. If it's shorting out like that, in firing, it could completely quit. In cardiac arrest, that's exactly what happens.

I went to visit a sister of mine while recuperating because there was less family strain that way. I could be away for while. There is a lot of family strain in our home and I don't know if this could have contributed to my condition — I doubt that it could — but definitely during recuperation you try to avoid all types of strain. I had complete quiet during the daytime because my sister works. I was there six weeks.

My family doctor monitored my blood pressure from time to time. He was in the hospital at the time I had the PCV's or premature cardiac vacillations and had to put me on some medicine to keep them from recurring.

After it's all over and you begin to feel good again, you feel that it didn't happen. You think, "I'm well again." I never really had thought I had a disease. It never occurred to me that having a heart attack was a disease or that there could be anything wrong other than a clot, or something. In fact, I'd had a toe operated on a month earlier which the surgeon thought was going to be nothing more than a nerve at the top of the foot, but when he got in there, it was actually a blood clotting situation in the vein and I thought, "Well, gee, this is probably what eventually caused the heart attack. He didn't get all of the clot out and it gradually worked up and that was probably what hit my heart." This was my own rationale and I figured the coumarin I was taking would keep the blood clotting down and I wouldn't have any more problems. It didn't occur to me that I had any disease.

It was by sheer accident that the doctor who met me at the hospital was a cardiologist. He was not the one who usually took our family doctor's calls. He only worked with me the first 72 hours and by then my own family doctor took over.

After the six weeks recuperation, I went back to work part-time and gradually increased it until, in about two weeks, I was working full-time.

On one of the routine visits to my family doctor, we were discussing my condition in general and he said, "Let's face it. You've got a coronary artery disease of some sort." Until that time, the word "disease" had never entered my mind. My doctor felt it would be good if I went to a coronary artery specialist and recommended one.

The fear was back. I thought that if I had some kind of disease it might be getting worse all of the time. In fact, the doctor implied it wouldn't get any better and I should see a specialist and get something done. My family doctor made the appointment for me.

The specialist did a preliminary examination and then suggested that I have angiograms of the heart itself so he could tell where there was clogging, where there was narrowing of the arteries. He suggested we do this as soon as possible and he also ran a complete blood test, maybe 40 different things controlled by your blood, a blood chemistry. He did inform me that I didn't have a cholesterol problem, that was within normal limits, but I did have a triglyceride problem. That's an intake problem. Cholesterol is made by the body itself but apparently triglycerides depend on what you eat.

"Did the doctor restrict your intake of alcohol."

I asked that question of my family doctor. He had me on Valium at the time which is a tranquilizer and said that if I was going out and going to be drinking, to knock off the Valium and let the alcohol be the depressant.

You really grasp at the things which are encouraging and anything that intimates you've really got something wrong with you, you grab onto that, too, so you have two hands full of straw.

Because I had a triglyceride problem, I thought, "Gee, this is great because at least I can control my intake, where if it had been a cholesterol problem I couldn't control that because the body itself makes cholesterol."

The arteriogram was the most interesting of all my experiences because they don't put you under an anesthetic to do it. They need you to be able to move at command. I remember lying there watching the doctor prep the artery in my arm, a "roto-rooter" operation.

"Was this a cardiac catheterization?"

Yes. He ran the catheter up my right arm across the chest to the heart itself. I really didn't realize that this would be such a difficult task for the doctor. After he cut that artery, he was trying to keep the bleeding down but every now and then, he'd get a squirt of blood on him and he was sweating and I thought, "My goodness, I didn't realize a doctor had to work like that."

He ran the catheter through and watched on a fluoroscope, I guess, as it went into each of the little branches and then every so often he flips that up and pushes something else and rocks you way up on your side and takes some movie pictures, x-rays.

I got tired of watching him because he was working so hard and I felt sorry for him so I lay back and looked straight ahead. All of a sudden I had one big pain, from my toes to the top of my head to the tip of my fingers. Everything hurt at once, just one solid pain. Just about the time the pain hit me, a man at my head said, "His blood pressure's dropped to zero." The doctor jerked back the catheter just a moment because I didn't have any blood pressure at all for a moment. I must have been in total shock but I didn't know it would be painful.

I had one or two more experiences during the catheterization that came close to that same pain, just sort of the starting of it. The catheter must have been going through some narrow spots. There's no pain with the catheter; you feel nothing going up except when it came to the bend at my arm, but when it got around the curve, there was no more pain. That really didn't hurt very bad, just a little pain.

Just as he was about to get it into the heart — he's still sweating and working — he told the nurse, "Get another catheter ready. This one's about wore out." And I thought, "Oh, boy, he's going to pull that one out and start all over." But it went on in.

He advised me ahead of time and showed me movies of what was going to happen. So I pretty well knew what to expect, everything except that blood pressure drop. I don't think the doctor expected that either. The movies explained that you would feel hot when the dye was released and how you would feel. He again advised me when he was ready to release the dye that I would feel a sudden flush of heat and it was just exactly as he told me. This was a very interesting experience, moreso than the bypass, because I was fully awake, fully conscious and able to communicate. It was an alerting experience because I was very much interested in what was going on.

I stayed in the hospital overnight and the doctor came in the next morning to consult with me. That was almost as though he had pronounced a death sentence on me. He drew little pictures of the heart itself and showed me that the artery to the left side of the heart was plugged up so far down that the capillary portion that bypasses on that side would not be of any benefit at all and he doubted that the right side bypasses would be productive. He said I should be seen by a cardiac surgeon and he'd make the arrangements.

From there, I went home, very much discouraged, really feeling that it was just a matter of time 'til they closed up completely and that would be it.

I got a call from the surgeon's office. He wanted to talk with me. This was a week after the cardiac catheterization. I went on in and my wife went with me. He explained the bypass method to us, what he thought he could do and what he didn't think he could do. He agreed fully with the cardiologist that the left-hand side of the heart was so clogged that he didn't think a bypass would do any good. But he said that on the right side there were two or three places where he could lay in those bypasses. Here there was some, but not nearly as much capillary damage.

I asked him what happens to the left-hand side of the heart. It gets worse and worse and worse and goes out of business, but he explained to me, "I've kept many a person alive for many years to pretty old ages with the left-hand side just lying there quivering. If I can keep the right side going strong, you'll be all right but I never know until I get in there how they're going to lay. After I get in there, I may change my mind again as to how I can get around some of the obstruction, even though I had the x-ray pictures ahead of time. The picture is one thing but the actual heart is another."

This was rather encouraging. He said the sooner the better because people have a tendency to put these things off, maybe get a little fearful of it because we will have to stop your heart, stop your breathing and put you on a heart-lung machine. We'll take veins out of your legs, out of the thigh on the back of your leg, and by reversing it, use it as an artery in your heart. I'd never stopped to think before that a vein would have to be reversed. It has flaps that keep the blood going in one direction. The vein has them going one way so you have to turn it around to make a vein function as an artery.

So we set this operation up for a month later, not long enough for me to worry too much about it. But then the doctor had to be away so the only time it could be rescheduled was a month and a half after that.

I reported into the hospital. He'd given me the choice of three hospitals. At first I said to do it any place but this one hospital, because the last time

I'd been there, for the cardiac cath, the room I had was sort of ratty and just wide enough for the bed. They were going through a remodeling program. And then I thought, "Well, how silly can you get? The room that I'm in after the operation really doesn't make that much difference." So I said, "Where do you work the best? That's more important than the room." Then he told me about two of the hospitals. "In both of those, I know where to kick the heart-lung machine when it quits working. Then there's a new one at Memorial Hospital. I haven't had a chance to use it but we could do it there if you'd want to." I told him I wanted to go where he knew the right place to kick the machine and start it up again if it quits.

I forgot to mention the difficulty getting blood for this. They have to have 10 pints of blood that match in more ways than just type. They have to match some other things that I don't know about. Generally speaking, it takes twice as many people as you need pints of blood. I had to rustle up the people to give blood: friends, people where I work and so on. Here is something which was embarrassing. I live about 20 miles away from the blood bank and several came from where my wife works and friends from around home and were completely refused, turned away because they had a cold, or were underweight or something. Of course, I was glad in a way that they were refused if their blood would have been wrong for me, but I thought to myself it was like someone offering you money. If they offer you blood and they're capable of giving it, you should go ahead and take it. You don't have to tell them you can't take it for this patient because they are there out of generosity, kindness of heart, or what have you. It could be used for plasma, or "straight-stick operations" or something of that nature. It was rather embarrassing for us to have people come that distance and then be refused.

The only thing I had a fear of, and I've had that fear all my life, is anesthetics. I've never been knocked out or fainted or been unconscious other than going to sleep, which I guess is the same, but I have a real fear of being given an anesthetic of any sort. I resist shots and fight off sleep like crazy. You remember they had to give me two shots of morphine at the hospital when I had my heart attack. I had full confidence in the doctor that he could perform the operation. I'd seen the scars of operations he'd performed on people so I was quite confident in the operation being successful but I was very fearful of the anesthetic. I voiced this with the surgeon ahead of time. I asked who the anesthesiologist would be. I'd met the surgeon and his assistants and the cardiologist and all but I didn't know, had never met the one who was going to put me to sleep. I didn't like the idea of being put to sleep by someone I'd never seen. So the surgeon said he'd have the anesthesiologist come up and talk with me before I went to surgery.

I was afraid that they might have to give me more anesthesia than normal because I'd fight it off and then when it came time to start that old ticker up again that it wouldn't go. That was the only fear that I had and I kept waiting and waiting for the anesthesiologist to come and see me. He didn't come the night before the operation but I slept well anyway and the next morning, I was still wondering where the anesthesiologist was. The boy came up and prepped me for the operation, they gave me the pre-op shot and started down to the operating room with me and I thought, "Gee, where is that guy? I'm not going into that operating room until I've seen him." But I was also thinking, "I don't have a whole lot of choice, strapped down on this stretcher and all."

Everyone was dressed alike and with the sheets being loose as they are, it was hard to tell males from females. They wheeled me down into a waiting room and I noticed that there were four people ahead of me. Then there were a bunch of people on the other side, about 15 people altogether. I thought I'd have to wait until the four people ahead of me were operated on but figured that wasn't so bad because I could have been fifteenth in line, waiting for the operating room. These other people were lying there chatting. Around the corner came this doctor, all suited up, his mask up and all, who came over to me where I lay and announced his name — I can't remember his name even now although I wrote to him afterwards and told him how clever and slick he was — and he dropped the mask he had on and I saw he had a full-blown beard. It was way down and then he reached up and took his cap off and he had long hair down to his shoulders. In a humorous sort of way, I thought, "Oh, no, don't tell me Christ has come after me before I even get in there." He looked like the pictures of Christ that you see. He was a very gentle person, a very clever one. He said, "I hear you have a fear of the anesthetics we'll be using." And I said, "You're right. That's the thing I'm really afraid of." I began to tell him that I was resistant to various things but I don't think he was paying much attention to me. He stopped me and said, "I'll probably be using sodium pentothal just to put you out with. That will keep you under and we'll be using various gases and things but I'll barely keep you under. I'll watch your fingers and if they go to moving too much or if you go to talking, I'll give you a little more, but I'll barely keep you under. So you really don't have to worry about an overdose and when we get ready to start your heart again, it'll start." That was good enough for me. All I had to have was that verbal reassurance. Then, he upped his mask and donned his cap and wheeled me on in, which was a surprise to me because of the four people ahead of me.

He stopped in the little hallway before we got in the operating room. "There's only one thing. You've had intravenous feedings before. I have to do the same thing in there but I can't put the needle in your arm, it has to go in the back of your hand and it's pretty big." He showed it to me. It look like a golf tee to me. It was about three inches long and as big around as a golf tee and plastic. He said, "I'll have to put this in and shove it up with the heel of my hand and it'll hurt a little bit." So he proceeded to do that, in my left hand, and I told him, "You're right. That hurts."

He was so clever to lay down two orange syringes on a pillow at my feet which I just knew was the sodium pentothal. I'm watching this like a hawk. They were crossed over, like Wilkinson's swords. Then he put the other needle in my other hand and wheeled me in, under the light. Of course, I was looking up and there were three lights. I always thought there were only two. He said if you stop to think about it, with three lights the surgeon's hands will never be in shadow.

I'm still eyeballing those needles because I want to know when I'm going to go out. I'm looking up at the light and all of a sudden there aren't any lights. Out. I never felt a rustle of cloth. No one touched me anywhere, no one touched the sheet I had over me, or my skin or any portion of my body. All of a sudden, I wasn't there. Instead of slowly blacking out, in fact, it wasn't black, it was gray. The room was suddenly grayed out. It didn't come in from the side, there was no time lag. It was just now I'm here, and now I'm gone. It was just that quick. No count down or anything like that. Now, how he got to me, I don't know. Maybe it was in those things he put in the back of my hand but if it was, it took a long time to work. I don't know how he did it and still don't know.

From there on, I don't know much, anything in fact 'til after the operation. Then we were circled up like wagons, all of us on carts. Those of us who'd had similar operations and had to be on respirators — is that what you call them? — that do the breathing for you. There was a nurse on the inside of the circle and a nurse on the outside of the circle, going around watching lights. I had been prepared for this by a doctor friend of mine. Nobody taking care of me had mentioned that I would be on one of these respirator machines but my friend had told me so I was not surprised when I woke up and found I had a tube down my throat and was hooked onto this machine.

But I think I had a psychological problem with the tube down my throat, primarily because of what my friend had said. He said that his felt like it was down too far and he had an awful time getting the nurse to get it up. So, I'm sure that's what caused my problem. I thought mine was down too far, too. My hands were strapped down but I could move them enough to get the nurse over. I would motion and she thought I was wanting it out. I motioned upward with my fingers as best I could with my wrist strapped down. She said, "Oh, no, we can't take it out. See those little lights? This machine does most of your breathing for you. When that light becomes green and stays green long enough, then we'll take it out." There was nothing I could do because she wasn't understanding. Then I motioned that I wanted to write and she brought a pad up. "This one thinks he wants to write" she said. She was right and I was wrong. I couldn't any more write than the man in the moon. My thinking was clear but my fingers wouldn't work. I could tell I was just scratching so I put the pencil down. Then I measured a small distance between my thumb and forefinger and also motioned upward, with an "out" movement of my finger. "Oh, you want it part way out. It's down too far." So she took hold of the tube and adjusted it and I was satisfied.

You stay in there long enough on that machine that by the time they put you in your room, you are really fully conscious. I felt like I was fully conscious when I first woke up but I'm sure I must not have been. When I got back to my room, even though I'd been through a heart attack, I had never before been hooked up to so many things as I was this time. Both arms had intravenous tubes running into them. One had the whole blood and also something else coming in and a little bitty joint below that, all three of them feeding into me. The other arm had just the regular, clear-looking stuff, saline, I guess. I was also hooked up to all of the monitoring equipment, the wires across the chest, an irrigation tube in the area where the doctor had done his work and I was catheterized. I had a tube in most every orifice plus two extra holes.

Then they arranged for visitors so my wife could come in. I said, "Oh, for heaven's sake, don't bring her in with me looking like this, it'll frighten her to death. I look like nothing but a manikin with all of these wires and tubes coming from me." They said they would tell her so she would know what to expect. She came in but later she said she did have a reaction to seeing me like that; she felt faint.

I was only there in that portion of the hospital about three days. Now, the only things that bothered me were two things. First, there was the irrigation tube. Every now and then the nurse would have to wriggle it back and forth to keep it from clogging. I kept telling her, "I think he's sewed it to the bottom of my heart and every time you pull on it, you pull on my heart and it hurts." The other problem was that I was required to cough. This was very funny when it was happening to someone else and very painful when it was happening to you. They'd have you breathe very deeply with the Bird *(positive pressure breathing)* machine, and afterwards, they would have you cough. And they wouldn't be satisfied until you coughed up something. So you had to try as hard as you could. I didn't know what to expect the first time because the nurse didn't say it was going to hurt. I let out a big cough and you literally yell because of the pain. Oh, man, it hurt. The most painful part of the whole thing is the cough.

The coughing we would have to do to try to prevent any build-up on the bottom of the lungs was painful when you were doing it, hilarious when someone else was doing it. Laughing hurt as bad as coughing. I was in intensive care at the time, so that's how I knew what was going on with the other patients. You could hear them, one by one, doing their coughing. They'd cough and scream, cough and scream. It was hilarious.

After three days there, the doctor came in and took out the irrigation tube, released me from all of the machines and I was taken to a private room. I'd requested a private room as a result of the experience in the hospital when I had my heart attack. I was in a semiprivate room then and I got to worrying so much over the other patient and trying to play doctor myself with him, so that after a while, my doctor put me in a private room where I wouldn't bother people. I was analyzing their condition and all, but I don't think it was bothering me as much as it was the other person.

I was only in the hospital six days after the bypass surgery. The doctor told me it would be a week to 10 days but it was not quite a week. They won't let you out of the hospital when you are discharged unless you ride in one of those wheeled chairs, but I could have walked just as well. I was walking up and down the halls of the hospital before I was discharged.

"Did the surgeon tell you the rate of blood flow through your bypass?"

I didn't know they could measure it other than do another angiogram where they can watch the flow of the blood.

"They have instruments now that can measure it."

Hmm. That's great. I'd like to know what mine is. I still may be fooling myself. I have the suspicion that I may be fooling myself, that maybe this bypass operation isn't all that great, you know. Subliminally, all the time I'm thinking maybe I'm just fooling myself. It didn't work all that well and I probably wouldn't have been a lot different with or without it.

But I feel great. I wouldn't take anything for this total experience, wouldn't trade it with anyone. This will sound stupid, I'm sure, but it was one of the best things that happened to me in my whole life, having the heart attack, having the angiogram and having the bypass. It did several things for me in other ways. It brought back what I would consider for myself, not necessarily for others, a new system of values. Many things which I had been overlooking for years now have a great deal of meaning for me. Life itself has more meaning for me, each day, each breath. Things which I had taken for granted for so many years are important; in fact, I find that they are some of the most important. It really doesn't matter whether a job gets done, or you're late or you're on time because if you don't take each breath, who cares? You're always one breath or one heart beat away from extinction.

"How does your family feel about it? How did they react?"

Well, to that one statement, I just made a reaction that is strictly from weird. And I agree, it probably does sound weird. But I think theirs is probably guarded concern. I know that the children's attitude has changed a great deal. I feel like I'm treated like a glass doll. There's still a lot of tension in the home but the fightin' days are over. In other words, there are no big fusses any more, very seldom angry words. I notice these changes and to me they're for the better. At the same time, I worry that maybe people don't have the outlets they once had. They have to hold it down because of the old man because if I do become emotionally upset, it does seem to precipitate these doggone PCV's.

"Do you still have them since the surgery?"

Oh, yes. I don't know exactly what causes this premature triggering of the heartbeat. The doctors give me medications, one to control the insulin output a bit and one which controls the adrenalin output. Apparently, nothing they did in surgery affects the PCV problem I have.

"Did the doctors give you a prognosis?"

After the operation, very little was said about this. Before the operation, I asked the classic question, "Well, what are my chances?" And he mentioned that across the country there was about a five-percent loss, which the surgeon said wasn't bad because there is a 2.5-percent loss with a simple gall bladder operation. But he said also, if it happens to be you lying there dead on the table when I'm working on you, it's a hundred-percent loss.

After the operation was over, I don't know that I got a prognosis in the sense that I was okay now.

"Did you expect that or ask for it?"

No. I asked at one time and I can't remember whether it was before or after the operation, "What can I expect after the operation, five years, 10 years or what?" He said that if in ten years or so these bypasses clog up and don't work, we could go back in and redo them, so this gave me confidence.

"Did the surgeon prescribe any changes in your lifestyle which might reduce the congestion or clogging of your arteries?"

Not the surgeon. After he took the stitches out, he more or less dismissed me back to the cardiologist. But the cardiologist has never given me any indication as to how well I'm doing. This interview has made me wonder what those bypass flow levels are now. I'll ask him when I go back this fall. He's given me a four-month break before I have to go back and see him. But I'm beginning to be curious why they haven't done another blood check of all these things.

Because the cardiologist didn't do much more than listen to me after the operation. I sorta get suspicious that I might not be okay but there isn't much they can do. I've noticed that I've become more paranoid concerning my health since this happened, particularly relating to the heart. I think maybe they know something I don't and they're not telling me.

But all in all, it has worked out the way I thought it should. By having talked with friends who had had this operation, I pretty well knew what to expect. I was entirely covered by insurance, with the exception of $127 difference in the room rate, so I didn't even have any financial surprises.

> *Of all the ailments which may blow out life's little candle, heart disease is the chief.*
>
> William Boyd (1885–)
> *Pathology for the Surgeon*

XIV.
Inside Story

Certainly it is by their signs and symptoms, that internal diseases are revealed to the physician. But daily observation shows that there is no uniform and invariable relationship between the extent and intensity of diseases, and its external signs. The prominency, the number, and the combination of these depend upon many circumstances beside the disease with which they are connected.

Elisha Bartlett (1804–1855)
Philosophy of Medical Science, Pt. II, Ch. 12

43. Diabetes

The judge. He is a tall, craggy-faced, brown-haired attorney who came from a small Midwestern town to the capital city to run for high political office in state government. Although he was unsuccessful in that attempt, he has never lost a campaign for district judge. He is an astute observer of human behavior, both from the bench and as a practitioner of politics. He is a Democrat, loves boats and fishing, lives in a new home in a development in the far-suburban fringe, miles from the courthouse.

- **Thirst**
- **Blurred Vision**
- **Urinary Urgency**
- **Diabetes**

I guess I was sick for a year before I knew I had diabetes. It came on when I was about 45, five years ago and I had a classic case but it was a long time before I knew what was happening to me.

I'd get terrifically thirsty and wasn't able to satisfy my thirst. I could be watching television, get up and drink a glass of water and be thirsty again before I sat down. And, of course, this meant that I had to go to the bathroom all of the time, which was embarrassing, but what was worse was that I couldn't hold it. When the urge to urinate hit me, I knew I had about a minute to get to the bathroom. Ordinarily, you can hold it, you can wait, but not when you've got diabetes. This wasn't too bad at home or at work but it could be a problem when I was downtown. I'll bet I've been in every bathroom in every store downtown.

Then I began to have blurred vision. One time when we were driving down to a football game my eyes began to blur and I couldn't read the billboards along the way. And when we got there I was unable to make out the numbers on the players' jerseys and you know how big they are. I couldn't read the scoreboard.

This prompted me to see an ophthalmologist but because this condition of blurred vision came and went, and I could see all right when I was in the doctor's office, he couldn't find anything wrong and, for some reason or other, he didn't think about the possibility that I might have diabetes and, of course, I didn't either.

Well, I kept getting worse. I had no energy, I was tired all of the time and I kept losing weight. Ordinarily, I'd weigh about 210, sometimes as much as 225 or 30, but I kept losing weight.

My memory started failing me. I found out later and, of course, I know now that lack of sugar in the brain affects your memory. I was run down. I had no energy whatsoever.

My wife and I went to a dance one evening with my doctor and his wife, who are our close personal friends although I hadn't seen him for a long time. I don't go to the doctor just because I feel bad. I think whatever is making me feel bad is going to go away. I've always thought that.

I don't even know why I did it; I just accidentally started telling him about these strange things that were happening to me. My doctor just took one look at me and said, "You be in my office Monday morning." I could tell by the way he said it that he knew what was wrong with me. He did. He told me later he knew then but he wanted to run some tests before he said I had it. He didn't want to jump the gun.

So I went ahead and took the tests and he told me to call him back. In a day or so, when I called him back, he said, "I have some bad news for you. The tests confirmed everything I thought. You have diabetes." I told him to go to hell, he didn't know what he was talking about, I didn't have diabetes and hung up on him. I didn't want to accept the fact that I had it because I knew diabetes was a pretty serious disease.

Anyway, I got to talking to him about it some more and he brought me into his office and told me about what diabetes was. He even told me a bunch of things about myself which I hadn't told him; about my memory; I hadn't mentioned that to him.

I accepted it then. I guess I accepted it when he told me the first time and I told him to go to hell. He's a very kind doctor. He told me then that there are different ways of handling it. He did a lot of explaining, which I appreciated. He explained the difference between the childhood thing and if you get it when you're over 40. He talked about the way the pancreas secretes insulin and gave me some things that I could understand.

He wasn't sure at that time what we were going to have to do. He said he was going to try to control it with Orinase, a medicine you take orally, a capsule, but it's not insulin, of course. Insulin you can't take orally. This is one of the big bugaboos about this disease. If you have to take insulin, you have to take it in a shot.

Now I take insulin but then he said some people can control the disease with diet, some with diet and exercise and others with these oral medicines they use to stimulate your own pancreas to secrete insulin.

We tried that for a year. I was determined that I wasn't going to take a shot. Shots don't bother me but for some reason or other, I just didn't want to give myself a shot.

So I took this stuff for a year and kept going down hill, down hill. I remember I drove back from a trip, maybe a hundred miles, and I sat down on the couch about midnight when we got home and I told my wife, "This is the end of the line. I can't get off this couch." I thought I was dying. I just couldn't move and told my wife, "This is the end right here. I'm on this couch for good." She called the doctor and then loaded me into the car and took me to the hospital.

"Were you in a diabetic coma?"

I think I was pretty close. I said I wouldn't go to the hospital but when you're at the point that you think you're going to die, you take a different look at it.

He said something that really amazed me. It was two o'clock in the morning and I was so sick I couldn't hold my head up. He said, "We're going to start you on insulin now and by morning, you'll be wanting to go home. That's how much effect this insulin will have on you." And, sure enough, it's true.

I had to stay in the hospital a week to "get regulated," so they could see how much insulin I needed and how I reacted to it. Once I got on insulin, it's really no problem. I take a shot in the leg once a day, every morning. It's not the shot now, at all. In fact, I have to take one disposable needle and the bottle to the bathroom because it's now so routine that I might not even remember that I took it unless the used needle is gone. Then, I know I've had my shot. And you can't take two shots.

The hardest part of insulin, if your diabetes is under control, is the regimentation. You see, I've never been a regimented person in my whole life, even though I was in the Army. But to have to eat three meals at about the same time every day drives me crazy. It still does.

At noon, I have to stop whatever I'm doing, whether it's work or play, and go eat. If I'm at work, I have to recess the court. By 12:30, I have to be somewhere that I can eat. And I have to do the same thing at supper, no matter what's going on. I have to or otherwise I'd go into insulin shock.

Diabetes has some drawbacks but you can live with it, especially if you have a good doctor who knows what he's doing and will communicate with you what's wrong with you, what you have to do and why, you see? That's one of the biggest problems because so many people won't regiment themselves and live by it. A lot of this has to do with the doctor. So many doctors don't tell you anything. They won't give you an answer. Sometimes it's because they don't know and there's not hardly a damn doctor in the whole world that knows those words, "I don't know." They'll give you an answer whether they know or not. I don't know how I could have handled this if I hadn't had a real good doctor.

But he takes good care of me and I watch myself pretty close but I lead a pretty regular life. I scuba dive, I do all kinds of things. But I can't drink whiskey.

Now, my doctor told me that I could fool myself if I wanted to. For a good 20 years, I'd have a drink when I came home in the evening. I'd sit down and have a scotch and water before supper and always enjoyed it. But he told me, and I believed him, that there is no way you can control diabetes using insulin and drink whiskey, too. I accepted that and quit right then.

Oh, you can take off so many units of food for lunch and so many for supper and save up the units to have one drink. But if you do that, (I tried that one time, after a year or two) and you have one drink after you haven't had any for a year, it just tastes terrible, it tastes like hell. It just isn't worth it. So I tried it about twice in five years and gave it up.

When you first go on insulin, they put you in the hospital. Of course, they put me in because I was so sick, but they also have to find out how much insulin is needed to control your diabetes. People are different, and there is no way for the doctor to know if you need 50 units, or 60 units, or 70 units, you see. They can't give you a shot of insulin and turn you loose because you might go into insulin shock. They also have to train you to give the shots to yourself.

The hospital had a very fine dietitian. She worked with my wife on this business of food units for my diet, what I had to eat. And she explained all about the diet to me and it made a lot of sense.

When I go to the doctor and a nurse comes in and takes my blood pressure, I want her to tell me what it is. A lot of them act like they don't want to tell you and that's crazy. It's my blood pressure. It's not hers.

My doctor is a personal friend so maybe I have an advantage that way. I'm not just a patient, I'm a personal friend, too, so I think we have a better rapport. I was very fortunate. I don't know how you would pick a doctor out of the yellow pages.

This is the only serious illness I've ever had. I've always been a very vigorous person, healthy and strong as a bull all my life. But I never have gotten my strength back and my doctor says I never will gain it all back. I used to weigh 210 but now I weigh 180; have for 5 years. Right before I went to the hospital I had dropped to 150 pounds. When the doctor put me on insulin, I started gaining, went back up to 180 and have stayed there ever since. I haven't varied half a pound in five years.

Before I had diabetes, I used to be a really big eater, used to like to eat but now I just don't care to eat. It's just not an attractive thing the way it used to be. The only time I'm hungry is when my insulin is high.

You have to watch it with diabetes, you know, because you are susceptible to other things that come along. You can have heart trouble, so my doctor gives me a cardiogram twice a year. Diabetes can affect your circulation and make things slow to heal. When I cut myself, it's very slow to heal.

During the four years I've been taking insulin, I passed out only one time. That was on Easter Sunday. I had laid down to take a nap and the family was there and they were late getting dinner on at noon. I woke up, got off the couch and walked in the kitchen. That's the last thing I remember. Apparently, I just passed out cold.

My brother-in-law caught me or I would have fallen. They laid me on the floor and gave me this special shot I can take under such circumstances.

The shot is a high concentration of sugar, which they put in the muscle. I was in insulin shock.

That was the only time I actually passed out but I've come close at times. Sometimes it sneaks up on you. First thing you notice is that you get a little nervous. Your hand starts to tremble a little bit. I can feel it. Oh, I know it. It's just as recognizable as anything in the world. I can recognize it immediately, but sometimes from the point that you recognize it 'til it starts really taking ahold of you, it can be a few minutes or it can come on real fast. Once I was driving down the boulevard, on a Sunday, and it came on me. I didn't have any candy available because I wasn't in my car; I always carry some sugar in my car.

I pulled into the curb. I had to get off the street because I could pass out just any minute, see. I was sitting there, about to pass out and I looked up. There was a grocery store that was open, a little grocery store, not any bigger than this living room. There was a lady in there and I thought if I can just get inside that grocery store I can get me something. I got inside and I was just at the point of passing out so I sat down on the floor in front of the counter because I didn't want to fall. I knew I was passing out. I said, "Lady, give me some candy." She went over and got me a Coke and two Hershey bars and gave them to me. I ate them and in a few minutes, I was fine. I said, "Lady, you sure got 'em to me quick." And she said, "My boss has got diabetes and I knew exactly what was wrong with you when you walked in here."

I have to watch it real closely. My kids never eat Snickers. I keep around Snickers for medicine. Any other candy bar, they'll eat it but they never touch my Snickers bars, which I leave laying around the house.

When I scuba dive — you just can't afford to pass out then — I take some sugar before I do it. That way I don't have an insulin reaction.

As I said before, I've got a damn fine doctor, who takes time with me. The thing you've got to understand about having diabetes or some other condition like this, if you can't communicate and you can't understand your disease, then you don't have any confidence in the medical help you are getting. The better the doctor explains to you, the better position you're in to abide by what he wants you to do. Especially with someone like me. I was a lawyer for 23 years before I became a judge. I deal every day with reason and logic and I can't accept someone saying, "Here, take this," or "Here, do this." I want to know why.

The better you can relate with the doctor and the people who are trying to help you, the better you can do. But some of them don't want to tell you. They want to make a big mystery out of it, for some reason or other.

If you don't get up some relationship with your doctor, then you can't tell him what's wrong with you. There are lots of feelings that are hard to put into words, especially if you've never had the feeling before. I had to explain things to my doctor which were a brand new experience to me, and I had nothing to compare it to. So if you can't communicate back and forth, and explain to him what's bothering you, how can he help you? It works both ways. If the communication is only from you to some stone face who won't communicate with you, it's bad. That's the reason having my doctor as a personal friend is such an advantage. I can tell him in plain old words what's wrong with me, where I hurt.

A lot of confidence and respect for doctors is lost because of lack of communication. Doctors are human. They can make mistakes even though some of 'em don't think so. If you can go to your doctor and say, "I don't think you did this right." and he can say, "Well, gosh, I believe you are right. Let's fix it," from the legal standpoint, I think you'd probably have a lot less malpractice suits. People don't sue Dr. Welby. Not Marcus. Of course, there ain't no doctors like Marcus Welby, not many anyway. But they wouldn't sue him. Not lovable Dr. Welby.

My Blue Cross policy covered my expense when I was in the hospital for a week. Now I have a group insurance policy through the state, that all the judges have. And it's a mess. Oh, it's a mess. They don't want to cover anything. They pay only parts of it. I just had a $130 bill on my wife the other day. I think they're going to pay $60 of it after all the yo-yo back and forth.

You *always* have to hassle with 'em. The only one I didn't have to hassle with is Blue Cross-Blue Shield. The other policies, it's always something with them. This isn't covered or that isn't covered. I'm a judge and I've been a lawyer, but it takes a Philadelphia lawyer to read an insurance policy, you know. Ordinarily, lawyers can't read an insurance policy. And the insurance companies are always looking for an out They want your money, but when you've got a claim, they're always looking for an out. It's always a hassle to get them to pay.

You buy the policy, see, and you don't know what all these medical and surgical procedures are. They may give $60 for a procedure but when you have it done to you, you find there's no doctor in town who does it for $60. It's a $180 procedure. You have no way of knowing what doctors charge so you think you're covered. Well, you're not at all.

We try a lot of cases in court involving medical bills. A lot of people say they can't get by the doctor's receptionist or his nurse to tell the doctor what's wrong. You've got to tell them what's wrong and then they'll tell the doctor and then they will call you back to tell what the doctor said. These people will tell you, "We never even got to talk to the doctor." Of course, I know judges who do the same thing, shield themselves from the lawyers who want to see them. I don't do that, but some judges do, so it doesn't apply just to doctors.

The biggest cryin' shame in this country — and I'm not soap boxin' — is that people who have good doctors are the ones who live in metropolitan areas. The doctors won't live in small towns, and there's a lot of good professional people in other fields in small towns. We have got to figure out some way to get the folks outside the metropolitan areas some decent medical care. I'm philosophizing now, of course, not talking about myself but the people in some of these little towns have no health service whatsoever.

Of course, I grew up in a town which is now about 40,000 people and there are some good doctors there. Even there, though, when it gets dead-dog serious they'll send you to the city. But they at least know enough to do it. For example, I know of one of the top ophthalmologists in my home town — everybody over there thinks he is — but he sends his patients who have something serious to a doctor here in the city. But the people in town think he's a top man, see. He doesn't attempt to do some things. He knows where to send them. So I guess he's pretty smart, at that.

The judge's wife is not usually accorded appropriate notice when she is first introduced by her given and last name. But when the introducer adds, "She is Judge Zachary's wife, you know," people go, "Oh, yes." and their faces light up with the glow of recognition.

But she is not the self-effacing shadow of the judge; she is her own person, affable, outgoing, capable. Affectionately known as the "Ad. Ass." (for administrative assistant) in the clinic where she works, she is half-Cherokee and fiercely proud of her native-American heritage. She is 40, has grey hair and the figure of a ballet dancer, which she once was.

• Diabetes: The Wife's Story

I really knew he was ill before he did. I could tell because his color was very bad and his energy was very low. You can tell by looking. It's like taking one of your children to the pediatrician and saying, "He doesn't look right to me," and he didn't. I knew he was ill.

"Did Frank know that you knew?"

No. Matter of fact, he began to drink so much water that I thought perhaps he was dieting on the water diet and not telling me that's what he was doing. He also began to lose weight. And his color was very bad.

Regardless of the symptoms I noticed, you can't live with someone and not know or pick up on the fact that they're not entirely well. So when he went to the doctor and the doctor told him he had diabetes, it was a relief to me and it was no surprise. I had suspected it might be worse, that he might have cancer or something else very seriously wrong with him, so when I heard that he had diabetes, he was very depressed but I was very relieved because I knew it was a controllable thing. I knew he could live a long, full life and have no problems. At that time, I had no idea what it entailed. I only knew it was a controllable thing.

In fact, the first meeting with the doctor after the diagnosis was made, he asked us both to come by. He talked to us about an hour and discussed the diet very extensively with me. I understood it completely and I did read the books on it. It seemed to me a terrible task, to regulate a person's intake to that degree.

At that time, the doctor had him on a weight-gaining diet; he'd lost 50 pounds. He had a big breakfast, mid-morning fruit juice, a big lunch, mid-afternoon snack, dinner and a sandwich at bedtime. I didn't fix all of those meals. I fixed breakfast but I had to send with him to the office the little fruit juices you can carry and things for his mid-morning and mid-afternoon snacks. Of course, I was reponsible for his dinner and his evening snack.

The doctor told me at the time that within a two-year period I'd be an expert on diabetes and it would be an absolute way of life. I didn't believe him. I thought I would always have that book in my hand, figuring grams and weights. I had to calculate everything. The book had the diets written out showing what would be proper, like a half a cup of peas, two ounces of meat, two starches, which would mean potatoes and corn, or bread. There's a certain amount of fat that goes with it, too.

I had to prepare a balanced diet and also dole out the right portions, and total it up to be sure he got the right amount by the end of the day. If he were short on something at the end of the day, he'd have to have a sandwich and a piece of fruit or whatever he was short on. The total day's calories had to add up to exactly what the doctor said he should have in every category, so much meat, so much fat.

I learned a tremendous amount because bacon for breakfast, for instance, is a fat. You'd think that was meat and although I'd had nutrition in school, I'd never really thought too much about it. So I had to learn first what categories foods fall into, in order to make up a balanced diet.

For a while, our meals were really very boring. We ate just about the same thing every day because that was the easiest way to calculate, you know. He still does eat pretty much the same thing for lunch every day; hamburger, french fries and a glass of tea.

One of the hard things about a diabetes diet is you cannot fix a casserole dish because there is no way to measure how much meat or noodles or other things. And it's very expensive. You have to have meat, vegetable, a couple of starches and fresh fruit — obviously, no sweets — every meal. You can't use leftovers. Those things are all out the window.

"Are you on a two-level system at your house? Do the kids eat anything they want?"

No. Everybody eats the same. When they put Frank on insulin when he was so very ill and he was in the hospital eight or 10 days, I had a meeting with the hospital dietitian every afternoon in Frank's room. She was a lady who had been helpful, much more so than the doctor who did not prepare meals and didn't know how to go about it. He could tell me what I needed but he couldn't tell me the nitty-gritty of how to do it. She was tremendously helpful to me.

She worked out about 20 menus for me and it was her advice that the whole family has to be on the diet. It's just too much trouble to fix two separate meals for the rest of your life. Oh, I do use some leftovers. If I have a leftover roast and make hash from it, I pick out enough meat and enough potatoes for Frank to eat like the rest of the family. If we have spaghetti and meatballs, I can put enough meatballs on his plate to make four ounces and measure the spaghetti, to a point. Or if we have leftover chicken and I make chicken pot pie, I can save a piece of the breast of the right amount for him.

"I can see why his weight hasn't varied a half a pound either way."

Well, his food is measured very accurately. The good thing is that I now can eyeball measure everything. I could put a half cup of peas on your plate and not miss it two peas.

The doctor was right. It does become a way of life with you. I serve my whole family from the stove. I served the same volume of food to everyone until it got to the point that my teenagers were so terribly slender. I have a teenage boy who is five-feet, ten-inches and weighs 120 pounds. My 11-year-old daughter is about five-five and weighs 90 pounds. However, my pediatrician tells me they are the healthiest kids he sees, much healthier than the overweight children. And they have absolutely no complexion problems. I do occasionally keep a cake for them, we usually don't have pie, and they have pop if they want it because their intake of sugar is so low.

Yes, there are side benefits. I'm a tremendously healthy person from the diet, my three teenagers have no complexion problems whatsoever and we have no weight problems. Everybody in the family is very slender.

If you're ever going to have a problem with your diabetes, it'll be when things are abnormal. As a rule, on the everyday average, I can manage very well. One of the hardest things is having the food there all of the time. You can't let your refrigerator get down to nothing. You can't go off on a car trip without a Coleman cooler, ice and sandwiches, candy bars and fruit. Food is with you everywhere you go. It has to be.

We own a boat and I'm never down there without food. The boaters we go with will run up to the restaurant and eat and never worry about food. It's the least of their worries. But me, I have to carry the cooler and food every place we go. If we go to a dance, I've got a couple of candy bars in my evening bag. You never know when their insulin is going to be up.

The only time we really had a problem, when Frank actually passed out, was on Easter Sunday. He'd been on insulin about a year. I got up and took the children to church, Sunday school. The whole family, my mother and dad and all of the aunts and uncles and their children were going to be at our house for Easter dinner. Frank had laid down on the sofa waiting for dinner to be served and had gone to sleep. It was about two o'clock and he hadn't had anything since breakfast. I got the food on the table, woke him up and he got in the buffet line. I looked up and he was just passing out. In the hospital, they had discussed with me the fact that Frank might pass out from insulin shock but they had not related to me what that would look like. I somehow thought he would slip into unconsciousness. I had no idea it would look like he was dying.

His eyes rolled up and everyone in the room, including me, thought he was dying. My brother-in-law caught him, I saw him as he was going and we laid him down. His face was simply white as a sheet and his eyes were rolled up but not shut. His hands were trembling.

I tried to get some orange juice down him but, of course, that just gagged him. They had given me an emergency shot to keep on hand to give him when he did this. They had also showed me how to use it on an orange, and that was fine in the hospital room with the orange but this was different when it was a person in an emergency situation. And I had to mix it. It was a powder and a liquid. I had to put the syringe in the liquid, inject into the powder, shake it up and then draw it back into the syringe. In the meantime, our daughters were trying to get the doctor on the telephone. Fortunately, we knew where he was, at another family gathering not very far away.

I got the shot mixed and the only place I could give it to him was the forearm because he was trembling and thrashing around so. So I gave it to him and pretty soon he came around. But he was very foggy and didn't remember anything that happened.

The people in the hospital had not prepared me for what happened. Now maybe they thought they had, but when they said he might lose consciousness, I had the idea he might slip into sleep. I'd never really pictured what that would look like. It scared me so badly that I couldn't function. I wouldn't have been so frightened if I hadn't thought he was dying on the kitchen floor with the whole family there.

My mother began throwing water on him and covering him up, alternately, so the first thing I had to do was fight her back so I could get to him with the shot. She was doing all of the first aid things. So I said next time this happens, the first thing to do is lock grandmother in the closet.

On Christmas morning most families have a light breakfast after they've opened their presents and have a nice, big meal about two o'clock in the afternoon. Those things are simply out for us. We have to get up and have breakfast, even though it is Christmas morning, before the present opening.

Frank's passing out on Easter with the whole family there was a dramatic experience so when we go to grandmother's for a holiday or any reason, she makes arrangements for him. If we are to have dinner at seven, there's cheese and crackers or something for Frank to begin eating at six. Everybody in the family, and the children, know that Dad has to eat at certain times.

When we go to mother's for the weekend, she has what he needs to eat, including Snickers. Snickers are medicine. He likes them and he figures that as long as you're going to have to eat something, it might as well be something you like.

It has been interesting to see how different people react to being married to a diabetic. Once you begin talking about your husband being diabetic, you meet many, many women whose husbands are. They react in various ways.

The R.N. who works for a doctor I see has a diabetic husband so if I get really stuck on something, I call her. She's an absolute expert on diet. Her husband has had diabetes for a long time.

There is no artificial sweetner that tastes like sugar. All of us have tried to fix desserts with it and it simply doesn't work. It's better to do without it completely. The dietetic foods are very expensive and now they have water-packed fruits, so I never buy any special dietetic foods. Dietetic ice creams are very fatty, so we just use regular ice cream, only one scoop. A lot of it has to do with quantity.

I fatten the children's diet up a bit so they get more calories. For instance, if I fix chicken and make cream gravy, the kids will have mashed potatoes and gravy but Frank won't eat any gravy.

A friend of ours is a brittle diabetic and one of the things . . .

"Brittle diabetic? What does that mean?"

That means that his pancreas secretes insulin at sporadic intervals. Frank's pancreas doesn't secrete anything, so the amount of insulin he gets in his daily shot is known and he is completely controlled. But a brittle diabetic will give himself an injection of insulin and sometime during the day his body may produce insulin, and at that time, his insulin will get too high. For a lot of brittle diabetics, this happens every single day.

They never know when it's going to happen and they're either on the sugar side or their insulin is up. They're never in control. And that's bad because a person whose insulin gets high gets nervous and they become very irritable. They say sarcastic things, you can even term them belligerent when their insulin gets high. The children can tell if their dad is very sharp with them. After a few minutes, when he has eaten something he'll be fine, he'll be Dad again.

"How long does it take for the sugar to change his mood?"

Not long at all. Hard candy, if you crunch it up with your teeth, works fast, in 15 or 20 minutes. At first, I would try to say to the children, "Dad's not feeling well," and I'd be in the middle. But I soon found that I can't be in the middle. They have to live with him, too.

For a brittle diabetic, this happens often, very often, and for our friends it was something they couldn't cope with. They had other marital problems but they did get a divorce.

Frank smokes more cigarettes and drinks more coffee now because that's his last stronghold in the vices. He can't have a drink. He substituted coffee for a beer or a drink after work. And, of course, he can't sit like you can in the evening and have a snack. He can't eat a package of Dorritos and a bucket of dip while watching television. He will get up and get an apple, but he does drink a lot more coffee and smokes more.

Other ladies who have diabetic husbands have gained weight, actually 20 or 30 pounds, as an empathetic thing. Your husband's weight is way down, he's on a weight-gain diet and you eat with him. I didn't keep up with Frank when he was gaining back his weight but now I keep down with him, so it has worked out fine for me.

When Frank got diabetes, we were on a sort of social whirl, where we went to cocktail parties, saw friends a lot. Now Frank can't stand cocktail parties and dances are a bore. It really changes your life.

"Why doesn't he like cocktail parties?"

Well, it's fine at the beginning but when everybody begins feeling their drinks, you see, things begin to deteriorate. The player piano begins to roll and people sing songs and he just isn't feeling that jolly. You have to stand around a long time and people aren't talking that coherently.

When we go to a dinner party, Frank has to have a sandwich before he goes. Of course, that takes the enjoyment out of it, because you go there to enjoy the food. Even when we go to a friend's house and they are aware that he is diabetic and needs to eat, you can't depend on them serving dinner at a particular time, it's usually nine o'clock or so. And you can't depend on hors d'oeuvres. They might not be enough.

But we avoid more of these affairs now or we go if we want to with the idea that if he gets tired, we'll leave. And this has been really a better way of life, I think. Frank will live to a ripe old age because he's very healthy, he exercises every day, doesn't drink and, of course, watches his diet.

I think our success has been because, in the beginning, the doctor told Frank he had to give himself his own insulin shot. A lot of doctors will have the wife give the shot and in some way that links you so closely with the diabetes. He is so attached to you, more so than he should be.

Some wives give their husbands insulin shots twice a day, and you can imagine how that hooks you up in order to have that happen. Frank will go to the lake by himself and stay four or five days so he's really independent. He can do for himself.

One of the female diabetics I have known is a model and she is just paper thin, reed thin, as models are, or ought to be. She regulates her own insulin which, to me, is like playing Russian roulette. If she's going to a cocktail party and wants to have a drink or two, she will up her insulin injection on her own. She is a brittle diabetic and she injects herself twice a day. Apparently, she's gotten it down where she has control of it but I can't see anyone regulating their own medication, up and down. Female diabetics have a harder time, strangely enough, because they regulate their own diet. They don't have someone to measure it out for them. And I think they have more trouble. The female diabetics I have known seem to be much less disciplined, yes. There is something about being responsible for someone else's health. In other words, I could mess up my health if I wanted to but I would not take the responsibility for ruining Frank's.

But I must say the responsibility rests rather lightly after a while. It gets to be a habit, having dinner at the right time and all. It's a way of life.

> *Man may be captain of his fate but he is also the victim of his blood sugar.*
>
> Wilfred G. Oakley (1905–)
> *Transactions of the Medical Society of London*   78:16, 1962

44. Gall Bladder Attack

A tall, grey-haired Virginian, he is in his middle 40's. An architect who received a graduate degree from one of the Ivy League schools, his planning responsibilities include the supervision of design and construction of buildings on the campus of a growing state university. He comes from a family of builders and thus has spent his entire lifetime immersed in his profession.

He is easy to be with, quiet and slow to express criticism but highly articulate when moved to do so. He likes dry martinis, history, good design. Every summer he spends two weeks as a soldier; his rank is major in the Army Reserve.

- **Pain in the Side**
- **Gall Bladder Attack**
- **Cholecystitis**

My sequence of events began on December 30 of last year. I remember that date because when the whole thing began to unfold, I realized that I wasn't going to go to a New Year's Eve party the following night. I found myself in the hospital instead.

That evening, December 30, I went to bed after a more or less normal evening at home and a normal evening meal. About two or 2:30 in the morning, I woke up with a very acute pain in my side, not only an acute pain but the feeling that there was a large, more or less solid mass in my right side above the belt line. The pain was so acute that when I became awake, it completely preoccupied my thoughts. My initial reaction was "I'm having an attack of appendicitis again." But I had had my appendix removed when I was 15 years old. The attack then, which led to the diagnosis of acute appendicitis, was of similar intensity of pain and slightly similar location in the body.

This time, below the rib cage, there was a very hard knot or lump. It was almost as though I had swallowed my fist. It was the size of a baseball or a small orange and it was very easy to put my hand on it. I tried to assume various positions in bed, or standing up, or walking around, or walking around bent over to relieve the intense pain. I finally found that by lying in bed on my left side and sort of suspending this hard mass in the space of the body cavity, I was as comfortable as I could get.

I spent a couple of hours walking around and sitting down and leaning over and applying pressure of the hands. I thought I must be having some very acute viral infection which involved the intestines. For a while, I thought it might be a violent attack of food poisoning.

Finally, when morning came, my wife awakened and began to ask what was going on. I said, "Well, I'm in very acute pain." I'd had a bowel movement but I had not thrown up. I'd sort of thought the intensity of the pain might lead to vomiting. My stomach was upset, but the vomiting didn't come. The pain remained as acute as any pain I'd ever had, with appendicitis or the acute phase of a viral infection. I've had things of that kind once or twice.

About nine o'clock, I made arrangements to meet my family physician at the hospital. It was over the weekend, as I recall, or at least it wasn't a regular work day. It was 10:30 when I met him. He had assumed from my description over the telephone that it probably involved the gall bladder. He made an examination and had me admitted to the hospital. I was sedated heavily.

The next morning, I was scheduled for a series of x-rays, which were accomplished. I'd been sedated to such an extent that I was no longer uncomfortable. I was just kind of out of it. I was floating.

That morning, they told me in order to take the kinds of x-rays they wanted to take, I couldn't eat. They started giving me some kind of pill that apparently tends to centralize in the gall bladder so the films they take will show what the situation is. The pills made me very ill and I found myself resenting the fact that I'd been left in the corridor on a stretcher to make the best of it. I tried to get across to the people that the drug I had been given was making me very sick and that I needed something to throw up in. This made a minimal, if any, impression on the staff of the x-ray department. I finally got up, after being told to be quiet and lie still, found a bathroom in the x-ray department and was quietly sick by myself for a little while. Then I got back on the stretcher.

What they were trying to do was to take a series of films over a period of time with maybe a 15 or 20-minute or half-hour break in between, so I spent three or four hours in the x-ray department.

Some lab work was being done concurrently so in the afternoon on New Year's Day, the day following the day I was admitted, a surgeon came to see me. My physician had told me earlier that he was pretty content that I had a defective gall bladder and in a brief, cryptic way indicated my need for surgery. I had some prior awareness of the surgeons in the community and I simply identified one that I thought would be acceptable to me and that one happened to be also in the mind of my G.P.

At any rate, the surgeon, when he visited me, seemed to convey the idea that the decision to have surgery had already been made and he was there to get the job done. My initial question to him was "Is there any other alternative?" His response was one of surprise or being caught off guard. We then discussed gall bladder attacks and after a while reached the conclusion that one of the alternatives certainly involved waiting through an initial attack and seeing if there were subsequent attacks and if so, at what frequency and what degree of severity. He left the scene, apparently having decided that my family physician and I should come to a further conclusion before his continued interest would be warranted.

I have a natural reservation about surgery but my real posture as a patient was one of not having information. I was being called upon to make a decision at a time when, first of all, I had no awareness of what the lab reports would show, if anything. My reservation personally was that, although my physician had indicated that my problem was a gall bladder problem, I was not sure that he had very much confirming evidence in terms of the x-rays and the lab work, since neither were available or at least had not been reported to me at that time. To put it succinctly and briefly, I had no data base. Very little information, a lot of supposition. And really, the supposition was a tendency to confirm the initial opinion expressed over the telephone before we'd ever reached the hospital.

In the late evening, my family doctor visited me and we discussed what the x-rays revealed. Apparently, my body functions were such that my body did not concentrate the dye material, or whatever it is that reveals the configuration of the gall bladder. The absence of the gall bladder dye tended to cast in doubt whether or not that was the central problem. I'm a little hazy on that point now but the lab work tended to show that the gall bladder, which had been malfunctioning the night before was, on a second test, functioning more or less normally. It was back on the track.

So this led us to conclude, at 8:30 in the evening, that I should be discharged from the hospital the following morning, since I expressed again strong reservations about having surgery. I asked to be discharged because I was no longer suffering from pain, because the very hard mass had dissipated. There was some superficial tenderness; there was some question about whether the cause of the problem was a flake, a partial stone, a chip or a small stone that had passed into the duct from the gall bladder, whether it was a transitory thing.

One of the things I haven't talked about at all is the kind of nursing care I received on the floor both times. I just have very good feelings about the quality of the professional staff in the community hospital in terms of their total . . . I'm not making a judgment about their professional capability so much as I am about their ability to deal with members of my family and with me and their response, the care with which they seemed to operate and the sensitivity with which they dealt with me as a patient. They dealt with me more as a person than a patient. For example, I had a medication problem that developed while I was in the hospital which led me to request a medication which the physician had not put into my chart and therefore they were not free to give me. They were reponsive about recognizing the problem, putting it in perspective and getting a good decision made.

The second admission was kind of a repeat of the first one. I was in 48 hours this time and most of that time was consumed doing parallel lab work. They gave me the dye, which I took orally at first, and they took a series of films and didn't get anything, so they had to give me a shot. The tablets I had to take the night before were very large; they were huge things and they didn't want me to drink anything so it was kind of like swallowing your thumb. And there were about 10 of them. And somehow I didn't have the capacity to ingest all of them within a half hour, so I was a minor problem for them on that score.

The surgeon did not make a second appearance so I guess my physician decided that before he went that route again, he'd like to have a firm commitment on my part that I was really inclined toward surgery. He's an individual who has a good sense of humor but it doesn't go very far when he's in the middle of a professional discussion. At any rate, without talking about it nearly as much as we did the first time, we kind of agreed the second time that I was not a candidate for surgery and that if I were going to have surgery that it would be scheduled for a time after I left the hospital. That was 10 weeks ago and I've now gone that long without any reoccurrence or any symptoms. On the second occasion, I guess the physician decided that a follow-up visit would not be a productive use of his time, so at the moment, I guess in his terms, I'm kind of in limbo, waiting for the bomb to go off again.

If I were to engage in kind of a "post mortem," I would feel that I was treated very well as a patient by the people in the hospital. I have a very high regard for my own physician's opinion and I think he's probably tried to speculate on the future course of events as they apply to me and tried to give me a fairly clear picture of what I can expect over a period of time. I also recognize that I have what I will characterize as a natural reservation to being involved in surgery unless I very clearly believe that it is the only good option open to me. I don't believe I'm neurotic or paranoid about having surgery; I've had two prior operations. I think there are some risks to having surgery and I personally would like to be convinced it is necessary and at the present time I'm not convinced. I think there is a chance that there's another solution. I'm aware that there is some unnecessary surgery performed and that gall bladders are a high-risk candidate.

The other thing that struck me, though, was that the community hospital was an unknown quantity when I was admitted there and I have good feelings about the way the hospital is administered and the way the people who work in it care. The caring is obvious, it's not just a superficial thing but an indication of professional dedication.

Subsequently, I talked with the dean of medicine, who is a personal friend and in almost a casual way he inquired about me and I expressed to him my interest in knowing something more about the general parameters of the problem that I was confronted with. He indicated to me that, without knowing the background or details of my case, there were certain kinds of normative data that indicated that the great majority, perhaps 90 percent of those who have surgery to remove the gall bladder, do very well postoperatively. Perhaps something in the range of five or six percent of the remainder have very minimal problems but have some continuing situations which seemed to reflect a lack of total resolution of the problem by the surgical procedure. Then an even smaller group, three percent or so, have some reoccurrence of symptoms and one percent have serious postoperative problems.

I asked him how you could have symptoms when the gall bladder was gone and he explained that there is a parallel to a pseudo-pregnancy, in which some conditions exist, in terms of the way the patient feels, that tend to be the same symptoms that led him to have his gall bladder removed in the first place. And yet he continues to have these symptoms, tending to indicate that maybe the problem has another origin or that there may be a psychosomatic component, I don't know. He really wasn't very explicit about this but this wasn't my central concern. My concern was to ascertain whether or not having one's gall bladder removed was a safe thing to do. The question is what is the function of the gall bladder and if it is removed, are there any accompanying problems. For example, does one have to be concerned about diet? The gall bladder has a function, presumably, and can the body accommodate to the removal of the gall bladder? It was in this context that he discussed the fact that the great majority of people are able to make a fairly easy accommodation. Because of the nature of the typical person's diet, the function of the gall bladder is incidentally involved and the body can adapt if it is removed.

After the first event, I was visited by a hospital dietitian who explained in her terms the nature of the problem and the things I ought to do for a period of time. The essence of this was to reduce fat intake for a period of time, for apparently the gall bladder's contribution to body function is greatest when a lot of greasy, fat or fried foods are ingested in a short period of time. So french fried potatoes, salad dressing and things that are heavy in cooking oils are the enemy of the gall bladder. But in discussing this with me, she said that there's a difference of opinion as to whether exercising this kind of dietary restraint really has anything to do with remaining comfortable.

So I followed the diet recommendations for about three or four weeks fairly carefully and have paid a lot less attention to them during the last 20 weeks, after the second episode. The drug therapy, though, I followed that through to the last tablet and the end of the prescription. I was on the broad-spectrum antibiotic 10 days the first time and 10 days or two weeks the second time.

At this point, I have a sense that I may very well have another attack, but I'm comfortable with the decision not to have surgery. Maybe I've avoided what will turn out to be inevitable. But at no time in this whole thing have I been told by anyone that there was a confirmation of the fact that my gall bladder was really not functioning. There were some short periods of time that it wasn't functioning reasonably, but the five tests done to ascertain gall bladder function, two of them taken when I was in an acute sort of condition, both indicated there was some sort of problem but three of them taken later indicated that my gall bladder was functioning in a reasonable way. Business as usual.

45. Hypoglycemia

The doctor is a blue-eyed redhead, slim, white-skinned, attractive. She is svelte now but not too long ago tended to be pudgy. Her hairdo has been updated, too.

A devotee of Weight Watchers, she avers that Americans are a nation of nutritional illiterates. She is working out a six-month rotation before beginning a straight internship in pathology at a 550-bed, church-sponsored hospital in a medium-sized Midwestern city. She is divorced, has one child, belongs to a liberal church.

- **Low Blood Sugar**
- **Hypoglycemia**

I was hospitalized four months ago for exhaustion. I didn't know what was wrong with me. That was when I was finishing up my senior year in medical school. My psychiatrist admitted me; we didn't know if there was anything physically wrong with me. I'd been tired for so long that all of the symptoms of weakness I had been having I just attributed to fatigue.

When I was admitted, the routine blood studies found that my blood sugar was low. Consequently, they did a five-hour glucose tolerance test which showed, in the third hour, that my blood sugar was 39. Hypoglycemia is determined below 60 and people will get symptoms below 60, so at 39, that was very low. I noted that on one or two mornings during the original hospitalization they took a fasting blood sugar which was 55. I commented that, "I feel this bad every morning." It wasn't unusual to feel this bad so it started explaining a few things to discover that my blood sugar was this low.

"Is a fasting blood sugar similar to a glucose tolerance test?"

In the fasting blood sugar, you just take the test before you have eaten. In the glucose tolerance test, you do not eat after midnight the night before. You get a fasting blood sugar initially. Then they give you a glucose load, it's about 100 or 150 grams of sugar, and they see how your body responds to it. In the test they gave me, they just measured the glucose curve, to see what your blood sugar does. In the third hour, my blood sugar went down to 39, the hypoglycemic state, and then it came back up. In the early part of the test, the first and second hours, the highest it ever got was 112. Normally, in a pre-diabetic, it will go over 160 in the first hour. So, there were still some questions. It was kind of an abnormal glucose tolerance test. At that time, they were diagnosing it as reactive hypoglycemia, which means pre-diabetic hypoglycemia due to abnormal insulin secretion. However, after I read further — in fact I just did a talk on this yesterday — I learned that usually it will go over 160 if it's pre-diabetic. In my case it didn't.

There are many kinds of hypoglycemia so the next step is to diagnose what kind. One of the reasons that you do the glucose tolerance test is to see if you have pre-diabetic hypoglycemia because it has a characteristic and they did not do the insulin levels. They decided, since there are six different categories of hypoglycemia, there are certain processes they need to rule out.

One is an insulinoma, a tumor which produces insulin. Ninety percent of them are benign. They are very rare, to begin with, as a cause of hypoglycemia. It's a rare tumor, but to rule that out you have to do a 72-hour fast, drawing blood every six hours up to 72 hours or until the hypoglycemic state occurs. In that test, only 50 percent of them are diagnosed. An additional test called the tolbutamide test, which is a dangerous test to do, will finish diagnosing up to 90 percent of these tumors. What it does is stimulate the pancreas to secrete insulin in a fasting state so you get an increased response. It is still being considered in my case to finish the studies for an insulinoma, but whether I have that or not, I'm still hypoglycemic, whether it's pre-diabetic or what.

Of course, it was helpful to know, after I was diagnosed, why I had been feeling so bad for so long. I was in the hospital for 10 days and came out with the diagnosis of hypoglycemia. As to the cause, that's still undetermined but it is most probably pre-diabetic.

The treatment for hypoglycemics is dietary management and weight loss if they are overweight but that wasn't the case with me. I am on a six feeding a day, high protein, low carbohydrate diet. The standard hypoglycemic diet I was given in the hospital was a 120 gram carbohydrate diet which is three breads, three fruits and three glasses of milk per day spaced over a six feeding span. There are usually three main carbohydrate feedings with two carbohydrate points. A glass of milk is one carbohydrate point. In between the three main feedings, you have three small feedings with one carbohydrate point. And you don't exceed that.

The timing is very important. You try to space the feedings three to four hours apart. Since I've had two tests now, and one showed the hypoglycemic state at three hours and one at four hours, the critical point for me is not over three hours.

"What does a hypoglycemic episode feel like?"

Usually, it's very gradual in its onset and you really don't notice it. Usually, you start getting into what I call trouble before you realize you are in one. There are two components of it; one is the central nervous system effect and the other is the hyper-epinephrine effect. Your brain functions totally on blood sugar so when you start getting symptoms from the central nervous system effect you begin getting blurring of the vision, decreased consciousness, weakness, you'll get confused, you'll have difficulty articulating, you'll have difficulty remembering things, you'll lose coordination. It's all very gradual and progressing. It's just kind of like falling off a hill. You don't notice it until all of a sudden, you realize you are really confused. You've already gone over and you are in trouble. That's why you become a clock-watcher.

I'll get up in the morning and eat my breakfast at six and then I know I've got three hours before I have to eat again. Now, I'm on a good routine and you have to do that. You have to be on a schedule from the time you get up and eat your breakfast until the time you go to bed.

That's the central nervous sytem effect, which can be very severe. You can go from a slight sense of confusion to total inability. There have been times when people ask me, "What did you do that for?" and I couldn't tell them. People in this state have been confused with being drunk. In fact, some of my episodes have been more severe than have ever been documented by my blood sugar. Anyway, people have watched me when I have been in the hypoglycemic state and I staggered. I can now tell when my coordination is going. I have to walk very deliberately, think very concentratedly in order to put one foot before the other and walk in a straight line. Sometimes I catch myself falling.

I catch myself holding on to walls. I have to concentrate hard just to pick up a form and move it. Also, there is a period in which you become almost hysterical when you get extremely hypoglycemic. Then, of course, you get into a depressed emotional state during the whole time. You have continued depression, as though you were depressing your brain. It has nothing to work on.

The second type of symptoms are the epinephrine responses because the body has a mechanism of increasing blood sugar by kicking out epinephrine or adrenalin. Okay, so when that happens you may get into an anxiety state because adrenalin causes increased anxiety. It causes vaso-constriction, blood vessel constriction, so it will cause extreme pallor.

"Does that also increase the heart rate?"

Yes. People can get into tachycardias. One thing I notice myself when I'm trying to decide if I'm hypoglycemic or not; I'll look in the mirror and if I'm blanched white, I know good and well. I used to think, "Susan, you are lookin' awful sick," and I even tried to increase the color of my make-up because I was going around pale all of the time. Now, I know. My color can change very rapidly because the epinephrine response can be very rapid.

In addition to this, your normal bowel system works on the parasympathetic nervous sytem. When adrenalin takes over, it opposes and does not have the normal bowel pattern. The musculature does not contract normally so often times in a severe episode, you will have severe abdominal cramping. That means, for me, that my colon will go into extreme spasm. I've had times when I've just missed a feeding, or gone over a feeding. Two weeks ago I was 30 minutes late with a feeding. Even after eating and continuing to have regular feedings the rest of the day, I had a severe spasm and it lasted 10 hours. My body never did get quite regulated the rest of the day.

"What happens during the night, when you are sleeping for eight hours?"

In the third or fourth hour after not eating, I go into the hypoglycemic phase. In the fourth or fifth hour, that's when the epinephrine response comes in to increase the blood sugar. So once you go to sleep at night, and you've slept three or four hours, the epinephrine will supply the blood sugar to keep it at a certain level for the rest of the night. But suddenly, you'll wake up. It depends on how well controlled you are, but it seems that I wake up every night about three o'clock which may be the time when my blood sugar is low. I go to sleep about eleven. This is about four hours and that makes sense because if that's when the adrenalin does come into effect, that would wake me up. I'll get up for a few minutes and then I'll go back to sleep. That could be exactly why I'm waking up because I've been doing that for months now, every night. It is always about the same time, between 2:30 and 3:30.

On the traditional hypoglycemic diet, which I followed very stringently when I got out of the hospital four months ago, I would occasionally get off my feedings by a half an hour. This clearly demonstrated to me that I couldn't tolerate getting off schedule. However, I found that even with following the schedule, getting a feeding every three hours, I was not controlled. I had many episodes, as many as two or three a day. Some days I would lose an entire half a day because I would get unbalanced. In fact, I'd go into a hypoglycemic phase and never really come out of it, no matter how I tried by continuing regular feedings. Actually, I could say I was no better physically than I was before I went into the hospital except that I knew what was going on. I increased the feedings and changed the proportions, which was a better adjustment than before but still, I didn't have that much response from the diet. I was still having as many or more hypoglycemic episodes and they were severe. I'd have at least one a day, sometimes two or three. Sometimes I would be extremely weak for several days in a row.

It is very difficult to differentiate hypoglycemia from exhaustion from depression. I have a history of depression and that is not unusual because there is a psychological component of hypoglycemia patients. I am able to differentiate now because I recognize that it is not in my mind, that I am hypoglycemic and this confusion is not exhaustion or depression. Weakness can be hypoglycemic or exhaustion or it can be both. And depression, well, it kinda gets caught in there all together.

But it is so difficult. If I look in the mirror and I'm pale, I know I *am* hypoglycemic. Sometimes, I'll lie down and then feel better, but that doesn't mean I wasn't hypoglycemic. It might be that my blood sugar came up while I was asleep.

"Are your episodes of hypoglycemia decreasing now?"

They weren't. In fact I was working harder and harder trying to get under control. Finally, about two and a half weeks ago, I had one of the most severe episodes I had ever had. I got off my feeding by 30 minutes, became hypoglycemic about one o'clock in the afternoon and stayed that way until I went to bed that night, despite regular feeding the rest of the day, and I had the most severe abdominal spasms I've ever known, which continued for about ten hours.

I was just desperate. I'd been having so many episodes; I was on call at the hospital every fourth night and I was just about ready to throw in the towel. I had done everything the book supposedly said to do and still couldn't function. I'd go lie down at three o'clock in the afternoon when I was at work in the hospital. I'd be totally exhausted after making rounds with the physicians. It was really becoming unmanageable and I didn't know what to do.

I finally realized that I was going to have to change that diet. I could tell, over that four months, that it took only a minute increase in carbohydrates for me to really go into an attack. So I decided, knowing enough about biochemistry, that if you decrease carbohydrate intake to almost zero, like the Atkins diet, and increase protein that you go into a glucogenic state where you produce your own blood sugar and you stay at a constant blood sugar level. So two weeks ago, I instituted a diet where I eat only meat, eggs, cheese and oils and no more than 35 grams of carbohydrate a day. This means about three cups of vegetables, like green beans, lettuce, etc., and one glass of milk a day.

"How are you doing now?"

Much better. I'm still having a lot of weakness. My psychiatrist agreed with my diet but I didn't have an internist who really . . . So few physicians know anything about diet and I just wanted to hit them when I heard what they were telling me to do because no one knew what they were talking about. They'd say, "Eat more of this, eat more of that." They'd say to eat some candy when you go into a hypoglycemic episode. They don't know anything about hypoglycemia. It may help the first attack but it is sure going to bring on the second. And so they really didn't know beans. I was really kinda furious and besides, I was very interested in weight control.

With this adjusted diet, I've had fewer attacks, although I've had a few. My tolerance is better. I have a little bit more leeway because now I can go 45 minutes past feeding time before I begin to feel weak. And the episodes are much less severe.

I went to a gastroenterologist last week and he agreed with me. He said that the hypoglycemic diet I was on initially was entirely too much for any hypoglycemic and that 60 grams of carbohydrate, just half of what I was taking before, was the most that I should take and even go back to the Atkins diet of zero carbohydrate.

Ketosis is a hazard of this diet. You go into a ketotic state which means there are ketones or acetates circulating in the bloodstream. What happens is that you're using protein up instead of blood sugar. I'm not exactly sure of all of the pathways. Usually when you are losing weight you are breaking down fat and when you are breaking down fat, you get acetates. But also, when you are using protein, protein and fat are both broken down into acetates and ketones which then go into the glycolytic pathway which produces blood sugar. These are acids, they cause acidosis and mess up your pH, your blood acid level. However, as the interns tell me, it's much better to be a little bit ketotic than it is to be hypoglycemic. So, you trade one for the other. You don't notice the ketosis, really, unless you get into severe ketosis.

Finally, I found someone who knew enough about it. The reason I went to this gastroenterologist initially was because I had become so exasperated and worried because I wasn't controlled by a normal hypoglycemic diet. I don't know how anyone who is not a physician can understand it at all. It is a very complex system. Being a physician and being sick and knowing precisely what is going on and still, in the confused state, not being sure, and rationalizing afterwards what happened to me, I don't see how a lay person would ever manage. Unless they were guided by an extremely well informed physician. But I have been talked to by many physicians who did not know beans. I've seen many patients mismanaged. Hypoglycemia is over-diagnosed. Severe forms like mine are rather rare. There are intermediate forms and then there are some that are very mild.

It is a very difficult problem for a person who isn't a physician to understand what is going on with them. It takes a well informed physician who believes his patient because these people are often written off as crazy, neurotic. I found this out through the psychiatrist's office. I'm not saying that all of my depression and anxiety was due to hypoglycemia, but a large component was. It certainly exacerbated what emotional problems I was having. In retrospect, I've had this symptomology at least two years. I'm not sure it wasn't longer.

Hypoglycemic people characteristically gain weight, large amounts of weight, quickly, in order to control their symptoms. I've had four episodes of weight gain since I was 18 years old. I'm 29 now. I'm not sure that the weight gain actually controlled my symptoms. It is hard for me to tell. I do know that two years ago I was as thin as I am now, 110 pounds, and I gained 77 pounds in six months. It was totally by eating sweets continuously and I mean continuously. It would control the symptoms, yes, because I was continually pumping sugar into my blood. But I was in a severe depressed state and the weight gain alone would cause that. I was under a lot of stress at that time.

There were a lot of psychodynamics involved because I'm involved with the psychodynamics of obesity. The obese personality handles a lot of emotional and stress problems by eating, usually by eating a particular type of food. However, anxiety stress is increased by epinephrine, which is one reaction to the hypoglycemic state. Also, it has been proven that a good deal of appetite is regulated by blood sugar. If the blood sugar is low, the hypothalmus gland reacts to this in their food centers and supposedly people want to eat. So it is not illogical that my own low blood sugar stimulated my satiety centers to say, "We need sugar right now. Eat a lot." So the components of the whole system could be, one, psychological obesity training, two, could be hypothalamic, low blood sugar, and, three, could be due to the high anxiety state, caused by the epinephrine which is caused by the low blood sugar. So it is extremely complex.

"What is your outlook now?"

Well, now I'm on this very stringent diet, which gets tiresome, but it feels awfully good to feel good again. I'm still having weakness but it is not nearly as bad as it was. My concern over my continual weakness has stimulated me to consult a doctor again for possible further work-up. Finally, I have confidence in this gastroenterologist. I have not had confidence in any physician I have seen up to this one because I knew more about diet than they did. I knew more about symptoms than they did. My internist who took care of me in the hospital previously was dubious about any pyschiatric patient, despite documented proof of my hypoglycemia. He did not consider my symptoms valid. He did not treat me seriously and he didn't know a damn thing about the illness. And he certainly didn't know anything about diet. So he was no help. I was my own physician in the hospital. I've been treating myself ever since I got out. And if I hadn't changed my own diet about two weeks ago, some idiot would have gotten hold of it and made me even worse. This internist would have increased the carbohydrate in my diet, which would have increased my weight, increased my tension and increased my depression. I was lucky enough to be a physician and say, "No, I think you are a damn fool." My body had been saying the doctors were wrong, but I couldn't find a physician to say it.

> *One of the chief defects in our plan of education in this country is that we give too much attention to developing the mind; we lay too much stress on acquiring knowledge and too little on the wise application of knowledge.*
>
> William J. Mayo (1861–1939)
> *Collected Papers of the Mayo Clinic and Mayo Foundation* 25:1105, 1933

46. Appendicitis

This ten-year-old girl has kinky blonde curls. She is bright, active and eager to talk. She lives with three full siblings and two step siblings on an acreage which is a goodly distance from the city. They attend a rural school, ride in a yellow bus every day to get there.

She describes the first of three episodes of suspected appendicitis, each of which had her doctor and her parents baffled. At the time these episodes occurred, things were in a turmoil at home and her parents were preoccupied. Later, when these problems were alleviated and the situation became tranquil again, her symptoms disappeared and thus far have not returned.

- **Abdominal Cramps**
- **Appendicitis**

Hmmmmm. It was about time for the school bus to come and it was Monday morning and I came up with the double cramps and I vomited.

"The double cramps?"

That's what the doctor called them. I vomited up my breakfast and I couldn't eat anything. I just lay down on the couch. My mother she said, "Well, I'll take you to the hospital after I'm finished eating. I've got to get the other kids off to school." So she took me to the hospital and they found that I had an appendicitis attack.

"Where was the pain?"

Uh . . . uh . . . the pain was right down . . . about where my appendix are. It was a sharp pain, a real sharp pain. It lasted about a day and a night. Tuesday afternoon it stopped, but Wednesday morning it started again.

When I got to the hospital, they took tests and everything. They took me into the x-ray room and took pictures of, you know. They took blood tests and other different things. I can't remember it all.

"Did they give you anything to help you sleep?"

Not really. They started lettin' glucose in me. I don't remember the other name.

"Glucose and saline?"

Yeah. There was a needle in my arm and it was coming through a tube. I slept for a while and woke up and watched one TV show, I think, and then I went back to sleep.

A sharp pain started comin' up, I think it was Wednesday morning or Wednesday afternoon, sometime in between there. My Doctor Wilson said he found out I did have an attack and next time that it happened he was going to have to take my appendix out.

"Did they take it out this time?"

No. The pain lasted a few hours but they kept me in there to watch me. I went home on Sunday.

There was one kid in my room. She kept having dizzy spells and headaches. She was in there before I was and she got out before I was. She was 12 or 13. We talked a lot in the afternoon. She'd go out for tests and then her mother and everybody else would call her and I had calls and I'd take her calls and take messages for her. Just like when I was out for tests, she'd take messages for me.

"What did you like about being in the hospital?"

Nothin', really.

Actually, I didn't like my arm stuck with a needle. I couldn't bend my arm or anything else. I could just barely color.

My roommate's name was Lisa and she was real nice to me. She gave me some comic books. I couldn't eat candy. She said whenever I was able to eat candy she'd give me a piece but I wasn't ever able to. I spent a lot of time coloring and reading books.

The first night I was really scared and had my mom stay with me but the rest of the nights I wasn't that scared because I'd got used to the hospital.

They kept wakin' me up and taking my pulse and taking my blood pressure and everything else. That bothered me because I really didn't want to be awakened. They did that every night.

I could get up and go to the bathroom but someone had to hold the bag thing (I.V. solution container) up. They had kinda like a hook thing, for those things, and they would put that on there. I could sit up and I could get up but they didn't want the blood from my arm running through the thing because most of the time when I stood up it drained a little bit of blood out of it.

I didn't watch TV much. I usually took naps because I was so tired. Lisa usually liked the TV shows I liked. We would only stay up . . . well, I'd go to sleep about nine and she'd stay up to about ten. She'd watch her movie she wanted to watch and I'd be asleep.

The nurses were nice. I got a penny bank from my Girl Scout troop and I remember saying, when most of the doctors and nurses come in, "Well, you can't stick a needle in me or you can't look at me or anything like that unless you put a penny or a nickel or a quarter or a dime in there."

"Did you collect lots of money that way?"

Yeah. I ended up with five dollars. My doctor put in . . . he came about three times and I remember he put a silver dollar in, a 50-cent piece in and a quarter. He's a pretty good doctor.

"I've never heard of the doctor paying the patient. The patient usually pays the doctor. Have you had any trouble since that time?"

No.

"Do you expect to have?"

I don't know.

"Was this the only time you have been in a hospital?"

Yeah. I would say so.

"You were probably born in a hospital but you probably don't remember that."

Oh, I remember that. First I turned blue, and then I turned red and then I turned white. Red, white and blue. Because I'm anemic. I used to take iron pills but I don't take 'em any more.

The last night I was there in the hospital this girl and I, we were neighbors across the hall, her name was Lora and she was the same age as I was. She was in the fourth grade, same as me, and she'd had an appendicitis attack, same as me. She and I, we would run the halls. We would walk up and down the stairs and call the nurses on the button things and play school. When we called the nurses, she would say, "Nurse, please bring me some orange sherbet." or "Please bring me some strawberry ice cream or vanilla."

"Would they bring it to you?"

Yeah. Uh huh. We ate six or seven cups each and got sick that night.

"What did you find when you were roaming up and down the halls?"

Nothin', really. All except people. I'd hold my penny bank with me because I didn't want anybody to come and get it. I'd set it down and people would come by and put money in it. So I ended up with more money.

We would do "pop wheelies" in the wheel chairs. We'd take a wheel chair, they had one right in our room, you know, and we'd pop wheelies in them. We'd sit there going like this *(demonstrates by leaning way back in her chair)* and then going like that *(leans forward)*. We had a ball that night. A wheelie, it's like you do when you ride a bike and lean back and the front wheel comes off the ground. This old lady I know lived in an old people's home, you know? She'd get in her wheel chair and pop wheelies all over the halls. They tried to stop her but she'd never stop. And one day she died.

While I was in the hospital I missed five days of school and church, but on Saturday, I didn't miss anything but work. I had a pretty good time in the hospital, all except the first three days when I had the double cramps.

"How do you like your doctor?"

He's a great doctor.

"Why do you say that?"

Well, he's the one who paid me the most money.

47. Polyp

Once I asked her why she works so hard to get ahead and she replied with one word, "Poverty." Actually, her family is not poverty-stricken by any means. Her father is a maintenance supervisor of the huge, automated presses in a large printing company and while they have a modest home, they are comfortable. She is single and still lives at home but she expects to move soon when she completes her second college degree. She has worked for more than ten years, putting herself through college majoring in economics. Now she attends night classes in computer science, in which she will get a baccalaureate degree.

She is brown-haired, comely, has perfect teeth and beautiful skin. She works as a secretary for a non-profit foundation concerned with health so she is familiar with medical issues. When she steps into the world of computers as a programmer, she will double her salary.

• Rectal Polyp
• Surgical Removal

I went in for my annual checkup to my local gynecologist and he discovered that I had a rectal polyp, which is not a serious condition. He referred me to a surgeon in a nearby building, so I went in, scheduled an appointment and had a little outpatient procedure there in his office. I was also referred to another clinic, a third physician, for x-rays, a barium series.

A polyp is a small, little growth of skin in the intestine, the mucous membrane. He didn't explain why they occur. He just said I had one and should have it removed, which made sense to me. They are benign as they are, but polyps can become cancerous if they're left in there for a long period of time.

I had the lower barium series, the G.I. series, to be sure there weren't any more farther up. The whole thing took about 10 days and I didn't even miss much work, maybe a day and a half.

The surgery was a little bit painful, a little uncomfortable. I went without food for a while. But it wasn't bad; I guess it was a fairly routine thing to go through.

What really made me mad was how much it cost and that my insurance didn't cover it. The impression I got was that if I had gone into the hospital, my Blue Cross-Blue Shield would have paid for it. But because I was healthy enough to stay outside of the hospital, they wouldn't pay. They paid $25 on a $250 bill. And I'd paid in hundreds of dollars in insurance premiums, either me or my employer had. And the first time I want to collect and have a legitimate complaint, they just fall through. There was just nothing.

The $250 was the surgeon's fee for that little procedure he did in his office and they wouldn't cover a penny of that. The x-rays were like $50 or $75 and they paid the $25 on that. And they would have covered more of the x-rays had I gone into the hospital.

My insurance was being paid for by my employer so I really didn't have much say so about the coverage I had. And in looking around at insurance plans, I didn't really feel like anything better was being offered. From what I understood, Blue Cross-Blue Shield was about the best you could get. And I still think that Blue Cross-Blue Shield is probably the best insurance plan available but I think that health insurance is geared wrong. It is not geared toward the patient. It's geared toward the hospitals and the doctors, who are the people who run it. It's geared for their benefit and the patients, we just kinda do what they want us to. They don't have our best interest at heart, obviously, because of the way it is set up. If it were set up right, outpatient procedures would be paid for more readily, perhaps, than hospital proce- dures, or just as readily, shall we say. Obviously, it would be cheaper to treat a patient, one who is treatable, outside the hospital than to put him in a bed. It is better for the insurance company and it's better for the patient. It is not good for the hospitals because then they have empty beds and their fixed costs are continuing to mount up. When their beds are not filled, they don't get paid.

I just don't think much of doctors in general. Most of them are in it for the money, not for the good of the patient. I guess the way society is geared, everyone is kinda money-oriented. But being a physician is a service profes- sion and in too many cases, the patient's welfare gets very little considera- tion, if any at all.

The particular gynecologist I had would really shuffle through the patients. In the first place, he wasn't available if you needed him. He was booked up two months in advance and if you happened to need to see him in a reasonable length of time, if an emergency had come up, he just couldn't work you in. At all. He had really what I call a cattle-car operation. He just moved 'em in and moved 'em out. You couldn't talk to him and he wouldn't explain a thing. He was supposedly very good. I guess.

Since then, I have been going to the family medicine clinic at the university and I have a little resident physician over there, perhaps not as skilled as this other doctor was, but a lot more available. And she takes a lot more time to discuss things. A lot of gynecologists have a paternal-type attitude. They don't believe their patients have a brain in their head or understand what's going on. I get the feeling that if a woman comes in com- plaining of pain, they just think it's all in her head and it's not worth taking any time with, at all. I don't know. They seem to make no effort to try and understand their patients.

The doctor I have at the clinic now is a woman, but there aren't very many women who are gynecologists. The one I have is in family practice but for me, that's fine. Someone like that can fill my needs real well. At the clinic, they offered me a list of doctors and I picked out the female physician. Then I quit going to my gynecologist altogether. He was real expensive, too.

"Do you think then that a female doctor has a much deeper understanding of your problems — you as a female?"

Oh, yeah. For sure. *(Laughs.)*
I think that the health care system is set up completely wrong. As I mentioned before, I think it is set up for the benefit of the hospitals and the doctors, rather than for the benefit of the patients. I still can't understand where we got the idea that doctors ought to be paid a fortune. And where they got such high status in our society. In other societies, they aren't any higher than lawyers or other professionals. How did they get all of this respect? How did they get these god-like complexes so that everybody bows down to their doctor? That seems to have arisen in about the last 30 years and I see absolutely no basis for it.

"Do you think more rigid control by the government would help to change the attitude toward doctors and the relationship between people and their doctors?"

No, I don't. It would probably just fix things in the pattern they're in now, just aggravate a bad situation. I don't think national health insurance is the way to go at all. I think the basic problem lies with the way we think of our health care system. It is geared toward being sick instead of preventing sickness. That's obviously one of the problems we have with costs nowadays. We have so many hospital beds that have to be paid for. You gotta have sick people to put in the hospital beds, so the whole industry is sort of geared to getting them into beds and incurring costs. The malpractice situation aggravates that with more and more tests being performed.

For national health insurance to be really effective, there would have to be a basic restructuring of the system toward a more healthful point of view, rewarding doctors and patients for staying healthy.

"Like the Chinese who, they say, don't pay their physician when they get sick but pay him only when they are well."

That sounds like at least as good a system as we've got now and probably better. Plus, we are so geared to the physician in our health care system. He is such an expensive person. To me, it would make much more sense to train three or four paramedical people for what we're spending to train one doctor. A paramedical person costs us less and provides for more basic type needs.

Particularly as the age of the population goes up. We need specialists but even more important we need people to help us with our basic health care. Someone we can see more often and who is cheaper than a physician.

All of us need help in gearing our lifestyles into a more healthful way of life. We need help to be well in addition to help when we are sick.

I read an article in a woman's magazine that said that the incidence of heart disease and stroke has gone down a significant amount in the last few years due partially to increased awareness on the part of patients and physicians that these types of diseases can be prevented or controlled with patient participation, by exercise, watching diet, and so forth. I think this is a trend in the right direction. There just isn't enough of it. We could all become aware of the things in our lifestyle which make us less healthy and try to correct those conditions.

Do you think people would go for a periodic checkup when they are healthy to a person who could give them a "prescription for wellness," improve their chances of staying healthy and out of the hospital?"

I don't think there is any question that if that type of service were available, it would be heavily utilized. There are all kinds of benefits to doing that. You would look better, you'd feel better, you would spend less money in the long run. All kinds of positive benefits.

Why can't we have wellness clinics, where you could go in for a reasonable amount of money — which insurance should cover — and talk over your lifestyle with an expert in that area, take a few basic tests and get a kind of prescription to stay healthy? The problem is that the people who run things aren't rewarded financially if you stay healthy. They get rewarded when you are sick. And you can't be just a little bit sick, you gotta be low sick.

Doctors are either revered as gods or vilified because they are ripping us off. There should be a middle ground, where they are respected as professionals, like anyone else.

Medical students are definitely geared toward the buck. I've known several, and without a doubt, each one of them was looking forward to being a rich doctor. They see medicine as first of all, instant status and second, instant money.

I don't date medical students any more. I don't like 'em. They're not interesting people. They are very narrow-minded. They have their own little world of medicine and, maybe, they have a hobby or two and that's it. They tend to be very conservative. They are just not very interesting people compared to other folks whose outlooks are broader and who perhaps think more about life in general.

The system is bad for the doctors, too, because they get locked into a role, particularly when they're going to medical school. They get certain ideas drummed into them. They get pushed into conforming with the current medical establishment. All of us have to conform to a degree but medical students must conform to a much greater degree. That's bad for them, too. Otherwise they don't stay in the fraternity very long. They either shape up or ship out.

Applicants to medical school are screened so that folks who are going to conform get in and folks who aren't going to conform never get in. The profession as a whole loses by being so strict in its standards and not allowing more freedom for its members.

After viewing the medical establishment as I have, I'm a big believer in staying well. Doctors ought to be an absolute last resort. If they aren't going to try to keep me healthy, then I'm going to try my best to keep myself healthy. I'll go to them if I have to, but, by God, I don't want to. I don't trust 'em any farther than I can throw 'em.

God heals and the doctor takes the fees.

Benjamin Franklin
Poor Richard's Almanack (1732–57)

XV.
Wires and Pulleys

Man is essentially a bulb with many thousands of roots. In him the nerves alone feel; the rest serves to hold them together and to move them about more conveniently. What we see then is the pot in which the man is planted.

Georg Christoph Lichtenburg (1742–1799)
Aphorismen (1764–1771)

Adapt or perish, now as ever, is Nature's inexorable imperative.

H. G. Wells
Mind at the End of Its Tether (1946), 19

48. Bell's Palsy

She is 17, a high school junior, has long brown hair and a bouncy personality. She is the youngest of two daughters. Her 21-year-old sister is married.

Her mother was divorced early and raised both girls by herself but has recently remarried. They live in a tract home in the suburbs of a medium-sized city in the country's heartland. She and her mother are very close, probably because her father was not around as she was growing up.

• Bell's Palsy

I was 10 or 11 years old when I woke up one day with Bell's palsy. I had noticed it before but nobody believed me. I couldn't say words like "people" and that's what finally made people like Mom realize . . .

"How did the word "people" come out?"

I just couldn't say it. There was no way.

Mother: And her smile. We noticed her smile. One side of her mouth wouldn't go up at all.

Daughter: It was blank, just blank. There were other words I couldn't pronounce either, but I don't remember what they were. Finally, my grandmother took me to the hospital. One side of my mouth just didn't move.

The doctor ran some tests. He would put salt on one side of my tongue and then on the other to see if I could taste it. He did a whole bunch of tests. Then he put me in the hospital and did some more tests and took x-rays.

Mother: They did some kind of a test on her brain to see if she had pressure. I forget what they called it.

Daughter: It was like a brain scan but it wasn't. I don't know how they did it but they did it. And they played around with my eyes, using sticks to see how far I could see on this side and then the other side. And then they tested me with different smells. I was in the hospital about a week.

The doctor said it would cure itself and it went away in about a week. But there was a lady down the hall who had it a whole lot worse than I did.

One of her eyes was completely swollen shut. She couldn't move one side of her face in any way. Paralyzed. It was scary.

"How did you get acquainted with her?"

I didn't; the doctor told me about her. I didn't see her.

Mother: Brenda was experiencing some paralysis, what they call the "lazy eye." She couldn't open one of her eyelids on the same side she'd lost the feeling in her tongue and her lip. Her hand and her leg were asleep, too, tingling. And the doctors would run this wheel-looking thing up and down for feeling sensations. So we didn't know how much paralysis if any she was going to have. That was one reason for putting her in the hospital. It was getting worse.

"But it cured itself spontaneously?"

Daughter: Yeah. The doctor said there was nothing that could be done for it, that they knew of at that time. Now, I'm supposedly okay.

Mother: There is the lip problem, though, with her smile. You don't notice it so much if you're just looking at her, especially if she's self-conscious about it, but in a couple of her school pictures if she is looking at the camera from the wrong direction, you can tell it.

"I can't tell which side it is. Is it the right side?"

Daughter: I don't remember.

"If you can't tell and I can't tell, it really doesn't make much difference, does it?"

Nope.

Mother: It made a big difference when we tried to get insurance for her. They asked if she'd ever had anything. I tried to put her on a hospitalization policy. Recently, the biggest problem was trying to get a life insurance policy. The doctor who treated her is since deceased and we had to get doctors' statements after going through a complete physical, which is unusual for a child of 16. And they still don't want to insure her. We had to get certification from two different doctors. We had to get a report of her old medical record from the hospital. And then they sent us a letter saying they were not going to issue the policy. Finally, our agent, who is a friend of ours and we have a lot of insurance with him, he called the company. I don't know what he said but we finally got the policy.

Daughter: They came out and interviewed me. It was a hassle.

Mother: They didn't make any exclusions on her policy, though.

"What did the doctors say was the possibility of recurrence of Bell's palsy?"

Mother: Brenda didn't hear that part then. We stepped out in the hall and the doctor told me that if she didn't have a reoccurrence of it by the time she was 16 or 17 years old, she probably would not have it again. But he said if she did have a reoccurrence of it, it would probably be much more severe and she might even have permanent paralysis. So he cautioned me to keep a good close watch on her and if I noticed any more the droopy eye or problems with her smile or her speech to do something about it immediately. But as far as we know, she's normal.

Of course, it's frightening for any child to go into the hospital, especially if they think it's something that's going to be of a permanent-type nature.

Daughter: I didn't like the hospital. We went over there and they thought I was going to be a little bitty baby and they had a "momma chair" in the room. I asked them to bring in another bed for my momma and they wouldn't do it. I didn't want her to leave me. They made her sleep in a rockin' chair. The nurses weren't very friendly at all. They were very rude and uncourteous. They were rude to Mom and that made me mad.

Mother: Usually, when a smaller child is in the hospital, they bring the mother a tray, but they wouldn't even bring me a cup of coffee, or a pillow, or a blanket or anything. And I wasn't about to leave her. She didn't want me to go. If I'd just step down the hall to the bathroom, she would be crying and petrified by the time I got back.

Daughter: They scared me once. Mom went to the bathroom and the guy came in to take me down for x-rays. He says, "You're goin'," and I says, "No, I am not," and he says, "Yes, you are," and I told him, "I'm not going no place 'til my mommy comes back."

Mother: They picked her up and put her on the cart, her screaming and crying and hollering. She didn't know if they were taking her to surgery or what they were going to do to her.

Daughter: Then one night, I finally got mad and told Mom to get in bed with me. I didn't want her sleeping in that old crookety rocking chair. But the nurses came in about midnight, I guess it was, and woke us both up and made her get out of bed and sleep in the rocking chair. I didn't like that. They weren't nice.

Mother: When I was first scheduled for my surgery last year, my doctor booked me into that same hospital and Brenda had such a fit that I called and asked him to change it. That's why I went to Memorial.

Daughter: They were screwballs. They didn't know what they was doin'. They didn't know how to give shots either; they hurt. You know, they give you those little menus so you can order what you want, but they never brought me what I wanted. The food was terrible. They always brought stuff I didn't like.

Mother: I think what she's trying to say is that they just weren't very considerate of the fact that she was young. Just because she wasn't sick didn't mean she wasn't scared.

I went to the head nurse on that floor and I asked her, "Why are you so upset because I'm staying with her? She's just a baby, my baby." To me she was a baby. She was scared and I was scared. Again, that was when I was single and didn't have much money. I could see all of these monumental medical bills building up and I was concerned about whether Brenda was going to be like this the rest of her life. I told the head nurse, "There's no way I'm going to leave her. Couldn't you make it a little more comfortable for me?" And she said, "No, we can't do that now. There's just no point in your staying. Just go home." And I asked her, "If that was your daughter, would you leave her?" She said, "Well, no," and I said, "What's the difference?" We got into quite a heated argument until I finally had to lower my voice, calm myself down and go back to the room.

The main reason that I shut up when I did and didn't carry it any further was that I didn't know how long Brenda was going to be there and if they got real pissed at me, I didn't want them to neglect her or take it out on her because her mother was a real grouch.

49. Dyslexia

The story of this boy's problem is told by his mother. He is now a teenager, in high school, but his trouble was discovered early in his elementary school years. His mother has spent countless hours helping him adjust to and overcome his handicap. She is an energetic 40 year old with constant good humor and friendliness. She has always pursued a career outside the home.

- **Difficulty Learning to Read**
- **Poor Reading Performance**
- **Dyslexia**

Up until the time when he began to learn to read, about age five, I had no indication at all that there was anything wrong. He was very normal, watched television, preferred to be outside. He went to a private kinder-garten where they began to teach him to read. He was rather slow but fairly normal. Then he began first grade and he learned to read fairly well.

The first indication I think I had was when he would bring home his math papers in the second and third grades. Unfortunately, Bill went to a kindergarten which was run by Christian Science people and although I feel now that they must have known or suspected, they ignored the problem completely because they didn't recognize any physical problems, as a matter of their religion. When I talked to them later, they still denied or would not accept the idea that they had any suspicions at all. Because they were teach-ing Bill a foreign language, I suspect now that they must have known that he had some difficulty.

His first grade teacher gave him a lot of special attention and taught him to read and he read normally.

Second grade was fine.

In the third grade, when he began to bring home his math papers, every problem would be incorrect because he copied the problem down wrong. He would transpose numbers. The problem itself would be wrong, particularly if he copied it from the blackboard. He'd mix up the numbers generally and, of course, if you get the problem down wrong, there's no way you can come up with the right answer. So I began to help him by copying the problems for him. Then he could do them.

When he was in the fifth grade, we decided to move into another school district which we heard was really good. They immediately put him in a remedial reading group, which meant slow learners, slow readers, slow everything. He was in this class all day long, every day, and he became very frustrated and his emotional state was very low. And my emotional state was exactly the same as his. He would come home with his shoulders hunched and mine would immediately hunch.

At that time he was playing baseball, a sport in which he excelled. That sort of kept him on an even keel; as long as he could excel a little bit he was happy.

So I decided to inquire around. First I took him to our internist, who checked him over thoroughly and really didn't find anything wrong except that he had rather poor nutrition. He's a "sugarholic," eats a lot of sweets. The doctor recommended a different diet for him. The doctor didn't suspect he had this reading difficulty and I didn't know it then.

My mother, who is a guidance counselor, had told me several times that she suspected dyslexia. She helped him with his school work and it was on her recommendation that I found this doctor *(Ph.D.)* who is the head of the reading clinic at the college.

In the meantime, while waiting for the reading clinic appointment, I decided to take Bill to an ophthalmologist to get his eyes checked. He was found to be a little bit nearsighted but they didn't find any other difficulty. No glasses were recommended. He doesn't see 20-20 but he sees well enough.

I remember that the appointment at the reading clinic was on Halloween morning. We had a brief talk with the doctor heading the clinic who explained to Bill that he would give him various tests. He said there wasn't any reason to be uptight because there wasn't any right or wrong answers. Whatever answer was acceptable to Bill was the acceptable answer. He would neither pass nor fail. He'd be very cool. I left Bill there and went home and Bill stayed there all day.

A week later, I discussed Bill's test with the doctor. He told me then he suspected dyslexia. He gave Bill all the I.Q. tests and he has an extremely high I.Q. except for this learning disability. He wrote me a five-page report that gave me hints about how to handle Bill, things I'd never really thought of before. For instance, I had always stressed his reading and his penmanship, which was atrocious and I made his life miserable making him try to make neat papers. He will never make neat papers. That's what the doctor told me. Do not stress his penmanship, which will never be any good.

The doctor described dyslexia as a perceptual problem. What you are looking at isn't always what registers. It gets scrambled some place between the eye and the brain.

Bill's problem is not terribly acute. I understand that there are children who see everything backwards. Those are the people you see in night clubs doing their act in which they write backwards. They see that backwards. But Bill's rather comes and goes. In other words, if he reads a sentence in a long paragraph, he will read the first part of it right and then get to the end and it will all sort of fade into nothingness. He'll not be able to understand or he will leave off periods. He doesn't dot any "i's," sees no punctuation, never wrote a comma in his life. Long math problems have to be done step by step, even if it means dividing the problem into three different problems and then adding them together. Rather than adding a column of nine figures, he has to do three and three and three.

The only way I can describe the meeting with the reading clinic doctor was one of real elation, because I thought the child was maybe incapable of good work. He made me see that his I.Q. was terrifically high and he was capable of anything he wanted to do. He called Bill in and said, "It's not my policy to tell people their I.Q. but I think you need to know yours. You've been stuck in remedial reading classes for slow people all day long, and you've looked out the window because you got it the first time around. They are boring you to death with their slowness and you've begun to think that you are slow, too." So the doctor told him what his I.Q. was and told him he could be anything he wanted to be. This just lifted a weight because Bill always thought he was dumb. He'd say, "I can't read it." And it breaks your heart when your child is getting taller than you are and he isn't reading.

Children with dyslexia are easily distracted. They have to concentrate so hard. Bill needs to sit where there aren't too many students behind him or to the side. The less distractions he has, the better off he is, so the back row on a corner where there aren't people behind him or around him is the best place for him to sit.

The doctor said to ask his English teacher to grade him on the basis of composition alone and to stop writing across the top "Bad boy — messy paper" or "Will not grade — too messy," which teachers are prone to do. So I did have conferences with his teachers and have had ever since.

Bill is very sensitive about anyone knowing that he has any difficulty at all, so I let him go, on his own, until the teachers begin sending notices saying his work is incomplete and he's not going to pass. Then I go, when it gets down to the crunch. I'm always torn between going to tell them first and waiting. But his reports are always on file in the office and all the teachers have to do is go look at them, but they never take the time. After I tell them about Bill's problem, they will go look, but before that, they never bother.

We moved out of the school system that kept him in the slow learners class and moved back where he could be in a small grade school, in a class of 20. The stigma of being in a class of slow learners was just killing him. And the school wouldn't consider taking him out. The fifth grade was very crowded and they told me they had no time for individual help. Bill just couldn't keep up without some individual help. At that time, the teacher had 35 students and said that every time she looked up, Bill was standing at her desk and she had no time to help him, which I thought was rather a sad commentary.

The children refer to the kids in a remedial reading class as "106 children" or whatever room number they are in. It's like being a "Section 8" in the Army, and if you are in that classroom, there is a great stigma involved. It implies that you are dumb, which Bill's ego could not take.

Every couple of years or so I get real lucky and find a teacher who is very understanding and will really help him. The fifth grade teacher in the smaller school where we moved was one of those.

He graduated from the sixth grade fine and went on to the seventh.

The seventh grade has a lot of reading — the classics — and he began having a lot of difficulty. That year, I decided he was getting to me too much. He was cute and funny and he was talking me out of our evening study sessions. We would spend our time laughing. They learn to be charmers, you know. They cover up all this other by acting like they don't care if they learn it or don't learn it which shows up as a discipline problem. So I decided to get Bill a tutor.

I hired a young English teacher to come to the house twice a week. We began with hour-long sessions. She helped him with math, English, all the subjects. After about two months she thought that 30-minute sessions were long enough. Then she would visit with him for maybe 10 or 20 minutes after the sessions. He liked her very much. She was very young and her husband was coach of the track team. She saw to it that Bill was not assigned to her English class. She was a teacher in his school.

As he entered junior high school, Bill began to be hyperactive, sort of "jitsey," nervous. His tutor didn't really help him with the actual reading. She helped with the English part of grammar. She made him learn his spelling words, which they required. He's not ever going to be a speller but the spelling tests counted a lot in his English grade and he had to take them. Every Thursday night she grilled him over and over, orally, on his spelling words for the tests they had each Friday.

I read the classics to him. I also cheated. I'd go to the college bookstore and buy little condensed versions of the book itself. I'd also buy him any comic books which tell classic stories like "Ivanhoe." He doesn't read anything all the way through. In fact, when we read novels together, I'll read aloud and when we come to an exciting part I think he'll enjoy, he will read it. He will skim over all of the description and just read the exciting parts.

I also got "talking books" from the library for the blind, but they didn't have much variety for younger chldren. This was three years ago. They're probably much better now. I haven't utilized them this year but I am sure they have a much better selection now.

Because he was so jitsey, so hyperactive, I still wasn't through with the medical men. I still thought there was something we could do which would make him instantly well. So I took him to our pediatrician who said that sometimes if you give hyperactive, nervous children a stimulant, it would work in reverse and make them seem very calm. So he put Bill on "uppers" but they just absolutely put him on the ceiling. He just went out of sight. That didn't work, so after a week of trying, the doctor told me to flush the uppers down the john, to go back to "cold turkey" in the classroom. We have never given him any downers.

By this time I had exhausted all of the medical men I knew. I'd been to a pediatrician, an internist and two ophthalmologists, so I began to realize there was no instant cure. He couldn't have an operation, or a shot or a pill that was going to immediately make him not be a problem.

The more I talked to educators, the more I realized that if Bill didn't have to read or write, he'd have no problem at all. He has good coordination; he's an excellent baseball player. He hits the ball every time it comes over the plate. He can dance, he can draw, he can paint. There aren't any fields he can't do, except reading and writing.

So we have kept him out of upper math but this year, in the tenth grade, I was not successful in keeping him out of a foreign language. He is going to fail Spanish; he'll never get it. I can't get it over to the powers-that-be that there are certain children who can never learn a foreign language.

Now that we're in the tenth grade, the work gets harder. He makes C's and D's. He does beautifully in science, biology, and in history. He told me that in a big test, on which he made 98, he learned the whole thing simply by listening to the questions and the answers given in class without ever opening a book, just from the worksheets. So you see what kind of a memory he's developed to compensate for his problem. He has to learn through his ears and through his eyes by what he sees in pictures.

We're still fighting the battle of teachers complaining about his messy papers. If I get them at home, I type them for him. And he's gone to printing. That way he gets less complaints from teachers and he can print almost as fast as he can write.

His morale goes down. He gets behind and the behinder he gets, the more frustrated he gets and the less he tries. I'm convinced that he can do anything he wants to do. If he's approached right.

We've thought about all kinds of careers for him. He's a certified scuba diver. He's thought about joining the Marines. He's interested in biology, lab work. I don't know whether he can pass college classes or not. I have no idea.

Speaking of consultation for parents of kids with this problem, in any good-size city, there will probably be a reading clinic. You can look in the yellow pages of the telephone directory or ask any teacher. An actual reading clinic is where they teach remedial reading to teachers or where they do testing of students. You have to keep calling until you find the right place.

"What is the incidence of dyslexia among children?"

I heard it one time and it's surprisingly high, something like three or four out of every hundred children have some sort of dyslectic difficulty.

The importance of seeking some sort of consultation is absolutely crucial. I'm all for getting a physical checkup, taking the child to the doctor first to find out if there is some physical problem that can be fixed. But if that doesn't work, that's not the time to give up. That's the time to find someone who can help. These people see dyslectic children all of the time and form very good opinions of how to help them. He said these children feel tense most of the time, tense about their work, tense about their studies. He said to me, "How would you like to feel on edge all of the time, instead of just once or twice a year, everyday, all day long?" When these children get into a school system which sticks them in a slow class it just defeats them because most of them have very high I.Q.'s.

I think any kind of menial work would bore Bill. We're going to send him to college to see if he can make it.

There was a dyslectic medical student who went through last year and made such high grades on the oral examinations. Of course, much of medical school is performance but you do have to assimilate the material some way. He had to have someone to read to him. And these people have to learn to type.

It is so important for these children to achieve in some way, anything they can do well, baseball, pool, anything at all. Anything that makes them feel worthwhile because a lot of times at school, no matter how hard they try, no matter how many sessions parents have with their teachers, they're going to feel defeated, put down. To hear Bill talk, everyone in the whole room understands and moves ahead and he doesn't. But, no matter how hard you try as a parent, you can't sit there in the seat with him and help him through every day.

I long ago decided to be a part of the solution and not the problem. The world seems to hassle a dyslexic and I try to smooth out the rough places.

Some time after this interview, this woman sent the following note:

I have succeeded since the interview in getting Bill out of a foreign language class forever and into some practical things like typing, business math, etc. I also have found a college specializing in dyslexic students with remedial work all the way through. It is most expensive, but we plan to give it a try.

50. Muscular Dystrophy

This physician is handicapped only in his ability to move about. He is a recognized expert in his specialty. In fact, he also has a satellite specialty which makes his considerable talents particularly valuable and sought after.

His medical problem inhibits somewhat his ability to render patient care, although he personally sees several patients each week. As a member of a single specialty group practice as well as an associate professor in the college of medicine, he spends most of his time teaching and consulting with the other doctors in his group and with practicing specialists in the community and the southwestern state in which he is located.

He has compensated somewhat for the slowdown which his disease has forced upon him by getting around in a battery-operated wheel chair and driving an "Ironsides"-type van which has hand controls.

- **Muscle Weakness**
- **Muscular Dystrophy**

The weakness first started when I was in my mid-20's, I guess. I had a physical examination and the doctor was trying to find normal reflexes and I didn't have any, anywhere. When he hit my knee with his rubber hammer, I had no reflexes.

This condition was largely ignored. It was my curiosity which led me to look further. I was in medical school then; now I am 39 years old.

So I went to a general practitioner friend of mine because of weakness, trouble getting up and down stairs, things like this. He examined me but he didn't know what it was. Then I went to the doctor who was chairman of neurology at the medical school where I was and he examined me. He didn't think too much of it but he did get an electromyogram, an EMG, which he felt showed old polio; in other words, a burned out, inactive process. And that was the end of that. That was my initial concern.

"When some medical students study diseases they tend to imagine that they have the disease they are studying. Did you ever think that your symptoms might have been psychosomatic?"

I never thought they were psychosomatic. They were too definite, too real. The thing that I wanted to know was whether it was amyotropic lateral sclerosis. It wasn't that.

"Is that Lou Gehrig's disease?"

Yeah. Same thing. I was convinced, almost from the outset, that whatever it was, it was not inactive. It was slowly changing, progressing.

After about two years, maybe three years, there was no doubt that it had changed, at least no doubt in my mind. And people who had known me and not seen me for a couple of years also knew I had changed. So I went back to the original neurologist, who was not impressed by any change. But he got another EMG which also supposedly showed old polio and as far as he was concerned, that was the end of it.

I was still convinced it was changing and by the time I was a resident, I felt it was changed even more. I went and saw two other neurologists. One didn't know what it was. The other one wasn't certain but thought it could be old polio and that it would change. How something inactive could change, I never found out. I then had a third EMG and also a muscle biopsy. I don't know how the EMG was interpreted; I don't think I was ever told. This was by now a fourth neurologist.

The muscle biopsy was inconclusive because the muscle was all pretty much gone so there was not enough there to really interpret. It was far-advanced, whatever it was, atrophy or dystrophy. Nobody had mentioned muscular dystrophy to me at that time, or other various entities, amyotonia congenita or Oppenheim's Disease.

Then I went out to see another noted muscle specialist at UCLA with my oldest son. We went out there on a very warm spring day so I could be evaluated for weakness in my legs. When we got to the medical center, there was absolutely nowhere to park except down the hill a considerable distance, the better part of a mile away from the doctor's office. By the time I got there, having made it up the hill to see him, it was *prima facie* evidence that I must not have been too bad because we had to walk all of the way.

We finally found his office and he came in and spent all of ten minutes, hardly examined either one of us. He drew blood on us and doing this to a child, my son, upset him to the point that he promptly threw up. By that time, the doctor had vacated himself from the office, so that we and the nurses were left to contend with cleaning all of this up. Then we had to walk back down the hill to the car and go back home. That was the account of our encounter with the famous muscle disease expert.

I took my son to see if this condition might be familial. This again was on my initiation. None of the doctors ever looked into the possibility of it being hereditary in any sense. Even in spite of the fact that many of these, especially muscular dystrophy, are genetically determined, this was never suggested to me.

We got the results of the blood tests and on me they were equivocal to abnormal and on him they were normal. And that was the end of that. I mean, there was no more. That ends that segment of the tale.

Then we moved to Florida and I went to a neurologist down there. By this time, I had gotten more involved in neurology and I was pretty well coming around to the idea that, no matter what they said, I had limb-girdle muscular dystrophy, a type of muscular dystrophy which affects the pelvic girdle and the limbs. The neurologist down there told me that he just didn't know anything about muscle disease and would not be of any great help. I appreciated that he was honest enough to tell me he didn't know.

By this time I was about 30 years old, after I had completed my residency. This had now dragged on for about six years, progressing very slowly. Although I could never convince them of that, to me there was no doubt.

One of the doctors thought I might have multiple sclerosis but that never proved out. I went to an orthopedic surgeon in L.A. who thought I might have syringomyelia or some other spinal cord lesion. He wanted to do a spinal tap, to which I told him, "Thanks very much, but no thanks." I couldn't see how that could possibly help.

We had a very noted muscle specialist from England visit the medical school in Florida and he examined me. He thought I had limb-girdle muscular dystrophy. By that time, I thought so, too, so at least we agreed. He thought that it was probably recessively inherited, not carried on the sex chromosomes but on the other chromosomes. There was no chance that it would be transmitted to my children.

I also saw another neurologist down there, number seven, who did an EMG and thought that I had another disease called Kugelberg-Welander disease. He also did nerve conduction velocity tests and it turned out that my problem was not Kugelberg-Welander disease. Still another neurologist did an EMG on me which he felt probably showed limb-girdle dystrophy. He also did an EMG on my son and he wasn't sure if that was normal or not; it may have been abnormal.

We then moved to the Southwest and the only time I was evaluated there was when they had another big ace come down from New York. His EMG interpretation showed "mixed muscle and neuronal abnormality" so I don't know what it is now. He didn't know if it was an autosomal recessive or an x-linked or sex-linked disease which I think shows an abysmal lack of genetic knowledge. If it were x-linked then it couldn't be transmitted male to male which is what I was concerned about. It cannot be x-linked, even though he thought it might be. But that's all right.

"At what point did you lose your ability to walk?"

Oh, that was after I broke my leg. That was really not related, *per se,* except that the cast was so heavy it immobilized me and the disuse atrophy took care of the ambulation. By the time the cast came off, the muscles had weakened from disuse to the point of not being able to regenerate. I was 32 when this happened. I was going through a heavy fire door and the person I thought was holding it for me let go and it hit me and knocked me down. At that time, I was walking with a crutch.

Before that I went to an orthopedic man in Florida because I was having difficulty walking. He fitted me with an ill-conceived brace which was an absolute joke. My left side was weaker than the right. He fitted me with a brace which was intended to stabilize the ankle; it came up from the shoe to just below the knee. The problem was that it was my knee which was weak and it would give way before anything else would. Then I'd lose my balance and fall down.

As I walked, the back and the top of the brace would go forward and hit right below my knee, having the effect of buckling my knee, just like a clip in football. If I walked too fast or didn't pay attention to what I was doing, this thing would come forward, hit my knee and down I would go. This happened three or four times the first day that I wore it. Without the brace, I didn't fall that much so I decided it was an absolute farce.

About a month later, I saw his name on a program giving a lecture on "Bracing in Muscular Dystrophy." I decided it wasn't worth my while to hear him because, for me, he had braced the wrong joint.

I knew that neurology is an inexact diagnostic science, as is medicine in general, but the thing that bothered me was that, given a reasonably educated, if not intelligent observer, a reliable observer, at least, a distribution of weakness that was fairly symmetrical and diffuse, that is, not just in one leg or one area, no other neurological symptoms, no sensory loss, no seizures, no twitching or anything like that and with a slowly progressive course, I think muscle disease would have been reasonably obvious. I felt I knew the diagnosis, to my own satisfaction, way before they came around to it. I was convinced and I believe they should have thought about it also.

"If you as a physician had this experience, wouldn't it be doubly frustrating for a lay person who knew nothing about such things?"

Oh, yes. I think this is true. Granted these kinds of diseases are not the easiest things to diagnose. The people I have known who have chronic neuromuscular disease have had a very similar experience; you know, people I have met through the MDAA *(Muscular Dystrophy Association of America)* Society. In Texas, we had a patient group that met every month and I would say that the experience of at least 15 out of every 20 patients there mirrored my own.

The time it takes to arrive at a correct diagnosis like this must be measured in years, not months, but years.

"What effect does this slowness at determining a diagnosis have on the treatment of the patient?"

None. There is, by and large, for many or most of these neuromuscular diseases, no treatment. It doesn't matter any from the standpoint of treatment. From the standpoint of peace of mind, and inheritance, it does matter. Many of these problems are inherited and you'd like to know that.

I knew, long before the doctors knew what I had, that it was muscular dystrophy. And I knew from my reading that there was no treatment. But it is my feeling that if there is any treatment which is not a great risk, I'd be willing to try it. Why not? What have I got to lose?

"What is the state of the art in muscular dystrophy research?"

They are doing a lot. The MDAA contributes millions of dollars and they are doing a lot. They are getting closer to an answer but they still have quite a way to go. They have opened up neuromuscular research institutes in a number of areas, Los Angeles, St. Louis, I think there's one in Houston, certainly one in New York, funded by the MDAA. The Jerry Lewis Telethon raised $22 million last year.

The problem is, though, if there is an area in neurology in which neurologists are weak it is the area of muscle disease. Play on words. Many of them just don't know anything about it and many centers are just not properly equipped to work up a patient. There is no point in doing a muscle biopsy if you can't handle it properly. And properly means not only regular pathology by someone who knows what the hell they're doing, which is not often, but histochemistry. There is a whole variety of enzyme stains, and electron microscopy. As well as the electromyogram. Often if you want it done right, you need to go to one of these MDAA institutes.

Many of the people I have met in the MDAA groups have the same regard in this area for neurologists that I do. They have been dealt with in an off-hand manner, at least according to them, not really well worked up. One doctor who examined one girl I know — I don't know whether or not he told her what she had — but he told her there wasn't anything they could do about it so not to worry about it. Of course, he didn't worry about it the moment he walked out of the room. *He* didn't have it. But she did. It is one thing to say "Don't worry about it" when you haven't got it and quite another thing to not worry about it when you have got it.

Everyone looks at their own problem as being the worst. If you say to them, "Wouldn't you rather have muscular dystrophy than be dead?" of course, they'd rather have MD, but they may still be very upset. Muscular dystrophy is going to have a significant effect on their life, not necessarily on the duration, maybe, but certainly their lifestyle. They cannot ignore it, they cannot forget it. It is there every minute of every day. For any doctor to say, "Forget it," or "Don't worry about it," is a joke. In a perverted way, I would like for some doctor to say that to me. He would not ever forget the reply.

The people whom I have met who deal with this kind of illness and for whom I have the highest regard as humanitarians are not the doctors at all. They are the physical therapists who are, with a few exceptions, very good people. They, and the people in the MDAA, the social workers or whatever they call their patient service coordinators, are real humanitarians, probably the finest people that I have ever met. Not the doctors, which I think is a terrible commentary on the medical profession.

How will society deal with the handicapped person in general? Whether the handicap is from Vietnam, from a birth defect, from an automobile accident or from disease, the handicapped may be the next great minority. But the problems are already here. There are too many things which are not dealt with now. Architecture is one of them. If a person who is confined to a wheelchair as I am goes on a plane somewhere, it is a major event. The airlines don't want to hassle it. Another example is the music center here in town. If I go at all, I must buy the most expensive seat because it is the only part of the hall I can get to. Somewhere along the line society is going to have to do something toward making things accessible for all of these people. There is no way, even if we had a mass transit system which was worth anything, that anyone who is handicapped can use it. The bus company gives a very low rate to handicapped people but few who are handicapped can get on the bus in the first place. So much for their discount.

One final point. It might sound as though I am not just terribly impressed over the general level of medical practice in this country in the way I was dealt with; that is true to a certain extent. However, I must add that I do think it is better here than any system that operates as a great socialized conglomerate. For all the trouble I had, in general the people were kind and were trying. If, added on to this trouble, I had had to contend with the bureaucratic red tape, inefficiency and dehumanizing aspects of a large volume welfare state system, it would have magnified the problems just that much more. I think any VA hospital would be a reasonable example. You notice that when Senator Kennedy had his son operated on, it was as a private patient, not as a clinic patient at a large government hospital. Who wants to be lost in a great crowd of people ensnarled in forms. Think back to your draft board physical, how dehumanizing. So, for all the problems I encountered, I still feel the system of private practice and non-socialized medical care is far and away the best way to do things.

> *In all important respects, the man who has nothing but his physical power to sell has nothing to sell which is worth anyone's money to buy.*
>
> Norbert Wiener
> *The Human Use of Human Beings* (1954), 9

XVI.
Germ Warfare

You have two chances — one of getting the germ and one of not. And if you get the germ you have two chances — one of getting the disease and one of not. And if you get the disease you have two chances — one of dying and one of not. And if you die — well, you still have two chances!

Anonymous

51. Bang's Disease

He lives in a large, white frame house which was once a farm home but is now totally surrounded by a medium-sized city in the Sunbelt. Although it is in sight of a divided expressway with three race lanes in each direction, it is necessary to skitter along a muddy road for a quarter of a mile to get to the house, which is in an area of widely-spaced, independently built homes.

He is 25, aggressive and intelligent. As a sales engineer for a prefabricated building manufacturer, he has prospered. He even pilots his own plane to visit prospective buyers. But now, he is off work, unable to pursue his career, waiting around for laboratory reports which will indicate to his doctors what they should do next. He is restless, disturbed, unhappy.

- **Nausea, Fever, Diarrhea**
- **Bang's Disease**
- **Brucellosis**

My illness, which I still have and which is undiagnosed as yet, started last October, five months ago, with symptoms of the flu: nausea, diarrhea, high fever. It was about the time everyone else was getting the flu. The fever continued and has continued to this date. At first, I just assumed it was the flu.

I went to my family physician, who is a general practitioner. He prescribed various antibiotics for about two months. He started out with penicillin which didn't do much good. He switched to amphycillin which seemed to work at first. The fever went away for a period of about two weeks and then came back again. He tried it again with similar results but the fever kept persisting after each treatment. He then prescribed Robyaxil — he called it his "big gun" — and I took that for 14 days without any effect on the fever at all.

After about two months of treatment, he insisted that I go to the hospital. I have a dislike for hospitals. None of us like to go to the hospital and I didn't feel sick enough to go into a hospital. I felt sick enough not to go about my daily activities, though. I'm a salesman and I have to be on my toes. But this low grade fever, having it this long, causes lapses of memory, dizziness, loss of orientation. I am also a pilot and was grounded because of this. The loss of orientation, getting lost while driving down the road, this sort of thing, is something I attributed to the fever. The doctors haven't said yes or no, but the two occurred simultaneously so I put them together. Anyhow, it has put me out of work. I've had to travel nationwide but I'm not able to do that now because I feel so weak, lost.

The fever is continuing. Very seldom does it drop to 98.6 degrees which is normal. It fluctuates on a daily basis. The lowest maximum it reaches in the cycle is about 100.1. The highest is 102. The fever tends to start about ten o'clock in the morning, peaks out about four in the afternoon and lasts 'til eight or nine when it starts dropping again. This happens every day, with about four days of high fever, two days of low fever and then four days of high fever again. They tentatively diagnosed it as brucellosis, Bang's disease, a micro-organism, a bacteria.

"I thought cows got that."

They do. Brucellis abortus is the name of the bacteria. It causes early aborting in cattle. Usually is undetected except the cow doesn't gain weight as quickly as she should and won't produce calves.

The diagnosis is not positive in my case because they haven't been able to cultivate the bacteria in culture nor has the titre, the level of antibodies in the bloodstream, reached a two-fold increase since the first detection.

The antibiotics they use for brucellosis are tetracycline and terramycin, both of which I'm allergic to. So rather than begin the massive treatments required to control brucellosis without having a positive identification, they're waiting for a four-fold increase in the titre level. They take a blood sample every couple of weeks to try to grow the brucellosis bacteria out and also to determine the level of brucellosis antibodies in the bloodstream.

The allergy I have to the antibiotics shows up as a rash in the wet portions of my body, in the mouth, under the arms, in the groin. So they want to stay away from that. They might cure the disease and kill the patient. And there's no percentage in that.

About 10 or 12 years ago, when these two were first introduced into the marketplace as common, broad-spectrum antibiotics, I had them given to me and broke out in this rash.

The amount of brucellosis bacteria in my body is apparently very small and the production of the antibodies occurs at a very slow rate. It will, over a period of three to five years, build up to a level sufficient to kill the bacteria. In the meantime, I'm just lying around having a fever every day. It impairs my ability to concentrate on what would be considered normal activities. As you can see right now, I'm breaking into a sweat.

They will probably use the antibiotics but it is sort of a Hobson's choice. I either have to put up with the fever or the rash. I'm supposed to know tomorrow if the diagnosis is really brucellosis.

I was in the hospital a week two months ago. They ran some tests, took blood samples for cultures every 30 minutes, tested for tuberculosis. Then I was in for two more weeks this month and they did the same kinds of tests only more extensively. This time they did lymphangiography where they inject dye into your feet to outline the lymph system. This is not diagnostic for brucellosis but may help identify the reason for this fever. I had the works. But after all of these tests, they're still not sure what I have.

I don't like hospitals. Hospitals are where people die and I was apprehensive about the outcome of my illness. I'd been in the hospital twice before, the first time for rheumatic fever when I was 16. I was in for about three weeks of bed rest. Then, when I was 22, about three years ago, I had appendicitis.

I thought the hospital I was in this time was excellent compared with the other hospitals I'd been in. Before, I was in an osteopathic hospital and a military hospital on an Air Force base. I think a private room is the only way to go. This hospital has only private rooms. But my insurance doesn't near cover all the expense of a hospital like this one. They charged me $83 a day but my insurance will only pay about $50. It covers the rest of it pretty well but I'll have to pay at least 20 percent of the bill.

It isn't the medical expense that bothers me; it's the fact that I'm losing my career. I've been incapacitated for five months now. I work for a construction company and do other paper work in this field on an independent basis. I've been a salaried employee for seven years and I had a very successful sales record last year and the company has been very generous. Despite that, it has eroded our savings, I know that.

In the hospital, the staff was excellent. The food service was a bit slow on occasion. There was one incident which irritated my wife and myself. After the lymphangiogram, I was weak and tired because I had been lying on that hard x-ray table for such a long time. My fever was up and when it goes up I automatically respond by drinking liquids. In the hospital, they have ice water so I started drinking ice water. About eleven o'clock it was pretty high, about 101 degrees, I guess, and I was delirious. I didn't know much what was going on. The nurse was asking me questions and my wife was trying to answer them and the nurse didn't like it and they had some words. It was a lack of communication. The doctor was trying to see what effect certain drugs had on my fever and the nurse was trying to find out but I didn't know this. We complained to the administrator about this nurse and he had the nursing supervisor look into it and after that, we didn't see that nurse again.

I've had four doctors consulting about me in the hospital and all but one deny that my fever could be brucellosis. One is an internist, another is a proctologist and one is an eye, ear, nose and throat man. I got a sore throat while I was in the hospital. The proctologist was called in because when I was a baby, my intestines were tied into a knot and the food wouldn't pass through and I had to be operated on when I was about three weeks old. This time, the x-ray showed some kind of enteritis at the base of the small intestine where it goes into the colon and they thought this might have something to do with the brucellosis. My family doctor just didn't know where to turn when he'd given me all those antibiotics and my fever was still there. He referred me to a specialty clinic in town and they put me in the hospital.

I don't see how that hospital pays its bills with all the people they have and their new building. People complain about their hospital bills but I know construction costs and I don't see how the hospital can make out with what it charges. They have good service. You don't have to wait more than 10 minutes whenever you ask for something.

My family doctor is someone we've been going to for years and years. He's an old gentleman in his 50's. I think maybe there ought to be a statute in which continuance is denied to doctors. I'm not saying the man is inept or incompetent but I think there's a stage in the game when a doctor should be retired. I think it should be after a general practitioner has served a certain length of time, perhaps 12 years. My family doctor may have caused the bacteria in my body to seclude themselves by the indiscriminate use of high-powered antibiotics. Had he taken the time to analyze me carefully, he might not have used all those drugs. I'm fishing for reasons but I've thought about it a lot. I think the family physician who gives patients antibiotics every time they come around may do more harm than good, may cause secondary infections to hang on because the antibiotics aren't effective when they're used too much.

There is so much happening in medicine today that if a man hasn't studied after he has been at school . . .

"What you are really advocating is mandatory continuing education."

Yes. A full year, back in the hospital, to learn the new things that are going on.

"Do you think there ought to be periodic reexamination and relicensing of physicians?"

I don't think reexamination is so important. It is just what the doctor knows about new ways to practice medicine. The doctors in the hospital were all younger and seemed to know more about diagnosing tough problems like mine. I know one thing. I'm not going back to my family doctor. And I'll tell him why. I wouldn't go back to him because I just don't have any confidence in him anymore. That may be a hard thing to say, but it may mean more if somebody like me comes right out and says it to him.

Why not put the surgical age of retirement for the attending surgeon at 60 and the physician at 63 or 65, as you think best? I have an idea that the surgeon's fingers are apt to get a little stiff and thus make him less competent before the physician's cerebral vessels do. However, as I told you, I would like to see the day when somebody would be

*appointed surgeon somewhere who had no
hands, for the operative part is the least part
of the work. Then, of course, many of us may
be, vascularly speaking, a little inelastic well
on this side of 60, or may remain in this
respect as youthful at 70 as are others at 50.
This is all a lottery of inheritance and
habits, and I shall be very glad, for one, to
have legislated to stop active work at 60.*

Harvey Cushing (1869–1939)
Letter to Dr. Henry Christian
November 20, 1911

52. Gangrene of the Foot

*It is night at the hospital. A low light provides a soft glow in the small, single
room.*

*She is a frail black lady, in her 90's, with sparse grey hair. She lies
quietly, occasionally shifting in the bed as she talks. It is difficult to get her to
discuss her condition; she seems to drift in and out of the present as she
recalls her life as a teacher. She married a Southern preacher early in this
century. She is devoutly religious and extremely well-educated considering the
opportunities available to a young negress in the late 1800's.*

*She is considerate and appreciative of all of the doctors and nurses who
care for her. While she silently endures her infirmity, her thoughts dwell on
the glories of the next life into which she eagerly awaits transformation.*

- **Painful Toes**
- **Gangrene of the Toes**
- **Amputation of the Right Leg**

My family doctor recommended that I be turned over to Dr. Tilson, that was
a couple of years ago, and I've been out and in. My regular family doctor
wasn't able to do surgery because he had been of the care-takin' himself; had

to have blood confusions and like of that. Dr. Tilson took hold of the troubles I had at that time which was connected with the colon and required surgery. It got better without hesitation and cured nicely.

This old foot was the thing that was giving me a whole lot of trouble recently. It gave me so much pain that it took all of the sweetness out of my mind. My doctor said that maybe my toes would have to be discarded. He said it was maybe either my toes or me.

That was last week and they completed the surgery. They had to take my right leg, right here *(points below the knee)*. This is the second dressin'. Dr. Tilson did the surgery last Tuesday.

"Are you feeling pretty good now?"

I'm feeling lots better than I did. They took off a portion of my limb. Now they take me to the place where you do exercises, by order of the doctor, twice a day.

"Physical therapy?"

Yes.

"What do they do in physical therapy?"

Well, now, that's like joyland. They're doin' first one thing and then another and it's marvelous to see how some people arc succeedin' on the directions that they give them, you know? Some have crutches and some have bicycles, some walkers. They were to put me on crutches yesterday, but they didn't. They're going to teach me to walk with crutches. That's one of the things they do. They do plenty things down there! It's a big room and different ones are doin' different things and succeeding. It's marvelous to see how one man learned how to walk, puttin' one foot behind the other. They had him walkin' naturally in no time.

I do well for my age. I've tried to make use of some little learnin' and I've tried to do as little harm to other people as I could, and in the meantime, take care of myself.

God gave me the ability to be a teacher and I was in the classroom for over 40 years, all grades. I was born in Georgia. I was sent to school without any knowledge of what learnin' meant and I had trouble, you know, right smart of trouble. We get other things from books but our wisdom comes from God. I had a secret place to hide in the garden where I could lock the gate, an old-fashioned garden gate so nobody could come in until I got through talkin' to God. I said I wanted to learn and I wanted Him to help me. I realized that He was the talent-giver. I said that if He'd help me learn myself, then I would teach others.

The record says I was one year old when 1880 came along so I must have been born in 1879. They didn't have birth certificates then.

I had good teachers who believed in honesty. And in what President Kennedy said — I can't exactly repeat it but — "not what my nation can do for me, but what I can do for my nation."

I spent the most time with the child that needed it most and I never had a minute's trouble with the boys and girls in the classroom. And I started some of them with their ABC's and they turned out to be doctors and lawyers. One of them panned out to be a doctor and he's in White Plains, New York. And I taught him his ABC's!

As a young woman I met a citizen of what they call Greater Miami and he took me, as a bride, to Miami, Florida.

"What year was that?"

Nineteen-hundred five. He was a minister of the gospel and I helped him. Where he went to preach, I'd go in the classroom. He'd go in the church. He'd preach and I'd teach. It was teamwork and we got along nicely.

"How long did you have this problem with your foot before you went into the hospital?"

I could feel somethin'. It's somethin' I can show better than tell. *(She brings her left foot from under the cover and lifts it up.)* My toenails grow so far and then they turn under, instead of growin' straight out. I believe I tore a portion of the nail off of that toe *(points to big toe)* and it turned black and began givin' me trouble. It started several months ago.

I want to be serious and not funny. My father was the father of eight children. I had one little sister that held me back gettin' to school. I stayed round home there 'til she got school age which got me behind.

I read my Sunday School lesson and learned that wisdom, knowledge and understanding must come from God. When I tarried in the garden He came; I won't say I saw Him but I heard Him. I was praying, tellin' Him what I wanted. And He said, "You want thus and so? Well, now, there are two roads." In a short answer, one led to hell and the other to heaven. He said what was at one end and what was at the other end, the opposite end. And He told me to make my choice. I made my choice. I stepped up on the royal right hand side. I told Him I wanted not a day's journey but a life journey.

This is what He said when I made my choice, "I'll meet you at the Jordan." When the Jordan billows begin to rage, He said He'd meet me there. And when I get there, all He'll have to say to the Jordan is, "Be still, be calm." And then we'll go over to the other side.

"How are the nurses and the doctors treating you here?"

Oh, everybody's just as nice and sweet, as they say, as a Georgia peach. Nothin' any better. Everbody's been nice to me.

I believe in that ol' time religion. If it's good enough for grandma, it's good enough for me.

"In a few weeks you will be out of the hospital and then you can go back to church."

There are lots of ways to go to church. I go to church anytime I stop to pray. I don't know when I'll be leavin' but other people needs this space here and they urgently needs to get rid of me as quick as they can. The family folks are talkin' and tryin' to get together and decide what can be worked out where I'll go. I don't know yet. They'll transfer me from this place to what they call medicare. I have been in intensive care and when they gets through with us with the exercises and everythin', we've got to move on.

I want to get on board His train, bound for Glory, when life's journey is finished. I want to hear Him call my name but you know what He told me? "Work back here." Maybe I had to talk to you. Maybe I had to talk to somebody else. He didn't let me in. He said, "Your reward awaits you. Work." When my day's labor in the vineyard is over, then I can come in. He knows more about when to tell me to come in. And I can't tell Him it's time to come in.

A physician can sometimes parry the scythe of death, but has no power over the sand in the hourglass.

Hester Lynch Piozzi, letter to
Fanny Burney, Nov. 12, 1781

53. Influenza

This story is told by the patient's sister, a retired college English teacher in her middle 70's. Her bearing is erect and commanding, undoubtedly as a direct result of example-setting for innumerable students over a lifetime of teaching.

She lives with another sister in a small town. Their home is a one-story white clapboard on the corner of two tree-shaded streets perhaps six blocks from Main. She raises flowers and thinks about the changes which have occurred over her lifetime. She laments the decline in standards of the performance of all professionals, educators as well as physicians. The current lack of emphasis on the basics of education is one of her major concerns.

● The Flu
● Influenza

This episode happened the first week in March this last spring. My sister living in the city became seriously ill with the flu. At that time, her husband was in the Veterans Hospital having a pacemaker inserted. Her family physician had died in December, and she had not yet established contact with a new physician. She was busy helping take care of her husband who is a diabetic, in serious condition, all organs affected, and she herself had worked with him, taking him back and forth to the hospital.

At that time the flu epidemic began getting pretty heavy and she caught it, somehow. A lot of people in the hospital were coughing and carrying on, she said. One night she was very sick and she called me up at seven o'clock the next morning for us to come and help her. We did. We took off immediately *(from a small town 70 miles away)*. Both of us live here.

We began giving her some of our home remedies, we took some medicine with us, standbys, you know, and I set about trying to find medical help for her. We gave her certain kinds of cold remedies that you hear advertised. These were my sister's standbys. I don't take any of them, so I don't know. We began trying to get some food down her because she hadn't been able to eat anything for two or three days.

Then I began calling, trying to find a doctor or somebody who could give us some help. She suggested that I call the county medical society. I did and the girl, the young woman or older, whatever, that was on the telephone, was indifferent about it. She couldn't do anything. We could take my sister to "emergency" and I said, "But she feels that she doesn't need to go to emergency. She feels that if she can have some medication to ease her, that would be helpful."

That story kept up all day that day, Tuesday. I called the neighbors and asked if they could give us any help. They tried their doctors and they would not offer any help. One of them suggested that we might go over to a nearby clinic because their doctor was over there. I called and the woman who answered was indifferent about it. I identified myself and the situation. In every instance, I went through the same story of what had happened because we weren't a case of someone being drunk, or out, or something like that. She was sick and we needed medical help. I tried to be as honest as I could in explaining the situation. Well, the girl over there said she didn't know what we could do except come to the clinic. I said, "Are there rooms over there where she could rest until the doctor can see her?" No, they didn't have that. I assumed that there would be facilities but, no, she'd just have to take her turn and wait there in the office which was full of sick people waiting to see the doctor.

I said, "Well, we can't do that. I cannot get her off this bed. She simply wants medication. She does not feel that going to emergency is what she needs." That was when the woman said, "Well, I don't know what we can do." At that point I was totally exasperated and I said, "I think I know. I think that we can prepare for death." She gasped and I hung up.

That wasn't the first calling. That was the seventh or eighth. I called 10 different doctors and organizations. When we reached that point, I was almost desperate. Before I had got to the clinic, I'd called the county medical society. The woman said, "I can't recommend doctors but I can give you the names of some doctors you might call and see if they'll help." The office personnel of these doctors again were indifferent, "No, the doctor does not make house calls." "No, the doctor will not be able to help you." "This is the doctor's day off and we have no way of getting hold of her. We have no idea where she is."

I kept on going, and calling, and crying. *Nobody* would give any help at all. No one. They didn't ask the doctor if he would help. They merely stated that he would not. These are office personnel, all of this time.

My sister said, "Let's try the physicians and surgeons exchange." I did, and went through the very same rigamarole. Every time it was of no help. No one was interested. No one would even call the doctor to the telephone to see if I could talk with him.

That's the way it continued all of that day. My sister's temperature was 104 degrees. She was so sick that she was almost in a convulsion. My other sister kept giving her this medicine she takes — it's a product you can buy off the counter at the drugstore and she thinks it is very helpful — but it made my sister even worse. It made her very sick at her stomach. It nauseated her dreadfully. She almost went into a rigor of some kind, convulsions.

All of this time we are getting no help but the neighbors are trying to help us and they are getting no cooperation either. The next door neighbor, who is a Catholic and attends the Catholic church there, said they had a nursing service up there and she said she'd see if she could get the nurse to come and give my sister a shot or something. We didn't quite get to that. We were about ready to call her but we decided to wait a little bit to see if we could get connected through the physicians and surgeons exchange.

Night came. We went through the night, badly. The next morning my sister said, "I think my pharmacist can help us. Call Joe."

He'd been her pharmacist for 25 years. "Maybe he can get us a doctor."

I called him and he said, "Yes, I can recommend a doctor over here. I've sent a number of patients to him that needed a doctor.

When I told my sister the name of the doctor he'd recommended, she said, "I believe that must be the same person who was in college when I was secretary to one of the officers of the college, long ago."

I called his office and his receptionist was the first one in all that long list of people I called who was even polite. I was encouraged at last. She said, "The doctor is busy but I'll have him call you." And he did, in about five minutes.

When I told him what my sister said by way of identification, he said, "Good God, that's 40 years ago."

I explained to him what we were trying to do and why she didn't have a doctor. He said, "I can do two things. I can put her in a hospital or I can call a prescription to a drugstore." I asked him to do the latter.

I went over and got the medicine and we started the medication. It was antibiotics. That was about noon on the second day and by night she was showing some reaction to the medication and she was able to settle down and rest a little. It was affecting her.

The next day she was better. Five days later, when she was improved enough, we took her over to the doctor's office. In the course of everything, he agreed then to take her case. He has her case now and she's very happy about him. He is reasonable and fine.

As I sat over there in the waiting room and looked around, and listened and watched, I noted that there are two other doctors in that complex. One of them is the woman doctor I tried to call whose office girl didn't know where she was and had no way of finding out. I didn't exactly buy that bill of goods, as you can imagine.

We spent an agonizing two days trying to get a doctor and it upset us terribly, and the neighborhood. I sat down and began writing it all down. I decided I had to get that out of my system and on paper. I jotted down all of the bits of information and what had been said to me. I said, "I'm going to write a letter to somebody."

I composed that letter and worked on it for about a week before I ever sent it off. I worked on it and polished it so that I thought it was reasonable and a fair and accurate statement. I made copies and mailed them to the county medical society, to the physicians and surgeons exchange, to the local clinic and to the doctors I'd called and to the two newspapers in the city. They both published it. They did, to my great surprise. One edited it slightly, omitted two sentences, but the other one published it exactly as I wrote it.

At any rate, I got the letter off to these people and appended a note to each one that I would like a response from the doctor, not the office personnel, and I have not heard from a one. Not one.

The idea is that if you don't have contact with a doctor that's strong, you don't get help. That's a problem you have to fight. It is a totally helpless feeling and so frustrating and disgusting. You get to thinking, "What is this thing of medical training doing for training doctors to be interested in their patients or in building a profession?" I think it's serious. And here is the hue and cry that we hear so often that we just don't have enough doctors. But we know three young men right now that cannot get into a medical school. They are worthy young men, through college, on other jobs, waiting for the word that they can be admitted to a med school. They're turned down right and left. One of them is the son of a doctor, who is a good one. Now, what is the problem?

It is difficult indeed for a layman in the city to find the right physician if he has been so fortunate as to have had good health until some emergency arises.

Robert Tuttle Morris (1857–1945)
Doctors Versus Folks, Ch. 3

XVII.
Head Trouble

Pain of mind is worse than pain of body.

Latin Proverb

54. Undiagnosed Psychiatric Disorder

She is 17, bright, vivacious, a college freshman. She is on her own, living on social security because her father, whom she adored, is now dead. He was a highly-paid research chemist.

She hates English grammar, loves accounting, wants to be a business executive and make a lot of money.

- **Suspected Mental Illness**
- **Psychiatric Treatment**

My mother has this thing about attention, she wants attention all of the time. So this one particular time, when I was 11 or 12 years old, she took an overdose of pills to get my father's attention. She wanted it to look like a suicide attempt but we all knew it wasn't real. My father was in the bathroom next to the bedroom when she took them and she told him the minute he came out so there was no more than a five-minute difference there. Well, they took her to the hospital and the whole shot and she wound up going to the psychiatrist, Dr. Schmidt.

They took me down there, and my father, we all went there because Dr. Schmidt wanted to talk to the family and find out what led up to my mother taking the overdose. He treated it like an actual suicide attempt although everybody involved knew it wasn't an actual suicide attempt. I knew, my father knew, my mother knew, the dog knew.

After my parents had talked with the doctor and with the psychologist who worked with him, Dr. Schmidt wanted to talk to me alone. He asked me, "What does 'A bird in the hand is worth two in the bush' mean?" So I told him. I don't know what I said now but everybody knows what these things mean. Then he said, "What does 'A penny saved is a penny earned' mean?" I told him that. "What does 'A rolling stone gathers no moss' mean?" I told him that.

He was your typical psychiatrist; he was German or Russian or something like that with a pronounced accent, beady little eyes and a bald head with a little tuft of hair on the top. The whole job. He would sit behind his desk, with his elbows resting on the desk and his fingers pointed like this *(demonstrates by placing both index fingers under her chin)*. And he'd stare.

He'd be slouched down under his desk and he'd stare, with nothing but his head sticking out and these two fingers pointed under his chin. He sat there and stared at me for a few minutes and I was getting more and more uncomfortable 'cause I was a kid, you know? Eleven or twelve. Finally, he said, "Step outside and ask your parents to come in here." After those three questions. Five minutes later, they had me bundled up in a car and on my way to the psychiatric center. Nobody had told me anything. All I was told was, "You're going to a mental institution" and, zip, I was on my way.

"Who told you that?"

My parents. And I was going, "Why?" you know. Anyhow, I didn't get to pack my clothes or anything. Nothing. Zip, and I was on my way, right from that psychiatrist's office to the place.

So we get there and I thought, "Well, the whole thing can't be that bad. It just can't be. It's just gotta be one big joke or something." Somehow, I knew that there were two kinds of wards, your open ward and your locked ward in most such places. And I thought, "I can't be any worse than open ward, for God's sake. I'm not a raving maniac or anything." They put me in the locked ward. I don't know why.

They had unbreakable windows and a guy in there went really nuts and tried to throw a bed through the window but it didn't even break the glass! The bed bounced right back.

There were several people in locked ward with me. There was Sharon, my roommate and a guy who called himself Beowulf. He had a little dog with him. His brother was a lawyer, good-lookin', too. Then there was the old lady going through menopause who would skip up and down the halls. She'd do that all day long. Then there was another girl named Sarah who was really nutsy. She ripped a towel bar off the wall and went after Sharon with it, like a maniac. Who else. Oh, yes, there was a lady named Bonnie but she was always in the room where they strap you down to a bed on a flat, low, leather-covered bed.

"Weren't you awfully frightened?"

Yeah, except that Sharon was normal and I really wasn't all that worried. Sharon took drugs a lot. There was nothing wrong with her mentally except that she couldn't get off of drugs. She wasn't schizophrenic and she wasn't psychotic and she didn't come at you with weapons and weird things like that. She wasn't an attacker. She just took drugs. We got to be friends and after I got out, we stayed friends.

It was like a hotel, kinda. It had a hall, with different rooms off the hall. Sharon was my roommate. In the locked ward, there were these rooms but everybody didn't have a roommate because there weren't that many people in there. In the open ward, they had a girl's room for six girls and one like that for boys, if you wanted to pay less money.

My parents didn't explain anything to me and I kept saying. "When am I going to get my clothes? Will you bring my favorite dress?" I was a kid, out for adventure and I wasn't really thinking about what was really happening. I was thinking, "God, I'm getting to get away from my Goddamn parents for a while. Oh, joy. Big vacation No school for a while. What fun." The whole shot, until I got there. It was a little different then.

I was really freaky because when I got there they said, "Okay, you're going in that ward there," and when I turned around to say good-bye to my parents, bam. Those doors were shut in my face. I didn't get to say good-bye to them or anything. It was really weird.

After I was in the locked ward for two or three weeks, Dr. Schmidt told me I could get in the open ward. So I went out there and was all settled in my new room in the open ward when he called me in to the conference room and said, "You're not going to be able to smoke any more." I said, "What?" I'd been smoking a long time. My parents had just bought me my first carton of cigarettes and I was really freaked out. I thought, "This guy's trying to take away the only thing I've got left in this place." You couldn't have your makeup because you might break the glass in your mirror and go after somebody, you know? So we had an argument about the cigarettes and he put me right back in the locked ward. And I didn't get my cigarettes there, either. I bummed them offa Sharon. Dr. Schmidt said I was too young to smoke. I told him that wasn't for him to say because my parents gave me permission and they were supplying me with them. "It's none of your damn business," I told him. He was there to take care of my mental health, not my physical health.

The locked ward was a lot different than the open ward, where they had occupational therapy. In the locked ward, there wasn't anything at all.

We could walk up and down the halls and when the nurses weren't looking, we could kiss the guys, you know? Biggy wow wow. Nothing to do so you do anything you can think of. Allen was my big heart throb. I got a big old crush on him, fell in love with him, my first heart throb. He was in the room across the hall from Sharon's and mine. Sharon had a crush on Allen's roommate so whenever . . . the nurse's station was positioned right on the corner and was glass all around where they could see into the recreation room and down this hall and the other hall. It was L-shaped. Whenever the nurses' backs were turned at night, we'd crawl across the hall like little snakes on our bellies. Sharon would crawl across over there and Allen would crawl across to my room. And we'd sit there and, you know, listen to the radio or whatever.

It was really rotten, though, because we had to go to bed at ten o'clock at night, all of us. They did bed check at midnight and by that time, all of us were asleep anyhow.

"Back in your own rooms?"

Yeah. What did we do for recreation? We sat there and stared at each other's belly buttons. We could read but there were no books. It was mainly the incidents which happened in there which kept us occupied. I had this brand new sweater. It was beautiful, lilac, kind of a middy, really neat. One day Sharon, who was much fatter than I am, wanted to wear it. Well, that was all right. It was a sweater and would stretch. She went out in the hall and the little old lady who skipped up and down said, "You can't wear that." And Sharon said, "Why not?" The little old lady said, "Because you don't look good in it." Sharon said, "I don't really give a damn." She was really snotty anyhow and they got into a fight. The little old lady tried to rip the sweater off of Sharon and Sharon was beatin' up on that little old lady and it was really weird but it was our excitement for the day, you know?

Once Sarah and Sharon got into a fight. That's when Sarah ripped the towel rack off the wall and went after Sharon, chasing her up and down the hall. And the nurses just sat back and watched. They didn't care. They just ignored most everything we did, unless we were trying to have a little fun. Then it was different. "You can't do that," they'd say.

"Did the doctors give you psychotherapy during this period you were in the locked ward?"

No. I saw Dr. Schmidt once or twice and his psychologist lady who worked with him, she came in once. We never really got to talk. The couple of times he did show up, he'd say, "Vell, how are you?" And I'd say, "I'm alive," and he'd say, "Good-bye" and walk out. Sharon hated him and she didn't even know him. And I wasn't on any medication except one little pill if I couldn't sleep at night, only on the nights I needed it.

I was in the locked ward about three weeks and then I got into open ward maybe two or three weeks. There was occupational therapy and we could make our little belts and tile ash trays and things like that. You could go outside, there was a volleyball court.

If you were one of the more advanced people in open ward, you could make a belt. You had to have your doctor's say-so because you had to use special tools and they were afraid you might attack somebody with the special tools.

Everybody in open ward, everybody, I mean the young dopers and the old ones, not old, but — you're going to kill me — about your age, ancient. They all went out for pizza because it was right next door, but I wasn't allowed to go. Nobody ever told me why. I'd ask and they'd say it was because Dr. Shit said so. I called him that because he was one big shit. He was.

In open ward you didn't have to eat the food if you didn't want to. And I lost a lot of weight in that place because they had really trashy food. I'm telling ya. You know, you go to jail and you get just as bad food as we got there. And they fed us lumpy, cold porridge in the mornings. The reason it was so lumpy and cold in the locked ward, they waited until the people in the open ward had already eaten. After they had cleared out of the dining room and the kitchen help had cleaned up the dining room, they'd take the oatmeal that was left over and bring it to the people in the locked ward.

Well, my God, by the time they walked from the dining room building to the locked ward building it was really cold. We just got what was left over. And we had to eat it. In my case, if I didn't eat it, I didn't get my cigarettes. The doctor said I couldn't smoke but the aides would give me cigarettes anyhow. I guess they knew what it was like to crave a cigarette. If I didn't eat my oatmeal, I wouldn't get my cigarette. It was kinda blackmail.

In the whole place, you're not allowed to have makeup. Come to think of it, in the open ward you were, but not in the locked ward. They keep it in a little tub, with your name written on it, at the nurse's station. They'd let you have it in the morning to put your makeup on and then they'd take it away from you. You could keep two or three things and nobody'd say anything so if you did that every day, you'd have it all by the end of the week. Well, if Sharon didn't eat her oatmeal, they'd come in and take away all of her makeup. If you didn't eat, you just lost out on whatever you wanted. You lost your privileges.

There was one time that Sharon said she didn't give a shit if they took her makeup away, she wasn't going to eat that shit. It was dinner that time and it was even worse than the oatmeal. It was some casserole which was really terrible. She said she didn't give a damn, so whenever she went to take her shower, they had a nurse stay in there the whole time she was showering and getting dressed and everything. She couldn't go to the bathroom without the nurse following her. She couldn't do anything. So she wound up eating. One way or the other, you'd wind up losing privileges or having some kind of discomfort applied.

After three weeks or so in the open ward, I finally got to go home but after that I had to go to group therapy in the doctor's office. There were about a half dozen other people in the group. One time when we met, Dr. Schmidt said before the whole group that I was illegitimate and that my mother didn't want me. Then he said I was a prostitute and a slut and a whore and all of these wonderful, lovable things. He said that I was worth less than a piece of shit and that my parents ought to put me in the garbage. Then he turned around and contradicted himself by saying that my natural parents gave me up for adoption. They kept my three brothers but they couldn't stand me and that's why they gave me up for adoption.

I didn't say anything in the group. I just kept quiet and went home and told my parents what the doctor had said.

"What did you parents think about that?"

My father was really pissed. I mean he really got mad. My mother didn't pay much attention because she doesn't think much about anybody else. But my father went down to the doctor's office and they had a big, blazin' fight and I didn't have to go back anymore. This happened maybe the second or third time I had been there.

There was a boy in the group who thought the KGB, the Russian police, were after him. And one time he wanted to go to the bathroom so bad his tongue was floatin'. The doctor wouldn't let him go but he decided he'd go anyhow and went to the door and started to open it when Dr. Schmidt grabbed his ears and started pulling them and made him sit back down again. He never did get to go until the group session was over. God, that poor guy. He was really frustrated.

I was convinced that Dr. Schmidt knew all along there wasn't anything wrong with me. He was just ripping off my parents by making them think he was doing them such a big favor by taking care of me. In fact, after this whole thing happened, my parents took me to another psychiatrist. Can you believe it? They still didn't believe I was normal. This other psychiatrist knew Dr. Schmidt and we had a little discussion about the whole thing and he said that just about everybody knew that Dr. Schmidt was like that. He said there was nothing wrong with me at all.

My parents adopted me when I was three or four years old and they didn't know what to expect. They didn't understand that 11 year olds are rude and rebellious and argumentative. At 11 years old, your average kid is like that. I wanted to stay out after midnight, wanted to go to girl-boy parties, wanted to go out on dates, wanted to wear the kind of clothes all the other girls wore, you know? They didn't understand all that, figured I was "tetched in the head."

Their friends didn't have any children that age either. My mother has always been a hypochondriac or an alcoholic or something. Always bidding for attention. She's never been good with people so my father never brought anybody home from the office. I think maybe three times in my whole life we entertained somebody at home. Since they didn't have any friends, there wasn't anybody to discuss the behavior of 11-year-old kids with. So they didn't know what to expect. They thought I was downright nuts.

My father never did want to take me to the psychiatrist in the first place. Nobody had to tell me that for me to know it. He was blazin' mad at my mother for starting this whole thing in the first place. Even though he didn't understand my behavior, he wanted to let it go for a while to see if I was really nuts or just being a kid. My mother, though, has a hang-up. She wants everybody to be crazy and go into nuthouses. She's been in, I think, two or three times. For some reason, I just think she wanted me to be crazy.

After my father died, I was into drugs for a while. I was takin' drugs because everybody was takin' drugs, you know. There's no reason why you take drugs, you just take 'em. (Laughs) I never took 'em every day or every week. I'd just take 'em once every three months for my big bango, my big night on the town. I took Elavils and Valiums. I took 'em because everybody at school was talkin' about how neat Valiums were and how hard they were to get hold of. And so here's my mother, sitting at home with a whole damn bottle full of them, for free. I didn't have to go out and buy 'em and I didn't have to worry about whether they were good stuff because they were prescription, you know? And, hell, right next to them there was sitting a bottle of Elavil. So I thought, "This is my chance. I'm going to hit it big with the rest of them." So I took a bunch of them and we went out to dinner that night. I could hardly get my dinner down and I passed out in the car on the way home. I took too many of them.

They thought . . . hell, I don't know what they thought. They took me to the hospital and the whole shot and let me sleep it off. My aunt told the doctor I'd been smoking pot and had passed out. You don't pass out from smoking pot.

The next week, I O.D.'ed again so my mother started putting two and two together. She decided, "Here's a good reason to call her crazy. She's takin' dope." I got loaded that weekend because my boyfriend and I had just broken up. I was pretty upset about it but not enough to do away with myself because Jimmy wasn't that hot stuff. But my mother decided I was trying to commit suicide so she sent me to stay the weekend with these friends of hers, another old fogey couple. Then she got ahold of this psychiatrist who talked to me for five minutes over the telephone and he says I ought to be committed. This was worse than Dr. Schmidt. A five-minute, over-the-phone diagnosis when I was on dope and he knew I was on dope and that I didn't know what I was saying. He asked me a bunch of dumb questions.

I don't know what happened after that. Everything's kind of . . . you see, my life's always been like this, so nutsy and everything, that I don't pay any attention to these odd things anymore. If you live in a haunted house, you forget about the ghosts after awhile.

Anyone who spends money on a psychiatrist should have his head examined.

Samuel Goldwyn (1882–1974)

A new definition of psychiatry is the care of the id by the odd.

Anonymous

55. Drug Addiction

It was late fall. We met outside the clinic door in a western mountain city. The clinic was closed so we sat on the grass in a tiny, triangular park across the street. The weather was unseasonably warm, the sun felt good.

She is 25, a slim, shapely girl dressed in faded blue jeans and a clean white sweater. She wears a short, beaded necklace from which hangs a small white bird which resembles a dove or a gull. Her blonde hair is a little stringy. She is learning drafting at a vocational school so she can support herself and her two-year-old boy.

- **Drug Addiction**
- **Methadone Treatment**

When I first came to the clinic, I was real strung out. I was taking about 60 milligrams of dilaudid intravenously every day, had been for two years. I had a friend who was on the methadone program and told me about it and I came over.

I was real sick. I hadn't had any drugs for about 24 hours and was very, very ill. It's like having the flu. You have a headache, cramps, you can't keep anything on your stomach. You're freezin' to death and you're sweatin' at the same time. You can't sleep, you can't eat, you have diarrhea. It's pretty bad. It's real bad. I understand alcoholism is worse but . . .

"If you had been using dilaudid for two years, where did you get it?"

From doctors. You can go to a dentist and be in some kind of pain or maybe none at all and tell him, "I'm visiting, I'm from out of town and I have this toothache and I just need some 'til I get back home where I can see my own dentist," and you can get a prescription that way. But I never got any drugs on the street. My boyfriend has back trouble and you know that's real hard to prove and he had a doctor who gave him 60 dilaudid a week and then he had another one who would do the same thing and I never had to pay for any of it.

When I went to the clinic, I was shooting as many as 60 milligrams a day. I started out with just a little and it built up. It got so I was shooting every couple of hours.

"Couldn't you take the pills by mouth?"

To the drug addict, shooting dope is the only way. That's the way you get a rush. I don't know just how to describe it, but as soon as the needle goes in you get a warm feeling all over. You feel wonderful. You might compare it to an orgasm.

I was in a situation where I had all of the drugs I wanted at my disposal. Most people get just enough to keep them from getting sick but for an addict, my situation was ideal. And that was my biggest problem. Even when I came to the clinic and got on the methadone program, I couldn't stay off of it. I had it around me. Now I've severed my relationship with my friends who were using drugs. I take my methadone every day.

"What motivated you to start on the methadone program?"

I have a two-year-old child and I'm on probation. I was threatened with losing him. So I came here one day when I was real, real sick. First of all, you have to prove that you are an addict. You have to show symptoms, needle marks on your arms and you have to give 'em "dirty urine" which is urine with drugs in it.

Then it takes about three days. They start you off with 10 milligrams and you work up until you're at a comfortable level. They substitute the methadone for the drugs completely. Only you don't feel anything, you don't feel any pain, it stops the pain of withdrawal completely. Once I quit cold turkey and my bones ached for months. The only problem with methadone is that it is equally as addicting as heroin or any other kind of narcotic.

You don't get the rush with methadone. It just stabilizes you. I'm not high right now. I just took my medicine. It just stabilizes you, makes you normal.

When you're taking drugs, when you're taking heroin, even when you're taking alcohol, it becomes a necessity, a part of your life, just like eating. Your body can't function without it. What methadone does, it just simply replaces it. It replaces an illegal drug with a legal one.

"Do you get it free?"

Twenty dollars a year.

"If methadone replaces dilaudid, does that mean you will be on it from now on?"

No. I started out at 60 milligrams of methadone and I'm now down to 25. I've been on and off methadone for a year. In other words, I started one time on a 21-day detox *(detoxification)* which is what they start you with. That will take you off the drug. Well, as soon as I got off, I started right back on again. Then about 30 days later, I came back and kicked again. As soon as I finished kickin', I went right back on again. This time, I decided I would stick on it. What I'm on now is called a maintenance program, where you can come off at your own discretion or you could stay on for the rest of your life if you wanted.

If you go on the 21-day detox program, you can get off the drugs completely and it's not as bad as if you went cold turkey. I've been on this decline program since April *(five months)* and I expect to be off completely in six more weeks. I'm starting what they call a biofeedback program which measures alpha waves. I'll be starting on that tomorrow. I've set six weeks as my goal to be drug free.

See, all right, let me explain the biofeedback program. You think, when do you want to shoot up drugs? When do you feel like you want to do it? When are you tense? What causes it? Then you think about what makes you want to shoot up drugs and you learn to control that urge, without the drugs. They have a room set up in the clinic for biofeedback.

"Suppose you felt like shooting drugs at two a.m. You are restless, alone and you get the urge, you want a rush. Do you think you will be able to utilize this biofeedback method without some way of measuring the alpha flow?"

What he told me is, you learn to control it without a feedback measuring device. It is a way of teaching you to be more aware of your inner self. We are living in a world where everything's out there and we don't pay enough attention to what we are actually feeling or how we are really responding. This is supposed to teach you to be aware of your feelings and your responses and things like that. At two a.m., it would be pretty hard to do anything about getting any drugs, anyway.

Of course, the first thing you've got to do if you're going to kick the habit is to get rid of the drugs and your friends. I've done both. I've had a lot of trouble, because I've been on and off. I've been clean now for four months, the first time I've gone that long. It's tough to kick your friends. They go hand in hand with your habit, you know.

My little boy is two and a half years old; his father and I are separated. He's really a little doll, real cute, healthy. He lives with me. I'm taking architectural drafting. I go to a school that teaches computer data processing, keypunch, and different kinds of drafting, things like that. I've been in this program two weeks now. So you see, suddenly, in just the past few weeks, a lot of changes have happened in my life.

"Do you get child support?"

No, I don't get anything from my husband. I'm on ADC *(Aid to Dependent Children)* and I have a grant, a $2500 grant from the government. It's not much.

All of my friends were into drugs. And when the supply diminished, the friends diminished. They quit comin' around. My boyfriend was their source of supply. That's the situation you find with most drug addicts. They're your friends when you've got a supply.

The way we got our drugs, we knew how much we were getting. There wasn't much chance of an overdose. There wasn't much chance of me having to go out on the street and sell my body to get the drugs. Heroin costs $65. I was on dilaudid all of the time. You can switch from one to the other 'cause it's all basically the same, but I didn't.

I came to the methadone clinic when I started needin' help. You get to the point where there's no amount of drugs that can . . . you know, you just need more and more. There's no end to it.

In my situation, it was basically legal. Immoral and unethical, yes, but legal. I wasn't on the streets.

"How many of your former companions have been able to do what you have toward kicking the habit?"

I don't know any.

Even a lot of the people who come over here to the clinic use drugs and they get methadone. Both! One thing methadone does, though. They try to get you on a blockading dose, which is 40 milligrams, and at that point you can't feel the drugs even if you shoot 'em. It kills the craving for a rush and if you want, you can get off drugs that way.

Now, I'm coming down. I admit I have a craving. I'd like to, but I have will power. I've come this far and I don't want to screw it up now.

One time I did some heroin and I O.D.'ed. I just went to sleep. If I was going to die, that's the way I'd do it. If I was going to commit suicide. I did it, I took the needle out of my arm and the next thing I knew I was being rolled around in the snow outside. When my friends revived me, I was loaded for at least 24 hours.

I have a terrific counselor at the clinic. He's very much involved in his work. There are some — I'm not too good with words — I think some of the counselors look down on you. I don't feel put down, but then, I'm more or less from the same background as a lot of them. I don't think I'm your average heroin addict.

"Are counselors ordinarily ex-drug addicts?"

No. None in there, no. I'd think that would be a little dangerous. Because there's a lot of people who come over here and sell drugs. You know, they'll catch somebody in a weak state of mind and sell drugs to 'em. You're never really cured, you know, that's what they say. Say a counselor had been clean for a year or so and he thought, "Oh, well, it wouldn't hurt if I did." He might go ahead and start again. On the other hand, I think it would be easier for an ex-addict to relate and also the clients couldn't pull the wool over their eyes which happens quite a bit, I think. But, basically, the counselors are pretty conscientious, concerned. The guy that does the biofeedback is really nice. He's really into it, helping people.

When you buy drugs off the street, you get mostly trash. You don't know what you're gettin'. What can I say? Most people have their connection, get it from the same person all of the time and that way they can be pretty certain what they're getting. But if you do get burned, if somebody does sell you bad drugs or something that's not even drugs at all, you can always go back to him and kill him. I mean, that's the way it is out there.

A lot of things are going good for me right now. I like drafting. There is a lot of need for good draftspersons, especially for women. You know, they have to hire a certain amount of women and there's only two girls in my class, out of 30. I have no idea where I'll go to work. I've only been in school two weeks. I have ten months to go.

The grant pays my tuition. It's called a B.E.O.G. grant, a Basic Education Opportunity Grant.

I've smoked marijuana and I like it. It does almost the same thing for you as three beers would do. A bag of marijuana costs anywhere from 10 to 25 dollars. I don't buy drugs at all, I never did, but I'll go over to somebody's house and they'll say, "Want to smoke a joint?" and I'll do it. But that's about the extent of it.

I started taking drugs when I was 14. I didn't start shooting drugs. The first thing I ever did, I sniffed glue. Then I got into my dad's liquor. Then I started smoking marijuana, taking LSD, speed, THC, you name it, I've taken it. Finally, when it gets to the point you'll do anything, you're a drug addict.

I didn't take drugs all that time everyday but you know, off and on. I was completely straight one time for two years. Early on, I wasn't shooting any drugs and I didn't think there was a thing wrong with smoking pot and I still don't think there's anything wrong with that. See, everybody was doing it. That was during the era of Haight-Ashbury when drugs were being introduced. That was the thing to do and I fell into that real easily. My parents knew what I was doing and they sent me to a bunch of doctors. We fought all the time at home over my using drugs.

I went out to California and lived right on Sunset Strip for a year and then moved up to Haight-Ashbury and lived right off there on Cole Street. I was by myself. I finished high school when I was 16 and I took off two days afterwards. And I've been on my own ever since, kinda. I went back home for awhile.

When I was pregnant, my husband was doin' real well. He was manager of the shoe department in one of the finest department stores here. I went into the hospital to have my baby, had a Caesarian and was in there a month. When I got home, he had quit his job because now I could work. He stayed home and took care of the baby and I didn't mind because I wasn't ready for motherhood. Except he wasn't doing a very good job. He'd sit home and pluck his guitar all day and have his friends over and they'd drink beer. He'd have the baby in bed all day so he wouldn't have to watch him, so when I'd get home at night, the baby would be wide awake and I'd have to clean up all of the beer cans from him and his friends all day long. I was working as a waitress, a cocktail waitress. It's good money.

When I was at Haight-Ashbury, I got all of the drugs I wanted free. I was young, healthy, rosy cheeked and had all my teeth and the guys gave me anything I wanted. It was easy. I used to like speed, amphetamines, the best. Speed makes you skinny, keeps you awake at night. That was the first thing I started shootin'. I can't describe the feeling; I don't know. I felt so good. It drives you out of your mind. It gives you a feeling of grandeur, like you can do anything. Other times it gives you a terrible paranoia, like you see a guy walkin' down the street and you just know he's a cop and he's going to get you.

You get sky high and I usually had to use something to come down, seconal or something. But the thing about speed is that the ideas you get while you're on it will continue after you've kicked it. The paranoia and all.

I've been smoking marijuana for 11 years and it hasn't done anything to me. Well, maybe it's hurt my voice a little bit. It's always been deep. I've noticed it lately because a friend of mine gave me a bag of weed the other day. I had a party so I could get rid of it. I don't like to have drugs around the house.

I say there is so much more in life that you can get high on. I don't think smoking a joint is harmful but anything you do in excess is going to hurt you. And I say, find something else that's interesting, a hobby, a boyfriend, anything.

"A baby?"

Well. I wouldn't advise that for a 14 year old. You always have to be using your mind a lot. You've got to be developing. Of course, we all have our period in life when we are stagnating. When people are bored is when they are most likely to use drugs.

I knew this guy once, he was about 30 years old and he was into speed. He'd kicked the habit maybe a year before but he was still paranoid. He thought people were talking about him behind his back. He was handsome, looked like you would imagine Jesus Christ looked. He was a great guy, great personality, talented.

One day he took some LSD, speed and something else. Then he took a shotgun, pointed it here *(points to her groin)* and blew himself all over the wall. He just couldn't get out of his head the things he thought when he was on speed. He couldn't accept the fact that it wasn't real. It's hard to accept the fact that you're crazy.

Thou has the keys of Paradise, oh, just, subtle and mighty Opium!

Thomas De Quincy (1785–1859)
Confessions of an English Opium-Eater, Pt. II

The Poppy hath a charm for pain and woe.

Mary A. Barr (1852–?)
White Poppies

56. Alcoholism

He is a man of considerable girth who wears black suits to deemphasize his weight. He is a consulting engineer, 56 years old, with expertise in nuclear physics and chemistry. Stimulated almost to logorrhea by controversial discussion, he has the educational background to argue politics, economics, religion and other subjects with disarming effectiveness. He is quite active in a one-of-a-kind liberal church located in a stronghold of fundamentalism. He smokes cigars.

- **Excessive Drinking**
- **Alcoholism**

Actually, I guess I was like many alcoholics in that my alcoholism was far from being a medical consideration. I consider I was really an alcoholic for five or 10 years but I drank a total of 17 years starting when I was 18-years old. The first part of my drinking experience was just ordinary drinking with the boys in college and this sort of thing. Drinking seemed to do more for me than for the average person and I used it more and more to relax and get to sleep at night. I rationalized this regular though fairly moderate drinking in my early years as just a coping mechanism, a little self-medication, the way many people use tranquilizers and sleeping pills today.

But it got to where I needed more all of the time. Of course, I rationalized that again, being a large person; I've always weighed over 200 pounds. There were lots of complicating details. I was concerned with my weight; I tended to be too heavy and knew that I was. I would try to diet and this sort of thing. The doctor was after me to lose weight and prescribed Dexedrine tablets as an appetite suppressant and a Dexamil tablet for the third tablet of the day which was supposed to not give me so much lift to where I couldn't sleep at night. After a period of time, I found this wasn't working too well. I was not losing weight and I was drinking heavily at night. In fact, it had gotten to be a compulsive drinking pattern. I mentioned to the doctor that I had gastro-enteritis and this was probably brought on by drinking too much and it might be better if I had a sleeping pill at night. He had tried to tell me to take a three or four block walk before going to bed and I tried that once and it didn't do any good. Anyway, we ended up with a prescription for a barbital of which I was to take one and then if that didn't work in a couple of hours, I could take another one.

It wasn't long before I found that it took one or two more to get the job done. Then I experienced drowsiness in the morning, so I would take two of the five milligram Dexedrine tablets to pick me up. So, I was trying to knock myself out at night and wake myself up in the morning with drugs. Uppers and downers. It was a typical self-medication effort that I see in a lot of alcoholics, medicating their tensions and anxieties with alcohol and other drugs.

I found that I could substitute a large, standard barbital tablet for about two ounces of alcohol. I proceeded to drink the other 10 ounces of alcohol every night. I wound up drinking a pint of liquor every night, half of that being alcohol, roughly, and taking the sleeping pills besides.

I started taking these sleeping pills early, about five or 5:30, before dinner, so I would get some effect before I ate. I was always careful to eat well, plenty of proteins and vitamin B and these good things because I knew that the damage from alcohol was largely due to nutritional deficiency, at least that's what they thought back in those days. They had found that they could achieve almost miraculous recoveries from the D.T.'s with massive injections of vitamin B, thiamine, B_1 or better B complex. So I was aware of the threat and I would eat well in the evenings, sometimes not so well in the mornings. I think I wanted to assure myself that I'd have something to throw up when I got sick.

We didn't party a lot. My drinking got well established because we worked a fairly long day and I'd come home, consume a half of case of ale, sleep eight or nine hours and then get up and go to work. I was using alcohol for fun and comfort and good taste and to go to sleep.

There were no visible ill effects at that time because I had time to sleep it off but I was establishing the pattern of increasing dependence. There wasn't any medical intervention at that time.

Later, I began drinking mixed drinks, distilled spirits, because it got to be too much trouble to haul in enough alcohol in the form of beer or ale. At that time, the state where we lived was dry so I bought my liquor by the lug, three fifths at a time, and the bootlegger made about two trips a week. I didn't care much for bourbon. I drank scotch some but I decided that since I was drinking it for the alcohol content, there was no use messing around. The cheapest thing that I wanted and that was not toxic was rum so I settled for that. Bacardi light rum has just as much alcohol in it as scotch or bourbon. Sometimes I'd get the dark rum but mostly I bought the light-colored kind. Now, for Christmas, I might order a case of Four Roses whiskey with a view toward entertaining or giving it to friends, but I would say that maybe one bottle of the case would be used for that purpose and the rest would just be part of my ongoing consumption.

Tying that much capital up at one time produced friction in the family over the question of whether we should put off paying the rent in order to pay the bootlegger cash on delivery. I was a young scientist and it was a financially significant expenditure.

With this much drinking, I developed ulcers and the doctor treated me for this. He characterized me as a high-strung intellectual. I had to go on an extreme soft diet, antacids and atropine-type chemicals to suppress the vegus nerve action. I'm sure I cut down on the alcohol at this time.

It's a funny thing. I drank beer as a chaser with this rum. I'd mix it to my taste and have one can of beer and another can with a little beer in it and half or two-thirds rum. I'd drink the stronger drink and chase it with the beer, but I'd also put a little rum in the chaser because it ended up tasting like distilled water if I didn't.

Of course, it got progressively worse. I was drinking more and getting sick more often. At least a couple of times I was taken to the hospital, thinking I had appendicitis and they'd take a white count and it wouldn't show anything.

My wife felt that the barbituates I took made me much groggier than the liquor. I discounted this but she was the sober one, so she was probably right. Anyway, she developed quite an animosity toward me because I took more of these pills than I was supposed to.

I always tried to make it a point to get in to work on Mondays. I'd read that it is a fairly good giveaway that you're alcoholic if you miss work on Mondays or after payday. Generally, I'd taper off on Sundays, maybe not have much of anything to drink on Sunday evening. Likewise with the pills. I didn't remember at the time but this one weekend I'd run out of pills on Friday and on Monday morning, I felt really bad. Double vision, heart palpitations, terribly nervous. So I took off work and went down to see my doctor. I told him how bad I was feeling and he measured my blood pressure, as he always did. I notice doctors never do that now, routinely. Well, he looked at me and I don't know whether my blood pressure was high, low or what, but he said, "Don't take any more barbituates! Please, don't take any more of them!" I promised him I wouldn't.

I think it must have been a withdrawal reaction from having taken close to an addictive dose of barbital for several weeks or months and then not having any for three days and cutting way down on the alcohol, too. But I didn't know what it was then. It wasn't like an ordinary hangover. I didn't have the nausea and the headache so much as this feeling that I couldn't see clearly, seeing double. I think I might have been trying to go into convulsions. That experience caused me to stop using the pills.

This happened maybe a few months before I decided to go to Alcoholics Anonymous. At that time I was consuming a fifth of rum diluted with three or four cans of beer. I did this five days a week and continued to work. I never did have any trouble with my employer.

"Was he aware that you had a drinking problem?"

I don't think so. I had no indication that he was, at least. The alcohol affected me so that I was feeling bad enough most of the time that I wasn't very productive. I'd be productive in spurts, you know? I'd get on a project, work long hours, cut down on the drinking, be enthusiastic, and turn in a good piece of work but the next time it might take twice as long as it should. The drinking was affecting my work performance. I was trying desperately to cover up and I was being passed over for promotion whereas before I had advanced pretty regularly. But it never came up as an issue with my employer.

It was a full-time job to maintain my posture as a non-alcoholic to my employer. I suppressed the symptoms. I never drank in public in a bar. I never drove after I'd had as much as one drink. My wife drove everywhere we went for the last ten years. I gave up being on the church board because it was too much effort to be there in the evening, talk to people, turn around and get a breath of fresh air and not breathe on them. I was consuming a lot of energy trying not to get caught, studying how not to be caught, taking the alcoholism journal to learn the giveaway signs of being an alcoholic. It consumed so much effort that my production was down and my enjoyment of life was nil.

And I'd get sick. I'd start out early in the evening to have four or five drinks and first thing I knew, it was two o'clock in the morning, I'd consumed a fifth of rum and I was going to be sick. It was so damned humiliating to a person as brilliant as I am, you know, to do this not once or twice but dozens of times. So when I went to AA and got the approach that alcoholism is an illness, well, I'd rather be nutty than stupid. Anybody who would do this over and over again had to have a compulsive drinking pattern. I could buy this.

The real problem was, could I buy staying sober? Could I stand to live without drinking? I was so dependent on this alcohol, you see, that I couldn't imagine trying to live without it. They said, "Don't try to imagine living your life without it. Just try living without it one day at a time."

"What inspired you to go to AA all of a sudden?"

Five years before I had been invited to an AA conference by the treasurer of our church. He invited me and the minister to go. He was an alcoholic who had been sober five or six years at that time. They were having a state conference and part of the purpose of the state conference was to invite lay people in to see what AA is like. It was just one long session of AA meetings, pretty much; individuals telling their story, that is, what it used to be like, what happened, and what it is like now.

We went to an hour or two meeting and heard guys describe their pattern of drinking, their coming to AA and their learning to live without drinking. They'd tell jokes on themselves and you really couldn't tell those who had been horrible alcoholics and ended up under the bridge from their family or friends. There were every kind, from bankers to filling station attendants. So I had this exposure to the live people of AA.

Also, once a year, our minister gave a sermon on alcohol and alcoholism and he'd end up saying that the people who had crossed the line into alcoholism, where they really had dependent drinking, should go to AA. So I didn't just dream this idea up all by myself, although it seemed that way at the time. But there was no particular catastrophic event which caused me to go to AA when I did. I was just getting sick and tired of being sick and tired. Well, there was one little thing that might have had something to do with it. I mentioned that I never drove when I drank. One evening we were over at an old drinkin' buddy's house, at a party. He lived only eight or 10 blocks from our house. When I got home that night, I realized I had driven home from this party and that was something I had told myself I would never do. So this was convincing to me, the crumbling of the illusion that I could control myself.

I frequently went by this friend's house on Saturdays, helped him work on his hi-fi set and we'd sit around and chew the fat. He liked to drink and he could drink himself out at a party and pass out with everybody around him. I never lost control myself so I'd go over and drink with him and about the time he was getting blotto, I'd suggest that we order another bottle from the bootlegger. I'd time it so that he would share paying for it but then he'd pass out and I'd get to drink most of it.

One Saturday morning, oh, I was hurtin'. I had really let myself go the night before. I was with this same friend who said that most suicides were committed in a hangover. I thought, well, I'd go ahead and drink some that morning. I had never done this before because you become alcoholic if you drink in the morning. I never before drank before four o'clock in the afternoon, even on Saturday. I decided to drink some this morning, though, to see if it would help my hangover, but I visualized that once I started drinking in the morning, it would be but 10 years until I'd be on skid row. It would really get me. I was feeling really rotten so I took a drink and then I took another drink and by the time I was feeling better, I was two-thirds drunk.

I knew I had limited time, anyhow, and I would put off suicide. I had contemplated suicide a number of times, figured up my insurance, calculated how things would work out. They wouldn't work out worth a damn. I felt a lot of obligation to my family, especially to my daughter and I put off suicide until she got out of high school. I had the idea that I could hang on for a while if I could just get enough to drink, make ends meet and survive in the job.

But here, all of a sudden, it was obvious that if I started drinking in the morning, it wasn't going to be 10 years until I was on skid row. It probably wouldn't be one. Because I had to get drunk to alleviate the pain of the hangover.

This was more of a catastrophe than you can imagine because I had the illusion I still had to drink in the mornings before I was a dead duck, a real alcoholic. The despair at that moment was like the guy who went before the judge for public drunkness, forgery, passing bad checks and the like. The judge said, "What do you think about going to AA?" And the drunk said, "You don't think I'm going to associate with that kind of people, do you?"

I really didn't go to my doctor for my drinking problem. I hid it from him. Even when I had other problems, flu or sore throat or anything, I was careful not to say anything about my drinking or have any evidence of it. I never went to him for help with my hangovers, which is not typical. Most alcoholics go through that if they have company insurance that will pay for it. But I suffered the tortures of the damned most mornings during the last five years of my drinking. It got to be unbearable. I either had to commit suicide or go to AA because it was getting worse. I was having to drink more and I was getting sicker and sicker. I had tried out mentally all avenues of not facing the full acceptance that I was dependent on alcohol and I would never be able to drink in a moderate manner. I'd tried it many times. I would maybe control my drinking at parties, my wife would drive us home, and then I would go ahead and drink on into the night.

I'd had a lot of "slips"; that's what we call it at AA, people who have an impulse to stop, go to AA and get some encouragement but then go out with the boys, have one drink and are right back on it again. Half of the people who come to AA go through this period.

But I didn't have such a period after I went to AA. I'd been through that before I ever went to AA, so that when I went to AA I figured that if I could get a little of whatever it was that made those real alcoholics stop drinking, I could then cut down to about a pint a day and I'd be all right.

So this is what I had in mind when I went to AA, to learn to control myself and not drink to excess. But everybody at AA talked about the various ways they had tried to control their drinking, switching from bourbon to scotch, or to wine, or drinking beer only, or drinking only after five o'clock. One attorney measured it out, one ounce an hour during the day and tried to get by that way. I thought, "How did these fellows know what I wanted?" But they all said they found out they couldn't control it that way and some of them had tried for years. Again, this jerked the rug out from under my illusions.

There was one doctor who showed up during those early weeks I was in AA. He had lost his license and gone back to work as a stock clerk in a drug company, went to AA, got sober and was readmitted to practice medicine. It turned out that my physician was one who had intervened to get him readmitted to practice at the hospital.

I kept getting this repeated story from all of these different kinds of people that the only way to keep from drinking to excess was to not take the first drink. And that was quite different from what I had gone there to find out.

So I went home and had several good belts of rum because I had promised myself that going to AA didn't mean I had to stop drinking. If I had not gone home and drunk some, I'd never have trusted myself again.

Later that week I went back to a closed meeting, just for alcoholics. It was more of the same from where I sat. Different people described the way it had been with them, their getting to AA, getting sobered up, and how it was now. And they were obviously real happy with how it was now. Those alcoholics could describe feelings and I knew exactly what they were talking about.

I went home that Friday night and again drank. I read the literature and made notes on the Johns Hopkins 34 questions that you ask yourself to see if you are alcoholic. And I even thought of three or four better questions they ought to ask.

The next day, my car needed work on it, I was trying to get out to the lab and I was so jittery and shook up that I couldn't get organized to do anything, so I thought, "Maybe I ought to get hold of that big book, *Alcoholics Anonymous*, and read it." The "big book" gives a general survey of how AA works and the last three quarters of it are stories of individuals, 36 of them. It is intended as a vehicle for new people to learn what Alcoholics Anonymous is about. This is the "holy writ," you might say. It was written and published in 1939.

The founder of AA, Bill Wilson, got the idea of calling on a "higher power" for help from a friend who had sobered up in the Oxford Group movement after consulting the psychiatrist Jung. He'd been treated for his alcoholism but had been relapsing so he asked Jung, "Is there no hope for me?" To which Jung said, "I've never seen a case as advanced as yours recover except through some sort of religious conversion." This man was desperate because he had gotten the best medical help that was available back in the 30's. He then got connected with the Oxford Group movement and Moral Rearmament group which had a self-examination program, sort of a confession-type thing. A lot of the principles, the 12 steps of AA, are an enlargement of the four principles of the Moral Rearmament movement.

I had met a guy at the AA meeting named Bud so I called him and asked to borrow a copy of the big book. He lived clear across town but he said he would bring it to me. Well, I was sitting there, about two o'clock in the afternoon, really hurtin'. Boy, I needed a drink. I was listening to *La Boheme* and that added to my pathos, you know. It added to the feeling of fighting to remain in control but not understanding, to this general feeling, "God damn, I've gotta do something." Boy, I wanted a drink but then I said to myself, "That's really something. You call up AA and then you can't wait 'til the guy gets here. You have to take a drink." And I argued with myself, "Aw, what's just one drink?" And then, "You really must be an addict if you can't do without one drink."

AA talked about calling on a higher power and I'd always thought that prayers were a ludicrous thing because the golfer prays for sunshine and the farmer prays for rain and they can't both win. I thought, though, that if I was going through with this AA program and trying to keep from drinking one day at a time, I maybe ought to call on a higher power. So I turned around, got down on my knees in front of the couch and felt like a goddamn fool, asking not to want this drink so bad. I waited to feel different and I didn't feel any different. So I figured I'd ask again and I did but still no particular sensation, no answer. Finally, a knock comes on the door and there's Bud, with the big book under his arm and a little pamphlet, "Alcoholism: Sin or Disease?" I guess they knew that the average guy might want to read the book but he would really read the pamphlet.

The biggest part of the AA program is to help somebody else, to carry it to the next guy if he asks for help. Even if it is inconvenient, it's really for your own benefit, not for his.

I went to a church picnic that night, Saturday night, and they had highballs and everything there, but I took two bottles of carbonated water with me and drank that all evening. I didn't drink any alcohol.

"Did you read any of the big book?"

Yes, I read the big book the rest of the day until time to go to the picnic. And it said, if you're going where there will be alcohol, take something else to drink so you won't get thirsty but don't drink the liquor. So that's what I've been drinking ever since, carbonated water. No calories, either.

"Did you have any withdrawal symptoms?"

No discernible reaction. My wife developed a rash, though, which she had for about six weeks. You see, when you start sobering up and attending to your responsibilities around home, paying the bills and participating in the family affairs, this causes a whole lot of adjustment and reorientation in other members of the family. The guy who was just lying around drunk every evening is acting different now. My wife thought it was the relief of pent-up tension which caused her rash. Or it could have been adjustment tension, you can take your pick.

This stepping over into sobriety gave me a tremendous sense of euphoria and satisfaction and I immediately got into AA work, helping other people who were in the same shape I'd been in. I've been at it ever since.

> *Drunkenness . . . spoils health, dismounts the mind and unmans men.*
>
> William Penn (1644–1718)
> *Fruits of Solitude,* Maxim 22

> *The more you drink, the more you crave.*
>
> Alexander Pope (1688–1744)
> *Satire and Epistles Imitated,* "Second Epistle of the Second Book of Horace."

XVIII.
Eating Apparatus

Taking food and drink is a great enjoyment for healthy people, and those who do not enjoy eating seldom have much capacity for enjoyment or usefulness of any sort.

Charles W. Eliot (1834–1926)
The Happy Life

57. Gum Disease

Her husband died of a heart attack a few years ago. She is in her 40's and alone because her two daughters have moved out to embark on their own careers, one in the Air Force and one in college. She has a new, short, curly hairdo and almost a new image since her life has changed so dramatically. She works for a professor of medicine, does secretarial chores, fears she will soon be "riffed," caught in a reduction in force.

- **Sore Gums**
- **Pyorrhea**
- **Periodontal Disease**

I always had problems with my teeth when I was a child, but I didn't know anything about gum problems or pyorrhea or anything like that. I'd gone to the dentist regularly all of my life and spent a lot of money. My dad complained about it all of the time. I complained about it when I was single and had to pay the bills. My husband complained about it and said he should have looked at my teeth before he married me.

Anyhow, when I was in my early 30's I started having abscesses. I'd had them before a few times and they were very painful and I even had to call the doctor. The abscesses occurred underneath my teeth; my face would become swollen and it was the worst pain I ever had in my life, much worse than labor as far as I'm concerned. Oh yes, much, much worse. That's the one thing I can say I'm glad I don't have any more, the pain. I can still think about it and almost make my mouth hurt.

I went for five years having continual abscesses in different places in my mouth. I would let them go, sometimes for a week until I couldn't sleep and aspirin, nothing would do any good. I would go to the dentist and he'd say, "We'll have to lance this," and the lancing was terribly painful. In fact, I remember this one dentist who was very cruel. I only went to him a couple of times and then I went to another dentist to have the abscess taken care of. I should have sued him, I guess. It was terrible because somehow he slipped and the needle didn't go in the right place and it hit something and I kind of went into hysterics which I'd never done before in my life. I just couldn't stop crying and he ushered me out of the back door and let me drive home in that shape. It took a couple of days for that pain to go away.

After they lanced an abscess, they would put me on antibiotics. We moved around a lot so I went to different dentists in different towns. I always got a dentist right away, even before I got a medical doctor. I had to. And none of them ever told me, until right before I had to have my teeth pulled, that antibiotics would not be good for me to take all of the time. I learned that six years ago, when I had my upper teeth pulled. That was when I went to my regular dentist. He said, "We can't just keep you on antibiotics." I just had one abscess after another and was in pain all of the time. I was irritable from the pain and it was affecting the family and me and everything.

He sent me to a periodontist. This man, I feel now that I look back on it, was just after the money. Maybe he was trying to do something for me and maybe he wasn't. He said, "Oh, I can save your teeth." It cost $700 to go through this very painful surgical process where they cut open the gums, scrape the bone and pack it with this horrible stuff and you can't eat anything. One year later, I had my teeth pulled after having this $700 worth of painful periodontal surgery.

The whole experience was very bad because I felt like nobody was really caring that much about the fact that I was going to lose part of my body and I felt like my teeth were part of my body. I really was scared because my teeth were so badly abscessed at the time they pulled them. I had a very good oral surgeon, a very kind, beautiful man whom I very much trusted, but he did tell me that it was a dangerous procedure because I had so much infection and it was so close to vital areas such as the brain. So I was scared. But he told me that. He was one of the few dentists who really talked with me. He was just a beautiful man, really.

Well, he was nice. But I had to go to another dentist. This is part of the problem with teeth that people don't understand, that I didn't understand. You go to a regular dentist, then you go to a periodontist, and then you go to an oral surgeon. I went to the hospital because he said it was safer that way and I'm glad I did that. They did all of the upper teeth at one time under anesthesia. In the meantime, I'd had my teeth made by another dentist. So, in a very short period of time, it involved four different dentists. And a lot of money, too. The money part could be taken care of, but it was the shuffling back and forth that was very traumatic. No one other than the oral surgeon seemed to be sympathetic with the fact that I was having my teeth pulled. The man who made my teeth kept saying, "Ha! You'll have all these pretty new teeth; no fillings and they're nice and shiny and you're just going to be fine." But he never did talk to me about the effects of losing part of me. I wasn't going to look the same and I also felt like it was going to have an effect on my femininity, and my sexuality. I felt people were going to say, "She has false teeth so we don't love her anymore."

"Do you feel that way now?"

Not very much, but sometimes. I think I have nice looking dentures, but I still feel uncomfortable about the fact that I'm not that old and I've always thought of people with dentures as old. I was only in my 30's when I had my upper teeth pulled.

When I had my upper teeth pulled, I had no more infections up there and no problem other than getting used to the teeth and the fitting of them. That was also not explained as well beforehand as it could have been. No one told me that I'd have to learn to eat all over again. So I didn't eat anything for a long time. I just drank things, soup, that sort of thing.

When I had my bottom teeth pulled about a year and a half ago, I happened to have an oral surgeon this time who didn't have that nice bedside manner. He has since then said, "Aw, you're just a vain woman." That doesn't help at all. I don't know whether it is vanity or what it is, but having all of my teeth gone was just that much more to go through, all over again. I did feel very self-conscious about having no teeth, even though I had no more pain other than the pain of having the teeth fit and that took six months to get used to. The psychological effect along with the physical pain needs to be explained.

I do think sometimes people must say, "I bet she must have dentures." which probably is not true. It only is inside of me. It's not so much a vanity thing, though. It would be the same kind of thing if I'd had an arm removed or a breast removed. But people don't think of teeth the same way; they're just teeth. But teeth are just as important as any part of the body.

People make fun of me still. I feel that is cruel of certain people, but they make fun of me because I'm slow in eating. I don't want to choke; I almost choked to death once because I couldn't chew a piece of meat and I just swallowed it and it got stuck and I was so damn scared. I thought "Never again. If it takes me six hours to eat a meal, I'll take six hours." I'm very self-conscious about it unless I'm with close friends who understand. And I still have some friends who say, "Aw, there's old Katherine, poking along with her food," or "Come on, eat a steak." which I don't do out in public because it takes too long. People are very cruel. If I had lost an arm, they'd be helping me in different ways, but it's not the same with teeth. I think people feel repulsed by people losing their teeth and maybe it's because they know some day they could lose their teeth.

"Did you lose some of your sense of taste?"

Oh, yes, definitely. Particularly when you lose your upper teeth. But I had more taste sensation when I still had natural lower teeth. Now that I have full dentures, I use a tremendous amount of salt and pepper and hot sauce. I ate Chinese mustard the other day, took a teaspoonful of it and put it in my mouth because it clears up my sinuses real good, and most people can't take that much in their mouth but I can because I'm protected. People kid me about that, too.

I guess it was six years between the time my upper teeth were pulled and losing my lower teeth. And I tried every possible way, because I was told by my dentist that lower teeth were difficult to fit and they were never really comfortable. The periodontist here was very nice. He is with the school of dentistry and he said he could save about four of my lower teeth and it would cost me a lot of money but if I wanted to, they'd do it and put separate teeth in between but he still couldn't guarantee I would keep the four teeth for more than a year. That convinced me. There wouldn't have been any point in doing that. I would still have abscesses with the remaining teeth and he said I couldn't continue to take antibiotics, penicillin, all of the myacins, the whole mess. And I did get worried about that because if I ever got sick and needed big doses of antibiotics, they might not have any effect at all.

I began to feel better after I had all my teeth removed. I didn't have a lot of achy pains and colds and things I'd had before. I don't even get the flu any more.

Before, I just didn't feel well because I didn't eat properly because my teeth hurt all of the time. So I can see the benefit of having my teeth pulled as far as my general health goes. But the discomfort and the psychological thing of wondering if I am still feminine still continues. I go through this when I meet new people, men in particular because I am single now. When my husband was alive, he was very supportive. He thought it was really neat, that my new teeth were beautiful! And that made a lot of difference. I had a lot of love and acceptance from him and it didn't matter.

"Do you get the impression that if you had gotten periodontal treatment early, it would have changed the outcome in your case?"

I think so. This is an hereditary thing, I've been told, and my parents both had it. My father didn't lose his teeth until he was older, but he had periodontal problems and my mother did, too. My sister had all of her teeth pulled, a few teeth at a time. I'm pretty convinced by that that it's inherited, but I still think with good periodontal care and more home care, things would have been different.

If anyone's going to a dentist now and thinks they have gum problems, but their dentist says he doesn't know anything about periodontal disease, that person should find another dentist, right away. They do know about it now and there is no excuse for them not treating it. As far as I am concerned, now there's just too much knowledge for a dentist to just slough it off and not be concerned. Just say, "I'm going to find myself another dentist," and then do it.

> *For there was never yet philosopher*
> *That could endure the toothache patiently.*
>
> William Shakespeare (1564–1616)
> *Much Ado About Nothing*, V, i, 35

58. Fractured Jaw

A *few people have had their jaws wired shut so they would not be tempted to eat. This is a highly effective way to lose weight and the same thing occurs, of course, when the oral surgeon has to wire the jaws shut to allow a fracture to heal.*

This 28-year-old law student was forced to keep his mouth shut as the result of a sports accident, and while his weight declined, his frustration titre rose.

He is an ex-Air Force officer, attending college on the G.I. bill to add an LL.D. to his undergraduate degree in business administration. He and his family of females (a wife, two tiny daughters and a pussy cat) live in a 50-year-old house, the interior of which he is gradually remodeling himself.

- **Broken Jaw**
- **Fractured Mandible**

The injury occurred during a basketball game. What happened was, I was going in to substitute for a guy and had checked into the game. I remember walking onto the floor and I'd started to play — I think we had gone up and down a couple of times — and the next thing I knew I was on the floor. The guys said, "Don't move." And I could feel a whole lot of blood on my head. I had been completely out, completely unconscious.

"How long had you been unconscious?"

They said I was out four or five minutes, something like that. I tried to stand up but they held me down. I could see that my head had been cut pretty bad, around the right temple. I really had no feeling in my jaw at all; I didn't realize that my jaw was injured, I just thought I had fallen and hit my head pretty hard.

This was an intramural college basketball game so they went over and got the intramural officials. A girl came over and gave me smelling salts which brought me around a little bit and then they helped me off the floor, called the University police and an ambulance.

They sat me down, put a compress-type thing on my forehead to stop the bleeding and that's when I began to realize that my teeth wouldn't match when I shut my mouth; they missed!

As I was sitting there, they told me what had happened. This guy had the ball and I had gone for it. He turned around and let me have it with his elbow, right in the jaw. It knocked me out in mid-air. The guys said I was unconscious before I hit the floor. I went straight down and that's when I cut my head, when I hit the floor. But the blow from the guy's elbow hit me right in the jaw. He happened to come across and catch me just right. It snapped my neck. The doctor said the break was up here almost in the joint.

My vision was blurred and I didn't feel like talking but the first thing they wanted to know was, which hospital did I want to go to. I had to make a decision, which I didn't want to do at that time. Also, the police wanted to know if I wanted to press charges against the guy who hit me. It was a real rough basketball game and all of the people we were playing were red-shirted football players. They were huge monsters and they were beatin' the heck out of us, physically. The police thought it might be a battery case but I said no.

I told the ambulance driver I wanted to go wherever they could take care of me the best. I didn't want to mess around. I knew that I had insurance which would cover it no matter which hospital I went to. Had I not had insurance, I would have had them take me to the University Hospital where the University would have paid for everything.

A couple of guys helped me walk to the ambulance but I didn't have to get onto the stretcher. I just sat there and held my head while they drove me into the hospital.

The first thing they did was take me straight to x-ray to have my head x-rayed all around to see what had happened. They had the emergency room interview-type thing and I told the guy I thought my jaw was broken. He said, "Okay. That's good. The oral surgeon is here right now. I'll go get him." It was eight o'clock in the evening and the local oral surgeon just happened to be there. That was really good that the doctor was right there.

He looked at the x-rays and could see that I had a fracture of the right jaw up close to the joint. He told me to treat it that he would have to wire my mouth shut for about three weeks.

The oral surgeon took over my case, sewed my head up and said he'd have to admit me to the hospital. The nurse asked me if I wanted a private room or a semiprivate room. When I asked her what Blue Cross normally paid for, she said a semiprivate room so I said, "That's fine." So they gave me a semiprivate room with this old guy. I don't believe he ever knew I was there because he was delirious most of the time. He'd had both legs taken off, he had diabetes and was in bad shape.

Nothing was done to my mouth that night. I had no pain in my jaw, really. My head hurt, I had a real bad headache, but my jaw didn't hurt except a couple of times I tried to line my teeth up and shut my mouth, which kind of hurt then. My main concern was my head, which was killing me. He'd put five stitches in my head and said he wanted me in the hospital that night to make sure I didn't have any bad complications, concussion-wise.

After I got settled in the room, the doctor came up and said there were two ways he could do the wiring of my teeth: take me down to the emergency room in the morning, give me a local and do it that way or take me to surgery and give me a general anesthetic. I asked him which way he would rather do it and he said he'd rather do it in surgery. I said, "That sounds fine," because I was chicken and didn't want any pain while they were playing around with my teeth. At that time, too, I thought they'd put pins in my jaw; I didn't know where the wires went. He explained that they would take little fine wires and wrap them around eight teeth, two on the top and two on the bottom on each side. Then they would loop another wire to each tooth where the wires were exposed and then turn it; tighten her down. You could still open the jaw by cutting the four wires connecting the upper and lower teeth. He scheduled the O.R. for ten o'clock the next morning. Later that evening, I asked the nurse to give me a shot for pain, which she did, and I went right to sleep.

The next morning before I was ready to go to surgery, they came in and gave me a shot of something which pretty well wiped me out for the ride down to the O.R. I was out pretty good. In the surgery room, I guess it was the anesthesiologist who gave me an I.V. and said, "The patient's going to sleep." I remember him saying that and the next thing I remember, I woke up in recovery and my mouth was wired shut.

I wasn't in pain but it felt strange not to be able to open my mouth. I didn't try to talk because I was still tired. Then they took me back to my room and I stayed one more night in the hospital.

I was climbing the walls by then. I felt pretty good. My headache had gone away but by the afternoon after the surgery, the wires began hurting my gums. I never had braces as a kid but I imagine they hurt the same way because those wires really hurt your gums a whole lot. About eight o'clock that night, I got a shot for the pain.

I don't know how they classify diets in hospitals, but all I could get was a liquid broth. Then they brought jello and there is no way I could ever have eaten jello. It was extremely frustrating to put a piece of jello in front of the tiny gap where your upper teeth overhang your lower teeth, and then suck it in. Later I learned to do it but I couldn't when I was in the hospital. I have a pretty good overbite but I could eat only whatever would go through the gap.

I was getting pretty hungry by then and told the lady I could take liquid jello but I couldn't eat this hard stuff. I could have eaten something more than just that liquid diet, some soup maybe, with a little more in it. No one could seem to understand that I had just had my jaws wired shut and didn't have to have broth because of my stomach or something. A milkshake, custard, pudding, anything would have been great.

In the recovery room, they put a wire cutter around my neck, strung there on a ribbon. They told me never to take it off, that it had to be there, but they didn't tell me the reason. I figured out that if I got nauseated and had to throw up, they'd have to cut the wires to keep me from drowning myself. I'd heard of that happening.

About one o'clock the following day, the doctor came by and as I said, I was climbing the walls, ready to leave. He said I could go so I got dressed real fast and called my wife to come get me.

When the doctor checked me out, I said, "Hey, do I need these wire cutters?" And he said no, so I took them off and laid them down. Later, when I was downstairs waiting on my wife, this nurse came running down from my floor, saying, "Are you the one with your mouth wired shut?" When I said, yeah, she said, "Well, you've gotta have these," and held up the wire cutters. When I told her the doctor said I didn't need them, she said, "Well, you're supposed to have them. You'd better come back up to the floor and ask the head nurse up there." So I got back on the elevator, went to the head nurse and said that the doctor said I didn't need them. I had to talk like this *(speaking with his jaws clamped shut)* and explain it all to her. She said, "I'm sure you are supposed to have them. You check with Mrs. So and So down at supply on the first floor." So I said, "Where is she?" and she told me where to find her.

So I took my wire cutters and went back downstairs and inquired where Mrs. So and So was. When they told me she was around somewhere and would be back in a minute, I said, "Okay," put the wire cutters in my pocket and left. I never did find Mrs. So and So.

The wires continued to give me pain. The doctor gave me some pills for the pain, capsule form, and what he told me to do was to take them apart, put 'em in orange juice and take them that way. I took those about four or five nights, I guess, because I just couldn't go to sleep with my gums hurting that way.

I was very frustrated about eating. It's unbelievable how frustrated you can become over food. The first thing I did was to fry a hamburger and then put some tomato juice in the blender and blend it all up but I couldn't get it in my mouth. The pieces were too big. You're really hungry because your stomach hasn't shrunk yet and I like to eat. So I started blending everything. If I could eat it, it was okay, but if I couldn't, we just had to throw it away. Lorie, my eight-month-old daughter and I were eating about the same thing for a while. We were going right after all of that pudding and stuff.

I could really blend macaroni and cheese all right and I could eat scrambled eggs by smashing them up with hot sauce. You want something in your mouth because everything tastes like creamed tomato soup, that's what I was eating most of the time. A piece of toast would have been nice.

"Did you lose weight?"

Oh, yes. I lost about 15 pounds. At the University cafeteria where I go every day, the waitresses would fix me mashed potatoes and gravy and try to figure out what they had that day which was soft enough for me to eat. And every day they would ask me if the wires were off yet.

I'm gradually getting my weight back now that the wires are off. I didn't want to lose weight. My pants were about to fall off, I lost so much.

A week and a half after surgery, the doctor saw me and said the wires could come off in about three weeks so I made an appointment with him to do that. I was living for that day, Monday, and all weekend before my appointment, I kept thinking about where I wanted to eat. I wanted to go to McDonald's and get a hamburger, more than anything.

I went to his office for my appointment and his nurse said, "He's not here today. He's sick." My heart went pow. "He's not sick. He can't be sick, I'm the one who's sick," I told the nurse. The nurse thought he had the flu and made me a Wednesday appointment. I was really upset.

When I called Wednesday to be sure he was in, the nurse told me he wasn't in and wouldn't be back for the rest of the week. She made me an appointment for the next Monday. Then I got to thinking that there must be someone taking his emergency calls and almost anybody ought to be able to take these wires off, so I called back to his office. The nurse said, "Oh, yes, you are the one with the broken jaw. Well, the doctor never takes those wires off in three weeks. They'll have to stay on for six weeks." I thought, "Oh my God. Six weeks." That took all of the wind out of my sails. I didn't know what to do. So I said, "Look, could I go to someone else?" And she said, "No, he would be very upset if you went to see another doctor."

The next Monday, four weeks after surgery, I went in for my appointment and he was there. It turned out that he did have the flu. I sat down and he said, "Well, you came to get these off." And bang, bang, bang, he took 'em off. He said, "Can you open your mouth?" And I said, "It is open, isn't it?" I had opened it about a quarter of an inch and it felt like it was gaping wide open.

After he cut the wires, I just didn't want to open my mouth at all, it was too sore. The muscles on both sides had not been stretched for four weeks and they contracted. He popped them open and then explained to me that the break had been so close to the joint that he wanted to open it early. Normally he does wire them shut for six weeks, but if you don't open ones like mine early, there is a possibility that you might not get the full movement back. He said there could be blood in the joint and it could solidify and bone form and all this kind of stuff that would not allow you to open your mouth all of the way.

He took the wires that were between the teeth and made hooks on them all around. Then he gave me some little rubber bands that he wanted me to put on at night to keep my mouth shut when I slept. And I wasn't supposed to bite on anything hard and I was to use the rubber bands for another week.

I had to take it slow because it was hard to open my mouth and hard to chew. There was soreness, that kind of pain. It took a week or two for that to go away.

"Did you have any residual problems?"

I sit around like this a lot. *(Demonstrates talking with jaws shut.)* And I grind my teeth a lot at night, but I've regained full movement and use of my mouth.

At six weeks, he gave me a local anesthetic, xylocaine or something, a topical anesthetic which he sprayed on my gums. I was sort of nervous about it. He said, "Now it's going to feel like someone pulling a piece of adhesive tape off of your arm. I'm going to do it real fast." so he just latched onto the old wire and jerked. It felt like kind of a dull sensation when he popped them out. There were eight of them. He wants to see me one more time, in three months.

"Did your insurance cover all of this?"

It has so far. High-option federal employees insurance. The anesthesiologist's bill was $80 and it paid that. The doctor bill was $200 but I don't have the hospital bill yet and that was over two months ago. I hope it won't cost us anything. That's why we have insurance.

"Were you able to brush your teeth?"

That's another thing. I use a Water Pik all of the time but ours was getting cruddy so I had my wife go out and get a new one. So I used a Water Pik, real gentle, and a little kid's toothbrush with real soft bristles to brush my teeth. When the doctor opened my mouth, it was real dirty. My tongue was solid yellow. It was terrible. I think that's why food tasted so bad those four weeks.

There is stuff on the market you can buy to eat when your jaws are wired shut. I used a lot of Instant Breakfast and there is also a powdered protein-type milk you can buy at drug stores which I got to be sure I was getting enough vitamins. Also, the doctor told me to get baby vitamins and squirt them in my mouth, the liquid kind.

One guy told me about a person who had to have a tooth pulled in order to get any food in his mouth at all. I talked to my doctor about people who have their jaws wired shut in order to lose weight. Apparently, he's done that but he didn't want to talk about it. He seemed real sensitive about that.

XIX.
Food Processing

To eat is human, to digest divine.

Charles T. Copeland (1860–1952)

59. Ulcerative Colitis

He is a sophomore in college now, 21 years old, a year behind his class because of the time he lost with his illness. The experience of serious illness at the late end of his teens has matured him well beyond his years and given him an appreciation of the preciousness of the moments and relationships of life. He is red-haired, quiet, considerate, handsome.

- **Chronic Ulcerative Colitis**
- **Pyoderma Gangrenosum**
- **Colectomy**

I must have been about, oh, 12 years old, pretty close to 13, when I started having problems. I didn't know it was colitis because it hadn't been diagnosed yet. It has been quite a while so it is hard for me to remember, but I think it first began with virus-type symptoms, vomiting and diarrhea. The vomiting went away, along with the fever and other kinds of things you have with a virus, but the diarrhea kept on.

It weakened me and I must have had some blood in my stools because I became anemic. After I became pretty weak and had lost some weight, that's when we decided to go to the family physician. I'd had these symptoms for longer than was usual, at least a month.

He ran some blood tests and the first thing he found was that I was anemic. I told him about my symptoms and he ran some tests on me, including a proctoscopic examination. That was very tough because I was feeling weak and sick at the time anyway and my colon and rectum were irritated. In the proctoscopic examination, they use a tube which they put up your rectum and that was irritating. That was a really bad experience.

After going through these tests, the doctor came to the conclusion that I had colitis.

He put me on some medication, Azulfadine and Prednisone. Azulfadine, I'm not sure what kind of drug it is, but I think it is used specifically for these kinds of disorders, colitis and whatnot. Prednisone is cortisone and it is used for various other kinds of diseases, also. My symptoms went away and I started getting better.

One other problem I had before I was put on this medication was inflammation of my joints, my knee joints and my ankle joints. It was extremely painful. The doctor said it was something which usually accompanies colitis. As I recall, the pain in my joints began to go away when I was put on the medication.

My appetite came back. That was one thing I lost when I had the diarrhea. I also had a lot of cramping, which made me feel nauseated. So I lost a lot of weight and became anemic.

"What grade were you in?"

The seventh grade. I had just started junior high. I didn't lose any school because I thought I had to go to school. I may have lost one or two days but I didn't let being sick get in the way.

A year or so later, I saw a specialist who deals with these kinds of problems and he thought I had Crohn's disease, which is a little bit different than colitis. It is basically the same thing but it sometimes creeps up into the small intestine. This specialist was not at all optimistic. He thought that a colectomy was pretty well inevitable later on in my life. I never knew this. My parents kept it from me. I had no idea what a colectomy was, simply because I hadn't been told. I thought I was going to be all right with the medication and the disease would go away. The family physician seemed to feel that this condition could be treated medically, with the drugs, and it could possibly go away. He seemed rather unsure about the whole disease in the first place. It is rather a mystery to most doctors who have studied it at all.

Anyway, after I began the medication, I progressively got better and the doctor tapered the Prednisone down to a very small amount, possibly five milligrams a day, and I was on that amount for quite some time, several years. He did keep me on the Azulfadine, also. I did go off the Prednisone now and then.

About the age of 18, I was off the Azulfadine completely and just on five milligrams a day of the Prednisone. When I did have diarrhea, I'd have cramping with it but I'd usually have diarrhea only after having caught some little virus or something.

In my freshman year in college, I seemed to be doing really well. There were times when I didn't take the Prednisone at all but that was only for a few days. The reason I was taking the five milligrams at that time was for my acne. I had a little acne and my dermatologist was giving me Prednisone for that. He sort of took over the treatment of my colitis. He had been in contact with my family physician who had turned the case over to him. The five milligrams was for both the colitis and the acne.

At that time, I was having normal bowel movements, no diarrhea at all and I was getting up early every morning and jogging. So I was really doing well physically. Then one morning, when I was jogging with my friend, I pushed myself really hard. When I got back, I felt nauseated but I got over that after about 10 or 15 minutes. At noontime that day, I started feeling sick again and by midafternoon, I started vomiting. I had completely lost my appetite and didn't go to supper that evening. I felt feverish and vomited all through that night at least 15 times. I was nauseated, sick at my stomach and had diarrhea and cramping again.

After a couple of days the nausea and vomiting went away but the diarrhea continued. Other than that, I felt fine again, but the diarrhea persisted for weeks. This was in late November or the first part of December. Several people on the floor of our dormitory had this virus, too, so it was going around. They had the same exact symptoms that I had, except that my diarrhea stayed with me.

As time went on, I got progressively weaker and the cramping was getting terrible. It was really hard to stand and it made me lose my appetite, so I lost weight and kept getting sicker and sicker. The cramping was worse than it had ever been. Sometimes it was almost unbearable.

By the time I got home at Christmas for the holidays, I was so weak that all I could do was lie around. It was during the Christmas break that I decided there was no sense going back to school because I was just getting worse, getting sicker.

One night toward the end of January, I noticed a funny spot on my leg. It looked like a pimple. I kind of picked at it, which I knew I shouldn't have been doing, but I thought it was just a pimple. The next morning, it had developed into a larger, ulcerated-looking area about the size of a pencil eraser head. Then, I knew it couldn't be a pimple.

I watched it for a day or so and it just kept getting larger and larger. It increased in size at an unbelievable rate. Each day it seemed to double in size. It was on the lower half of my right leg, on my shin.

When the ulcer got to be about the size of a silver dollar, I went in to see my dermatologist. It was round, too, like a silver dollar, almost perfectly round, black and red, like a rotten spot on my leg. The doctor took one look at it and two seconds later he said, "Oh, that's pyoderma gangrenosum." I sort of let that go in one ear and out the other because obviously I had no idea what he was saying. Apparently, he was looking for this kind of problem to pop up at any time because he knew it was something which is sometimes associated with colitis. I'm sure he was on the lookout for it and wasn't surprised at all when he saw it on my leg.

The dermatologist gave me injections of cortisone directly into the ulcer. That was just excruciating because the pain from this ulcer was bad enough anyway but to put needles directly into the ulcer . . . it was so painful I thought I was going to faint. It was the worst pain I had ever had. The cortisone just seeped out the top of the ulcer, it wouldn't stay in there, so it didn't seem to do any good. That is when he decided to increase my dosage of Prednisone to 50 milligrams. So I took the Prednisone everyday and just lay in bed. My mother brought my meals to me which I ate in bed and only got out of bed to use the bathroom.

The ulcer seemed to get better after a while and it looked like it was getting smaller. It really seemed to get better every day until one Sunday afternoon in April, when I noticed a little purple spot just like the first spot had looked when it started. A little purply, bruisy spot close to the top part of the ulcer in a part of the skin which had not been affected. I watched it and sure enough, later that evening, it broke open and a funny looking fluid came out. This new spot began to increase and spread rapidly just like the first one had, twice as big each day. The doctor increased the Prednisone but it didn't seem to do much good. Little spots kept breaking out all around the ulcer. They would break open and start to spread.

At the same time, I had deep cystic acne all over the upper part of my back. These cysts caused extreme pain. I couldn't lie on my back at all. The pain in my leg really increased when I put my leg down. The doctor ordered me to keep my leg elevated because he thought that would keep the little new areas from spreading. Consequently, I was in the bed all of the time.

The ulcer kept getting larger and larger until it was about six-and-a-half inches long and it covered half the width of my leg. It was getting completely out of control. I went to see my family physician again — an internist, not the one who saw me originally — and he said I should go into the hospital to see if they could treat me there. So he put me in the hospital.

They ran tests again, proctoscopic examinations, barium enemas, a lot of blood tests, things like that. The treatment they did for my leg was to irrigate it with clean, distilled water and some other kind of solution. I'm not sure what it was. They did that several times a day. Also, they were trying various other drugs to see if they would have any effect on my leg. They did increase the Prednisone and put me back on Azulfadine.

But no matter what they did, nothing seemed to help. They called in some specialists. One of these specialists did a proctoscopic examination and did some biopsies of my rectum and large intestine. He decided we had pretty well reached the end of the line and it was time for my colon to come out. That was the first time I had ever learned that I would have to have my colon out. He explained what a colectomy was and I was completely horrified. I wanted to die. I didn't want to have live with an ileostomy.

For the remainder of the time I was in the hospital, eight or ten days, I just sat around and brooded about the colectomy and I continued to get worse, regardless of what medication they tried. Finally, they said, "Well, there is not much we can do for you here." So I started thinking that it might be a good idea to go up to the Hanson Clinic (a well-known Midwestern medical center). The father of a very close friend of mine is a heart specialist who took his training at Hanson and a very close friend of his is an internist at Hanson, a gastroenterologist who specializes in these problems. He had suggested earlier that I see this gastroenterologist there.

After thinking things over, I suggested to my parents the possibility of going to Hanson's. We concluded that it was the only thing left to do so my dad called my friend's father and he made an appointment for me with the doctor at the Hanson Clinic. My appointment was late in May and my dad and I flew up there for the appointment. The specialist there ran more tests, more barium enemas and more proctoscopic examinations which were very, very uncomfortable for me because I was so sick and my colon and rectum were so irritated. That was a bad experience for me.

After running all of the tests and seeing the ulcer on my leg, he concluded that I did have colitis and referred me to the dermatologist there. They seemed pretty surprised at the extent of the ulcer on my leg, which was quite large and deep by this time. They put me in the hospital on the dermatology service late that afternoon.

They started treatment immediately, which was a clear, soapy-looking bath. They must have concluded that that wasn't very effective because the next morning they started potassium permanganate baths which is a solution of potassium permanganate mixed in clear bath water. I had a bath tub right there in my room so they could do these treatments conveniently. I sat and soaked in the bathtub each morning for 30 minutes. This solution, which was a real dark purple color, stained my skin brown and stained the ulcer a funny looking brown color. It seemed to help clean it out. That's really what it was for, to clean it out and keep staph and other things from growing in the ulcer.

The evening they put me in the hospital, the doctor who saw me in the clinic sent one of his residents over to do some biopsies of the ulcer itself. That was unbelievably painful. I thought I was going to faint from the pain because he used an instrument that looked like a belt punch, the kind that you use to punch holes in your belt for your belt buckle. He used this to remove little parts of skin in the ulcer itself and apparently they ran some tests on this skin but I guess that it came to no real breakthrough as far as a new diagnosis was concerned. I felt, later on, that that was unnecessary because they had already diagnosed the ulcer as pyoderma gangrenosum, which is an extra-colonic manifestation of the colitis itself.

They started me on an increased dosage of Prednisone, probably 75 to 100 milligrams a day. They also started me on Sulfapyridine. They had me on Valium every day, too. I didn't notice any difference in the way I felt from the Valium because I was in such excruciating pain all of the time. It had no apparent effect on the way I felt but it was given to me to help relax me and help me feel a little better. Apparently it is given routinely to most of the patients on the derm service. The nurse said it was a muscle relaxer. She also said, "We give patients Valium so they will like us better."

They also had me on some kind of narcotic. I didn't know what it was. The pain was so bad that it was hard for me to bear, so that's why they had me on narcotics.

After soaking in the potassium permanganate tub every morning, they wrapped my leg with a wet dressing soaked in potassium permanganate, which they changed every two-and-a-half hours, around the clock, 24 hours a day. They told me that the dressing helped to keep the ulcer clean and to keep things from growing in it.

It was a week or so before I could notice any improvement in my state of health. The dressings helped to debride the dead tissue; that's what they told me. Every time they removed the dressing, it was terribly painful because some of the dead tissue came off. At the end of the first week, all of the dead tissue had come off and I had a huge, open ulcer on my leg. I could see the muscle exposed on the right side of it. It was very, very deep. I don't think it got down to the bone, but I could see some tendon in there, it was so deep.

The air irritated it. Every time they changed the dressing, my leg would be exposed to the air, which caused extreme pain. So they would give me the narcotic painkiller about 15 minutes before it was time to change the dressing. It helped, but it didn't help that much to make the pain go away or keep it from coming on. It made my body feel a little better.

At the very first, I was really sick and it took at least a week and a half to get me turned around so that my appetite was a little better and my diarrhea was improved. Normally, I weigh 130 pounds. At my lowest, about the time I was first in the hospital up there, I weighed 95 pounds. They started me on I.V.'s when I went into the hospital.

Slowly, I began to get better. I gained a little bit of weight and I could notice a little improvement in my leg. But it was slow, very slow. All of this time I had to lie flat on the bed with my leg elevated. That sounds pretty uncomfortable, but it really wasn't too bad. I felt really relaxed after the pain got better. I could tell that the Valium helped keep me relaxed. I was able to get some sleep between dressing changes.

It took a week or so before my stools began looking more normal but occasionally I could have bleeding. It looked like someone had slit their wrists and held them over the toilet. It was bright red. The first time this happened to me was about a month before I went to the Hanson Clinic. One night I got up to use the bathroom, I had bad diarrhea and out came all of this terrifying blood. I was really scared to death. I had never experienced anything like this before and I thought I was having some really terrible internal bleeding. It was about four o'clock in the morning when we called up our family physician, the internist who was taking care of me then, and he said sometimes with colitis a small blood vessel will rupture and cause this kind of bleeding but that it really wasn't that serious. That helped to ease my mind.

After several weeks, my appetite was better, I was gaining weight and my bowels began to function more normally, but my leg, it was so slow to improve. I was in the hospital for 141 days. And at the end of that time, my leg was still not completely healed. They felt that it had reached the point where they didn't need to have me under close observation any more, though.

The doctors also treated the cystic acne on my face and back. These treatments consisted of hot packs of sterile water with Vleminckx's solution, which has sulfur and other things in it. They gave me a small stove and a stainless steel bowl. I'd mix the solution, heat it 'til it was boiling. Then they had this little gauze mask, a half inch thick, which I placed in the boiling solution. They gave me rubber gloves to wear because the solution dries your skin out and turns it yellow. I'd ring out the mask and put the damp, hot gauze on my face and on my back. That would open the cystic acne and help to drain it. I'd do that for 30 minutes, twice a day, morning and night. After a while, it began to burn my face so they cut down the treatments to once a day. The sulfur in the Vleminckx's solution smelled so bad but once I got used to it, it didn't bother me that much. There were a lot of paitents with bad acne and psoriasis on the derm service so the whole area had a smell of sulphur and coal tar, which people coming off the street noticed the first time they came to visit a patient.

"How did you keep from going 'stir crazy' during the almost five months you were there?"

I didn't worry about that because I was kept busy constantly, 24 hours a day. Every morning, I had the potassium permanganate bath, they wrapped my leg and then they brought in my breakfast and my pills. Someone was always coming in to give me pills or wrap my leg. The doctors and nurses were always around so I didn't have too much time to myself. I found it difficult to sleep because they changed the dressing on my leg every two-and-a-half hours. I was kept so busy I hardly had time to watch TV.

Each week they would photograph my leg so they could note the progress of healing of the ulcer. Also, on occasion they would have consultations on my case. The various doctors would all get together and talk about my case and try to decide what new things they should try.

From the minute I went into the hospital I got better until they changed doctors on the service and the new one decided it was time to reduce the Prednisone dose. As I recall, he reduced it 10 milligrams a day, which is a lot because Prednisone is supposed to be tapered very slowly. As a result, I had a big flare-up, my diarrhea came back and I had cramping and blood in my stools again. I was getting weak again and was not improving as fast as the doctor thought I should. The blood test results indicated I was really anemic so he started a blood transfusion. Just laying in bed as still as I could I felt sick and exhausted but by the time I got the blood, I noticed an immediate improvement. I felt a lot better.

Several days passed and they did more blood tests. In fact, they tested my blood about every other day because the Sulfapyridine had to be watched closely to maintain the proper sulfa level. The doctor gave me another pint of blood and I felt that much better. They kept slowly decreasing the Prednisone down to 50 milligrams. I'd have an occasional flare-up after that if they cut down the Prednisone too fast but I didn't have any more bad ones which required blood transfusions.

After about four months in the hospital, they started physical therapy because they were afraid that the scar tissue would leave adhesions and it would be hard for me to move my leg around. They started training me to walk again because I hadn't walked for 125 days. Each time I got up to use the bathroom, there was a bathroom in my room, I used crutches and kept my leg up. I practically had to learn how to walk all over again. My leg felt very weak although I was using crutches. It was very thin, having atrophied from being in a motionless position, elevated on a pillow, the whole time. It was much thinner than my left leg. I was on physical therapy for a week and a half or so. Then they sent me home. It was late October.

The entire time I was at the Hanson, there was the issue of having my colon taken out and the doctors had different opinions. The dermatologists seemed to feel that it would be dangerous to have a colectomy while my leg was an open ulcer. They thought there was a possibility of developing an ulcer at the incision site, which they felt would be really dangerous. They wanted to get my leg ulcer cleared up completely before beginning to consider a colectomy. They recommended tapering the Prednisone and sulfa down as low as possible to see how I did, to see if I could stabilize at a low level of medication. I got down to about 10 milligrams of Prednisone before I had a flare-up of my leg ulcer. And it seemed like whenever I had a flare-up with my leg, my colon would also flare up. It was kind of a chain reaction.

When I did get a spot on my leg, the doctor here put me back up to 50 milligrams of Prednisone for a few days and then dropped the dose back to 25 milligram a day. They could do this if you were up on a high level of Prednisone for only a short time. When you have been on high levels for a long time, it is dangerous to drop down suddenly. I stayed on 25 milligrams for quite some time. My leg healed right up after I was boosted to the 50 milligram dose for a few days.

Later I got down slowly to five milligrams of Prednisone and started having problems again so once more they boosted my dose up to 50 milligrams which I stayed on only a few days until my problem turned around.

After that, I couldn't go any lower than about 10 milligrams of Prednisone without having a flare-up of the ulcer on my leg. That's when we started to consider seriously the issue of the colectomy again. Obviously, I couldn't stay on 10 milligrams of Prednisone for the rest of my life and after awhile, even that wasn't enough. I had to go up to 15 milligrams or so. That's when I decided we had reached the end of the line, it was time to have a colectomy. There was no other alternative.

I made an appointment with the gastroenterologist I had seen earlier at Hanson and drove up there. He felt the same way I did: a colectomy was the only way to cure the disease completely, forever. He said that colitis is a disease of the colon and that when the colon is gone, the disease is gone.

He put me in the hospital immediately and they began preparing me for surgery. This was almost exactly a year after I went into the hospital up there the first time. I had a little spot on my leg and they wanted to clear that up before the operation so I was on the dermatology service about two weeks.

After the ulcer was cleared up, they began final preparations for surgery. About two days before the operation, they gave me enemas, I didn't eat, and they gave me a lot of laxatives to clear out my bowels. They also gave me shots of steroids and pills that supposedly cleaned out my colon as best as possible and got it ready to be removed.

The night before surgery, I took a shower with a special cleansing soap and that morning they shaved the hair around the area and inserted a catheter. The catheter gave me so much pain I could hardly stand it and finally after almost begging them to remove it, they did and said they would put it back in after I had been put to sleep with the anesthetic and before the operation.

I had some shots of steroids right before I went to surgery. They put me on a cart and wheeled me into a waiting area outside the operating room and I was lying there with some other people who were getting ready for surgery.

A receptionist there asked me a few questions. I felt pretty relaxed. I wasn't uptight because I had come to accept the fact that I was going to have it taken out. Really, I felt pretty good about it. I knew that they would give me the anesthetic and that would be it. Then I would wake up and it would be over with.

I waited there about 30 minutes before they wheeled me into the operating room. They had me put on a different kind of gown. The anesthesiologist came in, put the mask over my face and said the usual "Count to 10 backwards." I didn't feel myself gradually lose consciousness. I was counting and then I was out. It was just one thing and suddenly another.

Father: I waited in Tom's room while he was in surgery. They took him down about eleven o'clock and I left the room for a while for lunch but returned shortly after noon so that I could be there when he was brought back.

About one o'clock, one of Tom's nurses, an attractive, red-haired LPN, came to the door and motioned for me to follow her. At first, I had no idea where we were going or for what reason I was walking with her down the corridor. On the way, she explained that we were going to the next floor to the pathology department. When we arrived, I was escorted into a small room at one end of which were two cubicles. I was seated in one of them, at a counter-like affair.

Almost immediately, a technician from the department of pathology came out carrying a stainless steel pan. She seated herself on the other side of the cubicle counter and put the pan down. The pan was about eight-inches wide and 12-inches long, perhaps two-inches deep, and was covered with a blue towel. There was a card lying on the top of the towel and the card had a paragraph or so of typewritten information on it.

The technician began quoting the pathologist's report indicating, to my great relief, that there was no apparent involvement of the small intestine. We were afraid that Tom might have Crohn's disease which does affect the small intestine as well as the large bowel. Then she invited me to view my son's freshly removed large intestine. She said that it was not mandatory that I look at it because some people do not care to view such specimens but I could if I wanted to. I told her to go ahead.

She removed the towel covering the pan and there lay a gray mass of tubular tissue, sort of wrinkled, like a bloated snake, tapering down to the rectum. It had been cut along its length so that when she lifted and opened portions of the tube with tissue forceps, I could look at the inside of Tom's colon.

To say the least, this was a strange experience, knowing that this previously unseen piece of human anatomy had just been removed from my own son's body. It looked like all of the pictures in the anatomy books except that it was the wrong color. I didn't expect it to look so gray. I thought it would be pink and resemble cuts of meat you might see at the market. It didn't.

As the technician lifted portions of the colon to expose the inside lining, I could see areas of ulcerous tissue. Having never seen a healthy colon so dissected, I had no basis of comparison, but areas of the intestinal mucosa which she pointed to with her forceps did not look the way I imagined a healthy gut would appear. I was invited to ask questions but I couldn't think of any.

I left the cubicle with mixed feelings. There was something horribly fascinating about it all and yet satisfying. It was obvious that the technician in conveying the pathologist's report was convinced that the clinicians had made the correct diagnosis. Of course, there was never much doubt in our minds that the ulcerative colitis was present and, insofar as this unpracticed eye could determine, it was obvious when I looked at the specimen. I had no lingering apprehensions.

But all of this procedure was something totally new to me. Although I had been in hospital administration for 20 years, I had never heard of this procedure in which the family is invited to view the specimen removed from their loved one at surgery. Later, I discussed this with a pathologist friend of mine who said that Hanson's is probably the only place in the country where this is done.

Patient: The next thing I knew, I was gradually waking up. I was real groggy, in some kind of strange room and there was a light just above my head, shining brightly. I was incoherent, couldn't tell what was going on. I was on a cart in surgical recovery and everyone had left the room. I was beginning to wake up and the pain was just terrible. I remember trying to yell, trying to whistle and no one would come in. It was very frustrating.

Finally, after what seemed to be a long time, someone came in. It was probably only 10 minutes at the most, but it seemed like hours. They gave me a shot for pain. Then some orderlies and a nurse came in and they took me back to my room and lifted me off the cart onto the bed. I felt like a limp noodle. I had no control over myself at all. I was conscious for maybe a couple of minutes and then I was out again.

When I woke up again it was dark and I could tell it was late in the evening. My dad was sitting in the corner and that was a relief to me. My nurse was there, too, and they were talking. I said something and they realized then that I had finally awakened. They told me the surgery went just fine.

I was in this single room on the surgical unit, recovering for about a week. They had me on drugs and they had some drainage tubes leading from the incision site to drain the blood which would ooze out now and then. It was funny. They had two tiny tubes, a little wider than a wide pencil lead. They were inside the cavity of my abdomen and they came out parallel with each other. They attached a large syringe to one tube, squirted this solution into my abdomen and that helped to clean it out. But it stung, it really stung bad. I could hardly stand that either. The other tube was hooked up to some kind of suction which made a funny sound the whole time. It was kind of a slurping sound and sucked the blood that oozed out of the cavity in my abdomen. I guess so that it wouldn't accumulate and cause infection. I could see the blood flowing through the clear plastic tubes coming from the place where my rectum had been.

The operation I had was a standard colectomy. Prior to going to the Hanson Clinic, I read in a magazine about a new procedure which some doctors up there were performing as an alternative to the standard ileostomy. It was called a Koch pouch, in which they build a little bladder-type affair in the cavity where the colon was. They make this bladder out of small intestine. Then, through a tube that leads to the outside from this bladder, you can catheterize yourself as you need to, to release your waste. I thought about that because I thought it would be easier than the appliance used with a standard ileostomy but the doctor who performed the surgery had run into some complications with this new procedure, which they had only been doing for a year or so. He thought it wasn't a good idea for me to have this new procedure. He said if I decided later on that I wanted the Koch pouch procedure, I could come back and have the revision done.

I was real weak, of course, but each and every day I was getting better. First thing, they wouldn't even let me drink any water. Gradually, I could take very small sips of water and then they started me on a liquid diet. They gave me Coca-Cola, but that upset my stomach and I vomited that up several times. So they had to start all over again, with water and gradually get into the liquid diet. But by the time I was allowed to have solid food, I was feeling pretty good.

They took the tubes out and there was still quite a bit of bleeding so they had me wear a pad back there to soak up the blood. I had to do that for a week after I got home. In fact, it bled on and off, a little spot, for six months. My doctor here at home said that was to be expected because it is a hard-to-heal area. You are sitting on it. Immediately after the surgery, they had me take Sitz baths, where I would sit in a tub of warm water. That seemed to help to clean the area. I even did that at home and finally it cleared up. It took a long time.

I guess the worst part of having a colectomy is the emotional aspect of having it. The ileostomy is hardly any hassle at all, once I got used to it, but it's just the emotional part, losing a part of your body which you have had all your life.

They released me from the hospital and I flew home. As soon as I got home I had a big piece of cake and a glass of milk because I felt pretty good, but later on in the evening, I began feeling sick and I vomited and continued to vomit. I started having terrible cramping in my abdomen which kept getting worse and worse until the pain was almost unbearable. It was constant, 24 hours a day.

I called the doctors at the Hanson Clinic and they said that was just something which happens after an operation. They said it was normal but I was having excruciating pain, 24 hours a day. Finally, I contacted this physician here and he thought there was a possibility that I could have a bowel obstruction. He put me in the hospital and had one of his residents put a tube up through my nose and down into my stomach. He attached this tube to a suction machine and it sucked out all of the food and fluid which had accumulated in my stomach.

They thought that if I stayed really relaxed in the bed and had this suction to clear out my stomach that it might relax my small intestine enough so that it would unkink itself. They were hoping this would work and they wouldn't have to do any surgery.

I noticed immediate relief from the suction, which kept the cramping from coming on. I felt much better, but my bowels weren't really moving. We were afraid that the kink was still there. They decided that after no progress was evident, I was going to have to have surgery to correct this kink. I'd been on suction for two days.

They set up a time for the surgery which the doctor was going to perform late in the afternoon. Early that afternoon, they took me to x-ray to look at my small intestine, I guess as a routine procedure before surgery. All of a sudden, in the x-ray room, I noticed my bowels starting to move again. Apparently, the kink in my intestine had straightened out. What a stroke of luck that it happened when it did because I was only a few hours away from surgery.

They removed the suction, started me on water and slowly moved me into a liquid diet and later to solid meals. From there I seemed to do pretty well. While I still had some cramping, which the doctor said I could expect, it was not very bad and I got some pills for the pain, some antispasmodic medication which relaxed my intestine. After that, I had no problems.

The Prednisone was tapered slowly, at a rate of two and a half milligrams every two weeks, so it took several months before I got off of it completely. Directly after the surgery, I developed a slight kidney infection which the doctor said was a common occurrence after major surgery. Sometimes the catheter causes it. I kept in contact with a urologist about that and took an antibiotic for that. He followed me closely and the kidney infection cleared up.

After that, I slowly got stronger, gained back my normal weight and felt fine.

Ten months after the surgery I ran into another little complication. I'd taken a long bus trip, coming home from school, and hadn't eaten for over 12 hours. I guess my intestine must have shrunk a bit. I got home, ate a little bit and then began lifting weights. Then I noticed a funny kind of crampy feeling down around my abdomen, but I didn't think much about it because you have occasional cramping. But when it felt worse than ordinary, I took a look at it and noticed that my intestine had crept out of my abdomen about four inches. That frightened me a little bit but I knew that a hernia of the stoma happens occasionally. The stoma therapist at Hanson who helped me learn how to manage an ileostomy told me that it happens now and then. She gave me a booklet which mentions that, so I knew immediately what had happened. I really wasn't panicked. I knew I wasn't going to die. I knew the problem could be corrected but I thought it would have to be corrected surgically.

I went on over to the hospital emergency room. The doctor on call took a look at it and said, "Well, let's see if we can't get that back in there." He started pushing on it and pressing on it and finally got it back in to the normal length. He said I should be careful and not lift any weights until the area around the stoma got healed up and a little stronger.

I was trying to be real careful about that but it happened again about five or six days later. The doctor threaded it back in again at the hospital. He said I could do that myself, no problem. And it hasn't happened since.

From my experience, if I were to give advice to anyone who is diagnosed as having colitis, I'd say go ahead and have a colectomy as soon as possible because that way you eliminate the possibility of extra-colonic manifestations as I had, with the ulcer on my leg and the pain in my joints. If the condition has persisted for quite some time, of course. They say, and I've read some things about colitis, that something like only two percent of those diagnosed with colitis are completely cured of the disease and those who are cured have a much higher risk of cancer of the colon. If I had had a colectomy earlier, I wouldn't have had this scar on my leg and I wouldn't have had to go through the excruciating pain night and day that I went through with this ulcer. So I would say, if you've had colitis for any length of time, you should go ahead and have a colectomy and avoid the terrible complications I had.

The sooner patients can be removed from the depressing influence of general hospital life the more rapid their convalescence.

Charles H. Mayo (1865–1939)
Journal-Lancet 36:1, 1916

The stomach, the lungs, the liver, as well as other parts, are uncomparably adapted to their purposes; yet they are far from having any beauty.

Edmund Burke (1729–1797)
On the Sublime and Beautiful,
Pt. III, Sect. VI

60. Perforated Duodenal Ulcer

It was the end of office hours, well after five, but the doctor was still seeing patients. He stopped by his private office where I was asked by his nurse to wait, and he apologized for the delay. I waited for him another three-quarters of an hour while he completed his examinations and treatments. Medical books lined the tiny, windowless office. On his desk was a six-inch mannequin on which the acupuncture points were displayed.

The doctor is a tall, slim, grey-haired man in his late 30's. He wears a white coat in one pocket of which is a stethoscope. He is forthright and articulate.

After the initial amenities, he asked me for identifying credentials because, apparently, he was at first suspicious of my motives, perhaps suspicious of me. He also started his own tape recorder so he could have a file on this discussion. He was the only person interviewed who took these two precautions.

However, when his tape ran out he did not bother to reload his recorder, apparently convinced by then that his comments would be accurately quoted and properly used.

- **Abdominal Pain**
- **Perforated Duodenal Ulcer**
- **Surgery**
- **Sub-diaphragmatic Abscess**

I was on vacation and also attending a seminar on drug therapy in Hawaii. We had been there three days and I perforated. I'd had an ulcer since the age of 17.

"Stomach ulcer?"

Peptic ulcer. Duodenal ulcer. It had been giving me increasingly severe pain over the last several years and being chicken, I just wasn't ready to go for surgery for it until I had to, primarily because I had lost several relatives to that same surgery, the most recent one being an uncle about two years before that, who died on the table.

"Is it common to lose a patient during a gastric resection?"

No, it's not, but in our family, it is. I figured that when I went for surgery I'd probably not be waking up, so I put it off as long as I could. I fully intended to die, I was almost disappointed when I awoke because I was in agony, of course. I had a tube down my throat, a tube in my arm, a couple of drain tubes in my stomach and all that, you know? Couldn't have anything to eat or drink. If purgatory is any worse than that, it would really have to go some. If I go to hell, I really don't have to worry much; I can take it.

I was in intensive care for about six days and left the hospital in about 10 days and was feeling relatively well and appeared to be progressing satisfactorily.

I took the family, the wife and kids, to a display of camping vehicles. As I was lifting my little son up to see into one of these cars, I had a really sharp pain in my left side. I thought I had torn something. It kept getting worse, but I thought I was being a hypochondriac so I didn't consult anyone right away.

After a couple of days it really got severe, really intense, so I told the wife to take me back to the hospital. I wanted to go just about as much as I would have enjoyed having leprosy. I knew I had to.

They took x-rays and they told me I had some stomach gas, nothing more, which reassured me. The pain was easing up a little bit by then so I went on back home.

About two o'clock that afternoon, it began hurting really bad again. My bowels had not moved for a day or two in the interim so I thought, "Hell, this may just be constipation." So I found myself a chiropractor that had one of these colon irrigation machines and I went over there and had a colon irrigation. And it helped to relieve the pain a little. But that evening, the pain kept getting worse.

The next day, I finally just came back on in to the hospital and said, "There's something wrong. I know there's something wrong." They took another picture and again they told me I had gas under the diaphragm. They drew blood and found I had about 18,000 white count and decided, well, maybe there might be something wrong.

So they put me back in the hospital and I don't remember much of it because I was kept under sedation. I was in great pain and was given hypos for that. My wife could tell you more about it than I, but in the ensuing two-week period, my weight dropped to about 155 pounds from around 240. It was 240 when I perforated.

I kept getting worse and worse; my temperature kept going higher and higher. I finally told the wife, "I'm going down the tubes here and nobody is doing a damn thing about it." I had to practically twist Jim Tillerman's arm, the guy who was seeing me, to get him to start some antibiotics because the cultures were all coming up negative. As it turned out, the cultures were all negative because the organism was an anaerobe. It was not an aerobic bacteria and no one had bothered to grow anaerobic cultures. Furthermore, our radiologist had missed it, just flatter than hell, repeatedly. If I had not been a physician, I would have sued the livin' hell out of him, the hospital and everyone concerned. He can thank his lucky stars that I am a physician, that I intend to stay in this area, and that I am very forgiving by nature. Because I have a case and I could damn sure take them to the cleaners. They know it and I know it.

I spent 28 days straight in intensive care, which I sure as hell didn't like, and I was in and out of intensive care several more times. In total, I had four major operations. They went back in here for a second time. The surgeon thought that the incision had been coming unraveled, so he did a Bilroth Two, whatever the hell that means. It's a modification of the resection. He took several loops of bowel and formed a pouch which would function somewhat like a stomach. Apparently, they never did find the real problem which, as it turned out later, was a sub-diaphragmatic abscess.

In the meantime, I started hiccupping all of the time and the fever just kept climbing. Post-surgically, I kept getting worse, so at the conclusion of two and a half or three weeks more, I told my wife I wanted out of there. I said if I was going to die, I wanted a fighting chance. No one was taking me seriously. No one was doing anything. The cultures were negative so they were just going around wringing their hands. I was getting mildly perturbed, with what small amount of faculties I had left. From toxicity and drugs, I wasn't too sharp at the time.

This sub-diaphragmatic abscess was a complication of the surgery, hypothetically or theoretically due to a leaking of the anastomosis, where they take out the stomach. Somewhere along there it must have leaked a little and cornered itself up under the diaphragm, some anaerobic bacteria that I was unable to throw off set up housekeeping and began to increase and multiply. That was where the gas was coming from that the radiologist saw under my diaphragm. But he didn't interpret it as what it really was. He interpreted it as stomach gas but it was not. It was gas formed by gas-forming organisms. It was a plain case of, to put it bluntly, incompetence. It should have been diagnosed and it wasn't.

My white count reached 20,000 and my temperature was doing 105 and 106 degrees and they couldn't get it to fall and nobody was doing a damn thing about it. I finally badgered Jim into started an I.V. with some Terramycin on me. I said, "Hell, start the Terramycin now and if this doesn't start the white count and fever going down within eight hours, start the Chloromycetin and call in some specialists and let's get some things rolling. I don't intend to go out of this without a fight."

Well, I didn't get any better and so I told Janice to get me transferred to University Hospital. I thought I'd have a better crack at it over there because I'd heard a lecture by the chief bacteriologist over there and I was thoroughly impressed with him. I told my wife that if anyone could pull me through this, it would be him. He had more expertise in the field of anaerobes and bacteriological studies than any man in the region.

Dr. Jones *(the bacteriologist)* was kind enough to come out to the hospital here to consult first, which Janice asked him to, and he had me transferred to University Hospital. He got me in on the surgical service and they ran a needle in me, where I was swelling so badly and they drew off about 20 cc's of pus. This assured them of the diagnosis that I had already concluded. I knew what I had. No one would listen but I knew I had an abscess.

They took me to surgery within a couple of hours of the time I arrived at University Hospital and they took out a couple of quarts of pus, they put suction on me and left me on suction for about a week. They left the wound open, figuring they would have to. If they closed it, they knew I'd just make another abscess. I had private duty nurses around the clock and they lavaged it out with normal saline every few hours. During those times, I knew I was going to die and I wondered why it was taking so damn long. It just seemed like a cruel thing to have to go through so much misery.

The surgeon did an excellent job. He was the chief resident. You'd think I'd remember his name but I can't think of it, really. I blanked it out. He had a moustache. I get a perfect mental picture of him.

I had continual intravenouses. They kept me there in University about a month and finally sent me home, still with the wound open. I could look in and see my stomach and large intestine, spleen, liver, gall bladder, I could see all of that. It was just open. They had to. There wasn't any choice.

When I went home, I was given the privilege of stopping this normal saline lavage and simply standing in a hot shower and letting the water wash all of the crud out for half an hour, three times a day.

"Wouldn't the antibiotics touch the infection?"

The antibiotics helped but the infection was so overwhelming. I was full of pus. Two quarts of pus was not an exaggeration. I'm not exaggerating. That is the measurement of the pus they took out of me in surgery at the first whack. Plus, I don't know how many quarts that drained out later, and electrolytes, plasma, protein, whatever. I was in a hell of a shape. I was weak, I was hysterical, I would cry if somebody looked at me. I was broken. I had no semblance of manhood left. I was depersonalized, terrified, frightened, wishing for death, quickly. If I'd had the nerve and the strength, I would have jumped. We were high enough in the hospital that I could have done it. But I had neither. I couldn't get up out of bed and I doubt that I would have had the nerve to do it if I could. I had to have help to get out of bed.

After about six weeks at home doing this shower process and then going back to bed, cold all the damn time. I remember how cold I was. Always before, and now since I have regained my health, I am real hot-natured. Always sweating. Then I was always cold, shivering. And always on the verge of hysteria. Emotionally wrecked.

Anyhow, after six weeks of that, they told me things looked pretty good. The infection was down and I hadn't run a fever of any significance for a couple of weeks, so it was decided this would be a good time to attempt closure of the resultant hernia. So I went back in and had the hernia repaired and did famously that time. Got along very well. Got out of the hospital in a little less than a week, six days.

I did very well, recovered well, but of course, I was weak as a cat. I was up to the grand weight of 161 pounds; hardly any of it was muscle. I could walk about 100 feet and then I had to sit down.

"How old were you?"

I was 37. I still wasn't able to go back to work for another six or eight weeks. I actually came back to work way too soon. I really wasn't ready.

I had income protection insurance which kept me from really hitting the bottom. It wasn't like what I make here when I'm working but it paid $2500 a month total. It paid some for my salary and some for office overhead. Being a sucker, I didn't lay off any of my help, kept them all on, paid them. I had good hospitalization insurance which paid the whole thing off except a few hundred dollars. Financially, we had to pull in the belt a little bit. We had to give up a few things here and there, but there isn't a hell of a lot you want when you're laying around in bed 24 hours a day. Food isn't that expensive but you have house payments, car payments and the like, but my insurance policies were made up in such a way that when I was laid up I didn't have to pay the premiums. They had that clause in the policies. At the time I bought them, I didn't even know about it, but I'm sure glad it was there. Financially, it was no great hardship.

"How has this experience affected your general attitude, your philosophy, about your medical practice and your relationship with your patients?"

I think I go for my gun a little earlier than I did. I'm a little quicker on the draw when it comes to calling in special help. Any time a patient even looks like they're not responding like I feel they should, I call in consultation. I'm probably guilty of overdoing it now. I overtreat a little more than I ever did before. I'm inclined to use two or three antibiotics instead of one in a serious infection. If I don't feel right about a patient, I may call in more than one consultant, especially if I don't get an opinion I agree with. Not that they have to agree with me but if the patient still doesn't appear to be progressing very well, I'm not going to sit on my hands and watch him go down the tubes. To get help, I'll ship 'em a little quicker than I ever did before.

I have a hell of a lot less trust of our x-ray department. I look at a lot more pictures myself than I used to. I don't have any confidence in what x-ray tells me. I go more on my hunches than I do on lab or x-ray. I used to be more lab and x-ray-oriented. Now, I'm more hunch-oriented. I believe that all of us have an ESP ability if we develop it. I think that most of the diagnostic work that goes on in most doctors' heads goes on in the subconscious level whether they realize it or not. I really believe that. I believe that the subconscious brain or mind beams messages to the conscious brain and then we prove them by diagnostic surveys.

I have much more perception now than I've ever had before in my life. Many, many times now I'll walk into a room the first time I see a patient and I'll immediately know what's wrong. Then I proceed to let them tell me and I make tests and I'm right about 80 percent of the time.

I think I'm a much more sympathetic person now. I used to be a little on the hard-boiled side, maybe. I didn't put up with any sissy business. If they were bitching and groaning, I'd tell them to hush up, they were going to be all right, I'd do the worrying.

I'm more inclined to explain the situation to the patient and his family in detail now, than I used to be, because I remember the stark terror of not knowing exactly what was going to happen next. And I remember the aggravation, too. I try to alleviate the emotional distress because, I can tell you, psychic pain is a helluva lot worse than physical pain. Physical pain numbs you after a while, it can't reach you anymore. Of course, you'll scream when they hurt you, and all that, but when you are in continual, severe pain for days, weeks, months, and the only relief you get is that shot of morphine or whatever they decide to let you have if they think you're hurting bad enough, you get bitter, you get resentful and hostile, you certainly become addicted, which I certainly was. It was one hell of a time coming down.

"How did you kick that?"

It wasn't easy. Even to this day, I take a lot of tranquilizers, which I never did before. If I had my choice, tomorrow, of going through that and surviving or going under the knife and never waking up, I think I would choose the latter over the former. I certainly wouldn't choose to go through that again. I couldn't believe it was happening when it was happening. Every time I went through another surgery, it seemed like something else happened, some other complication just got worse. I'd get better for a day or two after surgery — they'd drain all of the pus out of there during surgery and that helped a little — and here started another complication. At first, I thought I was a hypochondriac. I thought, "Well, hell, I'm just a crock. I'm imagining this." The pain would come intensely and then it would leave completely and I would feel all right. But when I started running 103 and 104 fever, I knew that something had to be wrong other than just psychosomatic.

It was like a horrible nightmare but it was surrealistic. I'm sure that some of the emotional reaction was because I was under heavy sedation, morphine and whatever. I couldn't have Demerol because that made me vomit every time they gave it to me. Talwin wasn't enough to hold me, dilaudid didn't seem to make a dent in it, morphine was the only thing that would help. This made them all very suspicious of me. Nothing but morphine would do and of course morphine is the most euphoric of all of the analgesics. But, pardner, I'll tell you. When you've been on morphine for a couple of months straight, every four hours, and they are shooting it right through the I.V. tubing, it makes a change in your personality.

The morphine was pleasant. I looked forward to the pain shots. For just a little while then, I wasn't frightened, I didn't care, I was free of pain, floating around on that pink, narcotic cloud. Hell, that was the biggest thing in my life. I couldn't eat and I couldn't drink water. I could have ice chips. I could wash out my mouth with a wet rag. I could piss and moan and raise hell. But hell, I had a tube up my bladder, a tube up my rectum, drain tubes in each side and an I.V. in each arm most of the time, one arm all of the time, a tube down my throat and all that. The only bright spot in my entire existence for a period of weeks was the narcotic high which I won't deny, felt good. It was fun, it felt good and I didn't feel ashamed that I enjoyed it. Hell, I had nothing else in life to enjoy and I knew damn well I was going to die. They told me I had about a 20-percent probability of surviving when I arrived at University Hospital. The surgeon looked at me and said I had one chance and that was a slim one. And that was if they operated immediately.

He explained to me that they could not put me clear under for it because I'd had two anesthetics within the last month. So I was conscious during the surgery and it hurt like hell. They gave me some morphine and some nitrous oxide and oxygen. That's all they dare give me. They would have run a severe danger of destroying my liver if they had tried going with a more potent anesthetic agent.

So they just strapped me down and did it.

I was drugged of course, but I'm not going to tell you I am a brave man. I was screaming and crying and carrying on, as I believe most anyone would when someone starts cutting in there and pulling on your insides. I was sure glad that for the last operation I could have a general anesthetic. I didn't ever appreciate a general anesthetic so much until I went through a surgery without one. First the morphine helped the thing a little and they got me pretty drunk on the nitrous, but nonetheless, when someone cuts down into the peritoneal cavity and starts pulling the intestines over and probing around in there, you can feel it sitting up against your diaphragm. You are bucking and they're telling you, "Breathe easy, breathe easy," and you can't breathe any way. I remember screaming out several times, "Well, hell, just knock me out. Have mercy. Clip me one." But nobody would do it.

When I came out of surgery, Janice was standing there, and of course, I looked like death warmed over. She kissed me and held my hand all of the way down to intensive care.

When they finally took me out of intensive care and back to my room, I was really dejected and depressed. I had asked my wife several times to bring me a gun. I'd rather finish it, not drag it out, haggle it. I checked on the insurance policies and they paid. I had them over two years and they would have paid, regardless. She wouldn't bring me a gun. By the time I had the strength to jump, I was better and I changed my mind. I decided I was going to try and live.

The whole thing was a mess. When I first perforated, I was staying in a hotel in Hawaii. On some of the islands, it is almost like going back into the 30's as far as facilities are concerned. The hospitals don't have inside plumbing. It's incredible, it really is. Their staff was some natives they put uniforms on. They have a couple of G.P.'s or so on each staff who play God. And they have some foreign medical students or interns who don't speak English, Japanese, Korean, whatever, and they don't know what in the hell is happening. They treated me like some kind of narcotics addict when I came in there, all doubled over.

I knew when it happened, what had happened. It hit me just like thunder and lightning. It was just like having a hot poker shoved in the middle of me when I perforated. The acid hit the peritoneum and I just fell out, fell right down on the floor.

Janice drove me over to the hospital; they call it that. I told them I had perforated and said I needed some morphine to get me back to the States. Apparently, they have a lot of addicts in that area so the student, or doctor, or whatever the hell he was said the only way they could give me any relief would be if I checked into the hospital. Well, hell, they didn't have anything there to do it with. I said all I wanted was something to give me relief until my plane left in two days, but to get anything, I had to go into the hospital.

"Couldn't you get an earlier plane?"

I already tried that. They wanted $2000 to charter an airplane, that is, if we could get one and there was none available for two days. The plane I was scheduled on left in two days, anyhow, so we decided to go back on that.

When I left the hospital they gave me two syrettes of one-quarter-grain morphine, for the three hour bus ride to the airport and then the plane trip home, which was ridiculous. I couldn't talk them out of any more. The doctor was pissed off that I wouldn't let him get out his knife and go to work. He couldn't seem to understand. I said, "Doc, I know I'm going to die of this and I'd rather die at home. I'd rather die under the hands of a surgeon than a G.P." That really pissed him off. He was very uncooperative, to say the least.

I knew I had "walled off" because after the first surge of severe pain, the first eight or 10 hours, it started localizing up under here *(points to diaphragm)*. At first, it felt like fire all over and then it was just a little burning, a little smoldering up under the diaphragm, up where the pit of the stomach is. I told Janice, "I've walled this off." I knew it had sealed and there was no great urgency for surgery to the point that I had to submit to this.

At first, before I decided to go into this little hospital, we drove into one of the large towns on the island and went to a hospital there. I told the guy there, the little extern or little jerk who was interviewing me, the story and he was resentful that I had diagnosed my own case. He told me, in his opinion, I was a drug addict, trying to get drugs. I wanted enough morphine to get home. I didn't want Demerol because I knew damn well it would make me vomit and I had Talwin with me and it didn't help. I'd had a hernia surgery about a year and a half previous to the ulcer perforation, which was the only other time in my life I was ever seriously ill. That's when I found out I couldn't take Demerol and it was also my first exposure to morphine. I knew that would work, it would stop the pain. I knew damn well I wasn't playing with them and it burned me up that I couldn't get it. They were putting it this way, "Either you play my game or I'll take my marbles and go home and you won't have anything. You can just suffer." And that's exactly what happened.

After I left the hospital and started on the bus ride, I took the first shot and by the time I got to the airport and on the airplane, it was four hours. I took the second shot and it lasted for two and a half or three hours. I had freedom from pain that long and then it began hurting and kept hurting. I remember bits of the trip. I was bathed in sweat and in agony. Frankly, there was no other way to put it. I drank every bit of milk on that airplane, actually, no exaggeration. They didn't have a drop of milk left when the plane got into San Francisco.

When I got to the airport here, I drove my family home and drove myself on down here to the emergency room of the hospital. I told them I needed something for pain right away. I was in a hell of a shape. Then I had them call the surgeon.

"How did you select the one to call?"

I had used him as a referring man for a long time for my patients and I knew he was able to do an adequate job. I felt reasonably safe in his hands and I didn't plan on survival, anyway. I just wanted to get home, I don't know why. When you're really sick, your brain doesn't function as much as your emotions.

"Do you refer to him any more?"

Yes. I really don't feel it was his fault. He's not a radiologist. He was relying on the information he was receiving from the radiographic reports and the laboratory reports. He was confused. And, not to put the man down, when things really start getting tough, he yellows out. He just hides his head in the sand. He let Jim Tillerman manage the case and Jim is an anesthesiologist. He just threw up his hands. Jim sat on his hands and watched me ripen. If I had been sitting there, with all of my faculties about me, watching a friend of mine go down the tubes, he would have been shipped out of there a good week, maybe a week and a half earlier. When things start going sour, I'd want to get my patient into a bigger institution with more facilities and more help.

I don't have anything to do with Jim anymore. We used to spend a lot of time together, our families — to the club for dinner and dancing — our wives and kids are still good friends. But I can't feel close to him anymore. He's friendly to me. I may be wrong, probably am, but he failed me when I really needed him. Oh, I've forgiven him but I don't ever want to depend on him again. I'll never put myself in a position again in which I even remotely depend on him.

The surgeon, I'll use, but with caution. I don't wish to sound braggadocious but I always retain the right and privilege to write orders on any chart for surgery. And he gets pissed off occasionally, and when he does, I say, "If you're really pissed off, I'll quit using you, if that's what you want." As long as I am referring a case, I am not relinquishing my authority over that case. And if he ever presses me on it, I'll just tell him, "I don't think you are a competent doctor. You are a good surgeon but I don't think you are competent for after-care." I think that I am better qualified to handle complications post-surgically than he is. I try harder. I'm not a loser. I'll cheat before I'll lose. I'll call in everybody I can call. Pick brains. I'd pick shit up off the floor to save a patient.

"How do you think about your experience compared with a patient who has no medical knowledge?"

If I'd had no medical knowledge, I would have been even more terrified, probably. Or maybe not. I'd seen some people go down the tubes. I'd scrubbed on surgeries. I know what's happening. When I went to sleep I knew what was about to happen to me and I knew what was going to happen to me when I woke up and I knew I was in for a hell of a time. In that way, you are more frightened. You know exactly, and in detail, what's going to happen. You don't just wake up with a bunch of bandages on.

I knew that when they were giving me these seven or eight different antibiotics at one time that I had a fairly good chance of winding up with impaired hearing, which I did. My hearing is moderately to severely impaired. I don't hear well. I have to see people, usually, to understand them. Fortunately, the loss occurs over 2000 cycles. Anything over 2000 cycles, I don't hear it. Anything under that I can hear fairly well, as long as there is no background noise. I can hear all of the heart murmurs, all of the rawls, which is a real break. I ought to be thankful, really thankful, that my professional ability was unimpaired. But as far as stereo, and really enjoying music as I once did, that's gone. The high notes I just don't hear. It's aggravating and inconvenient but, hell, it's a minor loss compared to being able to go on breathing, walking, working.

"How was your experience in the hospital as far as the rest of the patient care was concerned?"

I wouldn't be able to comment on that because my situation was a little bit different. I had a private room from day one until the last day I was in there. I had private duty nurses 24 hours a day. I remember there were some of them that I really hated. There was one bitch I would really love to kick down the hall. She was a sadist; there is no other way of putting it. Every time she did anything that could hurt a little bit, she made sure it hurt all it could. If the doctors left orders that I could have ice chips ad lib, she'd make sure it was just a teaspoonful every 30 or 40 minutes. No more. Just barely come up to the letter of the order, that's all. I had to put up with her for about three days until I could get her off the case. I couldn't get any other nurses.

Then I had some others who were just incompetent, bless their old souls. They tried the best they could, but they had the mentality of a fern, the intellect of a squash and the hands of a brick mason. Really and truly, there are some really incompetents running around in our profession, both as physicians, nurses, whatever. Everybody knows that. But I became acutely aware of it.

I know now that when I write an order for something, it ain't necessarily going to come out that way, unless I'm right on top of it. And I do check it. Now, instead of writing an order for a shot of antibiotics every so many hours and figuring it's being done, I go by and count the holes in my patient's butt. If it comes up wrong, I raise hell. I'm considered an asshole by some of the nurses on the staff over here but let them consider it.

There was a time when one of those special duty nurses forgot to give me my antibiotic injection for six hours. It was six hours late. That could have been it, right there. I was on a razor's edge. My white count was 20,000, I was running 105 to 106 degree fever. At that moment, they had me on four antibiotics and she forgot to give me the one that was given intramuscularly. The ones which were being given intravenously, thank God, were being taken care of by the charge nurse out at the desk, piggy-back, or I.V. push or whatever.

At any rate, I was really disillusioned with my profession. I'm not very happy with it now, to be very honest about it. If I could make a good living doing something else, I think I would. I think I'm a better doctor than I was but I feel impotent. I don't feel like I can deliver what I should and I don't feel I deserve the trust that the patients give me. But I must have that trust in order to help them. If I don't have their confidence, I've lost half the battle. At least 70 percent of the good a doctor does his patient is psychological. If not psychological, metaphysical, call it what you will. The will to get well or the desire to help a person, faith healing, psychic healing, psychic energy, whatever you wish to call it.

There are some doctors who can walk into the room of a patient that is really going bad and put their hands on him, some of them don't even have to put their hands on him, be with him a few minutes, and that patient rallies and gets better for no scientific reason. You must simply have their confidence. But you don't deserve it. I don't deserve it nor does any other physician because we don't know what happens at that hospital when we go home. We think we know, but we don't know.

"Do you believe that some patients, through psychic energy, can change the outcome of their metastatic disease?"

Yes, I know it. I'm very much into that right now. I'll use anything that works. I don't care what it is as long as I see a benefit for someone, I'll use it.

I don't care if it's immoral, I don't care if it's sacrilegious, if it'll help someone, I'll use it.

I wouldn't even have picked up an acupuncture book before. I thought we had all of the answers. I know damn well we don't now. I've read most of Edgar Cayce's work concerned with psychic healing. I'm quite sure that our race of people was evolved to a much higher degree at some time or other on the planet than we are at this time. I think most of the answers to most of the mysteries of our lives are probably tied up in the Great Pyramid of Gizeh, Cheops Pyramid. I don't know if you have read anything about Atlantis. A lot of people think I've lost my mind since all of this has happened because I've got different answers now than I used to. It has changed me. My personality is not the same, I'm not the same person I was. I used to be very pragmatic, cocksure, a little cocky, absolutely confident. And I'm not any more. I don't feel like I know everything any more.

I think I'm a better doctor for it, but I'm not as happy at it. I was in an ignorant, hog's paradise before. I didn't realized that I had mud all over my clothes. I thought I was dressed in shining white garments, raiments of finest linen, on a white charger coming up to save people. Now, I know I'm not.

Many people claim there is no such thing as psychic healing but I happen to know that there are men in the Philippines who can open the abdomen and close it without an incision and take out cancers. I have case records of hundreds of them that have been done. I'm going to the Philippines as soon as I can save enough money to go and I'm going to study under one of these psychic surgeons. I don't think It's quackery. I really don't. I used to. I used to scoff at it. Have you read a book about Argo, the surgeon with the rusty knife? He did cataract surgery with an old dull pocket knife, a rusty one at that. His results were far superior. He hardly ever had a complication, never had an infection, always got some improvement of vision. He performed surgery on a board with a rusty pocket knife, hunkered down in a squat, and got better results than the finest trained minds in this nation are getting with $50,000 worth of exotic equipment. To me, that indicates something that we don't have and we need and I'm searching for it. If I find it, I'm getting out of this and I'm going into that.

I honestly believe that cancer is a psychosomatic illness, just like an ulcer, colitis, certain types of dermatitis. I'm quite sure in my mind that all disease starts here *(points to forehead)*. I'm laughed at by most people for these opinions. I know that all disease starts in the mind. I was sick of soul, sick of spirit, sick of mind when my ulcer perforated and I'm still not well, but I'm getting better. I think I'm looking in the right direction.

"You are not talking about Christian Science, are you?"

No. They are looking at it from one angle, faith healers are looking at it from another angle, pyramid researchers from another angle, metaphysical parapsychologists are coming at it from still another angle. Somewhere, there is an overall picture that will all come together and fall into place. I really think we are in the dawning of a new age. An age of Aquarius, whatever you wish to call it. I really believe that in our lifetime, we'll have a cure for age. I think we'll be able to reverse it.

Maybe we are not just as far along as we think we are. I'm looking for the answer. I'm not a very religious person at this time. I believe you'd call me an agnostic. I believe in God. I know that God has to exist. The universe follows a logical pattern of laws. There's logic in it. There's logic in astronomy, there's logic in astrology. I think that astrology is a valid science. Astrology is the residual of the super-science which was available when Atlantis was actually flourishing, before it fell into the sea. I think most people would disagree with that but they are becoming more and more aware of it.

You can look at the effect of the moon on an ocean. If it will raise a tide, billions of tons of water, 28 feet twice a day, why would it be impossible to believe that it would affect the biochemical and bioelectric processes going on within the brain cells of a human being? Why do women have 28-day cycles in their periods? It's just peculiar. I think a lot of what we call pseudo-science now, when it's fully understood, will be recognized as lost information.

Since I've gone through all of this crap I've gone through, I feel that on at least two occasions, I've brought people through who otherwise wouldn't have made it. One of them was a massive coronary in a friend. His prognosis was nil. The whole back side of his heart had infarcted. The cardiac specialist who was taking care of him said, "We'll do the best we can, but it doesn't look too good."

That man never left my thoughts. He had a setback, went into congestive failure, went back into intensive care for a week. I visited him at least twice a day, every day. When he was real bad, he wouldn't know I was there, but I'd put my hand on him and ask God to let some of my life force, some of my energy go to him, to use me as a conductor and pour it through.

I'd always feel drained at the end of this period, as though something had gone out of me. I'd go home all tired, exhausted, wouldn't even want to screw, and for me that's very unusual because I've always been oversexed. But for a period of two and a half weeks, I didn't even want sex. It seemed like all of that was drained out of me at this man's bedside.

He and I are very close, to this day. I'll never know for sure — that's something you can never be sure about — but I really feel that when I really and truly, with all my heart and all my soul, want someone to live, I believe I can make them live. God will help me let them live.

I really feel that medicine, as we know it, compared to what it is going to be is as primitive as trephining holes in cavemen's skulls in prehistoric times.

I am not a remarkable person but I have been through a remarkable life so far, to me. It has not been exciting or anything anyone else would be interested in. I was born to parents, neither one of whom had been through high school. I was the first one in our family to complete college. It always was my dream, but I don't know how I ever got to be a doctor. I should be out busting rocks. But it was what I always wanted to do. Even when I was a little bitty toot, I wanted to be a doctor. I think that's because everybody looked up to doctors. You can't be sure why you want something. Maybe your parents hypnotized you or brainwashed you into wanting what you want. All of us are a conglomerate of happenstance, whatever genetic makeup happened to fall into our hands when the cards were dealt and the set of circumstances under which those cards are played. We have some control over it, our own destiny, free choice, free will, and so forth but we certainly aren't the absolute governor of our own fate.

You cannot be a perfect doctor till
you have been a patient.

Stephen Paget (1855–1926)
Confessio Medici, Ch. 7

Index

About the Author

Robert C. Hardy has spent more than a quarter century in the health field serving sick people in a variety of ways.

A health planner and consultant since 1966, Mr. Hardy began his career as a pharmacist in the Army Hospital at Los Alamos in 1945 and later managed the pharmacy at Delaware Hospital in Wilmington. He was also involved with the beginnings of the Hill-Burton hospital construction and licensure program in Georgia.

In the early 1950's, Mr. Hardy studied hospital administration at the University of Chicago under Dr. Arthur Bachmeyer and Ray E. Brown. After a residency at the University of Alabama Hospital in Birmingham, he became administrator of the City of Memphis Hospitals, the teaching facility for the University of Tennessee. A decade later, he headed the University of Arkansas Medical Center Hospital in Little Rock.

Mr. Hardy currently lives in Oklahoma City.